Rethinking the Public Fetus

Rochester Studies in Medical History

Series Editor: Christopher Crenner
Robert Hudson and Ralph Major Professor and Chair
Department of History and Philosophy of Medicine
University of Kansas School of Medicine

Additional Titles of Interest

Childbirth, Maternity, and Medical Pluralism in French Colonial Vietnam,
1880–1945
Thuy Linh Nguyen

The Birth Control Clinic in a Marketplace World
Rose Holz

Health Education Films in the Twentieth Century
Edited by Christian Bonah, David Cantor, and Anja Laukötter

Cancer, Research, and Educational Film at Midcentury: The Making of the Movie
"Challenge: Science Against Cancer"
David Cantor

Save the Babies: American Public Health Reform and the Prevention of
Infant Mortality, 1850–1929
Richard A. Meckel

Female Circumcision and Clitoridectomy in the United States:
A History of a Medical Treatment
Sarah B. Rodriguez

Medicine's Moving Pictures: Medicine, Health, and Bodies in
American Film and Television
Leslie J. Reagan, Nancy Tomes, Paula A. Treichler

Shifting Boundaries of Public Health: Europe in the Twentieth Century
Edited by Susan Gross Solomon, Lion Murard, and Patrick Zylberman

A complete list of titles in the Rochester Studies in Medical History series may be
found on our website, www.urpress.com.

Rethinking the Public Fetus

Historical Perspectives on the Visual Culture of Pregnancy

Edited by Elisabet Björklund and Solveig Jülich

UNIVERSITY OF ROCHESTER PRESS

First published 2024

University of Rochester Press
668 Mt. Hope Avenue, Rochester, NY 14620, USA
www.urpress.com
and Boydell & Brewer Limited
PO Box 9, Woodbridge, Suffolk IP12 3DF, UK
www.boydellandbrewer.com

ISBN-13: 978-1-64825-071-2
ISSN: 1526-2715

This book is published with support from Lund University Library and The Sten Lindroth Memorial Fund. An ebook version is openly available under the Creative Commons license CC BY-NC-ND.

Library of Congress Cataloging-in-Publication Data

Names: Björklund, Elisabet, 1983– editor. | Jülich, Solveig, 1966– editor.
Title: Rethinking the public fetus : historical perspectives on the visual culture of pregnancy / edited by Elisabet Björklund and Solveig Jülich.
Other titles: Rochester studies in medical history ; v. 53. 1526-2715
Description: Rochester, NY : University of Rochester Press, 2024. | Series: Rochester studies in medical history, 1526-2715 ; 53 | Includes bibliographical references and index.
Identifiers: LCCN 2023030350 (print) | LCCN 2023030351 (ebook) | ISBN 9781648250712 (paperback ; alk. paper) | ISBN 9781805431404 (pdf)
Subjects: MESH: Pregnancy—psychology | History, Modern 1601– | Fetus | Feminism—history | Ultrasonography, Prenatal—history | Public Opinion—history
Classification: LCC RG551 (print) | LCC RG551 (ebook) | NLM WQ 11.1 | DDC 618.2—dc23/eng/20231025
LC record available at https://lccn.loc.gov/2023030350
LC ebook record available at https://lccn.loc.gov/2023030351

A catalogue record for this title is available from the British Library.

This publication is printed on acid-free paper.

Printed in the United States of America.

Contents

Acknowledgments

This project started as an international workshop on the "public fetus" at Uppsala University in May 2019, organized within the research programme "Medicine at the Borders of Life: Fetal Research and the Emergence of Ethical Controversy in Sweden." We are very grateful to everyone who attended this workshop and would especially like to thank Barbara Duden for her inspiring keynote lecture, her enthusiastic participation in the discussions, and her warm support for the project.

We are also deeply indebted to the two anonymous reviewers of the manuscript for their careful readings, insightful comments, and constructive suggestions on how to improve the book. Jessica Dandona, Annelie Drakman, Rose Holz, Nick Hopwood, Mariah Larsson, and Manon Parry gave valuable feedback on different versions of the introduction and conclusion and deserve a special thank you.

We would like to thank the artists, photographers, and other rightsholders of the images included in this book for giving permission to publish their work. Rosalind Petchesky generously provided us with the picture of her and her fellow panelists at the Beijing Fourth World Women's Conference in 1995. We also wish to especially mention Lars Björklund, Annelie Drakman, Monica Englund, Bee Hughes, Lennart Nilsson Photography, Sarah Maple, the Monica Sjöö Estate, the MYA Network, the National Partnership for Women & Families, the family of Núria Pompeia, Liv Strömquist, and the family of Dea Trier Mørch. Photographer Malin Thomas Nilsson provided excellent service with preparing the images for print.

"Medicine at the Borders of Life" was funded by the Swedish Research Council (registration number 2014-1749) and hosted by the Department of History of Science and Ideas at Uppsala University 2015–2021. The Ragnhild Blomqvist Fund supported the workshop at Uppsala University in 2019. Funding for the open access publication of the volume was provided by Lund University Library. The Sten Lindroth Memorial Fund supported the costs for proofreading and image permissions.

Rethinking the Public Fetus

An Introduction

Elisabet Björklund and Solveig Jülich

Today, images of fetuses and pregnant bodies are ubiquitous. We encounter them everywhere—from ultrasound pictures of expected babies in family albums to childbirth scenes in reality television shows or on social media platforms. Images of fetal bodies are also frequently seen in antiabortion campaigns. The capacity of fetal photographs and ultrasound images to both stir up strong emotions and be interpreted as scientific truth has long made them one of the most effective tools of persuasion for antiabortion activists. Yet, while their pervasive presence in today's visual culture is of course connected to the expanding media landscape and contemporary struggles over reproductive rights, visualizations of pregnancy and fetuses have a much longer and more varied history.

An important aim of this volume is to counteract the conception of fetal images as depictions of a universal truth about pregnancy in contemporary culture and reproductive politics. In abortion debates, these powerful images are often used as evidence of the "personhood" of the fetus, even though they—as all images—must be understood as representations. That is, they show certain things, leave out others, and are created from specific perspectives, with certain technologies, and with particular audiences in mind. Moreover, embryos and fetuses have not always been associated with abortion. Indeed, the connection between fetuses and abortion is not natural or inevitable but rather the product of a specific cultural and social situation in time and space.[1] Consequently, in order to deepen the understanding of the power of fetal images in visual culture, and sharpen the critical analysis of today's antiabortion campaigns, we find it essential to further unpack and denaturalize "embryos" and "fetuses" as historical constructs.

---

1 Lynn M. Morgan, *Icons of Life: A Cultural History of Human Embryos* (Berkeley: University of California Press, 2009), 4–5, 160–61.

It is therefore timely to revisit the influential concept of the "public fetus." This was a term that feminist scholars—most notably political scientist Rosalind Petchesky and historian Barbara Duden—started to use in the late 1980s and 1990s to describe the growing dissemination of fetal images in the public domain. In these scholars' works, the breakthrough for the public fetus was often connected to Swedish photographer Lennart Nilsson's pictures of human embryos and fetuses published in *Life* magazine and the book *Ett barn blir till* (*A Child Is Born*) in the mid-1960s as well as to the increasing use of the obstetric ultrasound. This development, it was argued, threatened to undermine women's reproductive rights, as the way the fetus was represented in these images constructed it as an autonomous person, separated from its mother, that could be claimed to have a "right to life." Since then, many have analyzed the consequences of this change and how images of fetal bodies have been used in antiabortion campaigns, especially in the US context.[2]

The present book seeks to revitalize this scholarly discussion by exploring the emergence of the public fetus from an interdisciplinary and *longue durée* perspective. In recent decades, historians have demonstrated that visualizations of pregnancy and fetuses for broader audiences can indeed be found much earlier than the 1960s and that the assertion of novelty in discussions on the public fetus thus needs to be qualified.[3] Moreover, much previous research has been focused on the United States, while other cultural contexts have been less explored. Therefore, this volume brings together international scholars from several disciplines, including history, anthropology, and film

2   Rosalind Pollack Petchesky, "Fetal Images: The Power of Visual Culture in the Politics of Reproduction," *Feminist Studies* 13, no. 2 (1987): 263–92; Barbara Duden, *Disembodying Women: Perspectives on Pregnancy and the Unborn*, trans. Lee Hoinacki (Cambridge, MA: Harvard University Press, 1993). For a historiographic account of the public fetus and a discussion of the "maternal erasure" theory, see Jülich and Björklund in this volume. For Nilsson's pictures, see Lennart Nilsson and Albert Rosenfeld, "Drama of Life before Birth," *Life*, April 30, 1965; Lennart Nilsson, Axel Ingelman-Sundberg, and Claes Wirsén, *Ett barn blir till: En bildskildring av de nio månaderna före födelsen: En praktisk rådgivare för den blivande mamman* (Stockholm: Bonnier, 1965). The first American edition of *A Child Is Born* was published in 1966 by Delacorte Press and the first British edition in 1967 by Allen Lane/The Penguin Press.

3   Morgan, *Icons of Life*; Nick Hopwood, *Haeckel's Embryos: Images, Evolution, and Fraud* (Chicago: University of Chicago Press, 2015); Raymond Stephanson and Darren N. Wagner, eds., *The Secrets of Generation: Reproduction in the Long Eighteenth Century* (Toronto: University of Toronto Press, 2015); Tatjana Buklijas and Nick Hopwood, *Making Visible Embryos* (online exhibition), 2008–10, http://www.sites.hps.cam.ac.uk/visibleembryos/index.html (last accessed May 6, 2023).

studies, to explore visualizations of pregnant and fetal bodies across different geographical and national contexts, from the eighteenth century to the present. We approach the public fetus as a flexible analytical concept rather than a historical object with a fixed meaning. The key is to analyze how fetuses and other reproductive phenomena have been materialized, mediated, and used in public settings for many purposes and by various actors over time. In addition, we draw on the notion of visual culture rather than, for example, the media, in order to include a wide range of representations. Hence, the chapters harness a wealth of fascinating and previously unknown or underused empirical materials, including wet specimen preparations, papier-mâché models of the pregnant uterus, obstetrical machines, films on childbirth, menstruation art, and Lennart Nilsson's early photographs of the living fetus in utero.[4]

Taken as a whole, the goal of this book is to advance the discussion about the history of the constitution, uses, and meanings of the visible "fetus" (including its construction as blastocyst, embryo, baby, child, individual, person, citizen, and patient) as well as the imaged reproductive body, pregnant and not. Moreover, it aims to demonstrate the relevance of historical scholarship to a more qualified and nuanced analysis of our contemporary visual culture of pregnancy. For instance, academic and professional discussions will profit from the contributions in this volume on such issues as the uses of human fetal remains in contemporary medical museums and why the same fetal image can acquire different meanings in different national contexts. By shedding light on visual rhetoric and past strategies, we provide critical tools for understanding the power of reproductive representations today.

Challenging the Icon of the Universal Fetus

As a critical term, the "public fetus" not only refers to an increased number of fetal images in public but also captures the emergence of an abstracted idea of the universal fetus that is created in many of these images. For example, single pictures of late-term fetuses have often been used to stand for all the stages of human development from conception to birth, thus symbolizing "life" in general. At the same time, these symbolic pictures have often been presented and interpreted as objective, biological "fact" rather than depictions of particular bodies and circumstances taken from certain

---

4   For copyright reasons related to the open access publication of this volume, we were unfortunately not able to include some central illustrations, such as Lennart Nilsson's photographs in *Life* magazine in 1965.

perspectives.[5] Building on insights from earlier scholarship, this book further challenges the very notion of a universal, objective fetus that exists without context. There are four aspects in particular that we believe deserve deeper consideration.

First, we give many historical examples of how visualizations of fetuses and pregnant bodies were shaped by and promoted notions of gender, sexuality, race, class, and disability in a wide range of domains. Gender obviously matters a great deal. Crucially, the visibility of the fetus in the famous photographs by Lennart Nilsson and followers such as American photographer Alexander Tsiaras was achieved at the cost of the maternal body's invisibility. It diverted attention from the labor of the female body and the economic and social situations of pregnant women.[6] Since the advent of Nilsson's photographs, the invisibility of pregnant bodies has been challenged in many representations, not least those during feminism's second wave, when many artists explored women's experiences of pregnancy, childbirth, and abortion (figures I.1 and I.2). However, other types of erasure—or veiling—of the pregnant woman have also appeared. It has been shown that in current blogs about transnational surrogacy, expectant parents often post ultrasound images alongside images of the belly bumps of pregnant, sari-clad Indian women whose heads are usually cut out of the picture.[7]

The European and American histories of colonialism, slavery, eugenics, and medical racism have influenced representations of pregnancy and fetuses in many ways. For instance, eugenic conceptions of race, class, disability, and nation were interwoven in many early medical photographs of pregnant women.[8] Most fetal images have depicted the fetus as White. A telling

5   This argument was put forward early on in Barbara Duden's publications, see for instance, "The Fetus as an Object of Our Time," *RES: Anthropology and Aesthetics* 25 (1994): 132–35. Also see Monica J. Casper, *The Making of the Unborn Patient: A Social Anatomy of Fetal Surgery* (New Brunswick, NJ: Rutgers University Press, 1998), 18. For an analysis of the rhetorical strategies used in contemporary antiabortion arguments, see John Lynch, *What Are Stem Cells? Definitions at the Intersection of Science and Politics* (Tuscaloosa: University of Alabama Press, 2011), 53–57.

6   Carol A. Stabile, "Shooting the Mother: Fetal Photography and the Politics of Disappearance," *Camera Obscura* 10, no. 28 (1992): 196; Morgan, *Icons of Life*, 218–21.

7   Sayantani Dasgupta and Shamita Das Dasgupta, "The Public Fetus and the Veiled Woman: Transnational Surrogacy Blogs as Surveillant Assemblage," in *Feminist Surveillance Studies*, ed. Rachel E. Dubrofsky and Shoshana Amielle Magnet (Durham, NC: Duke University Press, 2015), 150–68.

8   Sandra Matthews and Laura Wexler, *Pregnant Pictures* (New York: Routledge, 2000), 123–31.

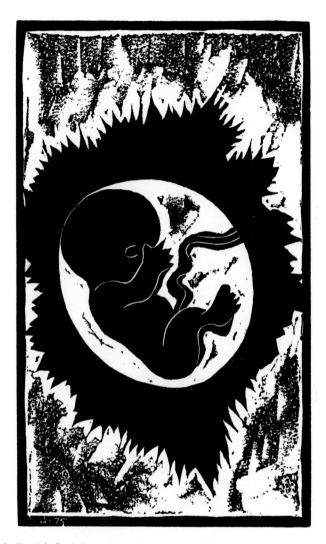

Figure I.1. Danish feminist artist and author Dea Trier Mørch explored the theme of pregnancy and labor in her best-selling novel *Vinterbørn* (*Winter's Child*, 1976), which was richly illustrated by her own graphic art. This reproduction of a linoleum print of a fetus in its amniotic sac and surrounded by the placenta clearly resembled Lennart Nilsson's photograph from the *Life* issue in 1965 that became known as the "Spaceman." Trier Mørch's picture was, however, placed in the context of a narrative of a diverse group of women at an obstetric ward together with many other images of pregnant and birthing women. ©Dea Trier Mørch/Bildupphovsrätt 2023.

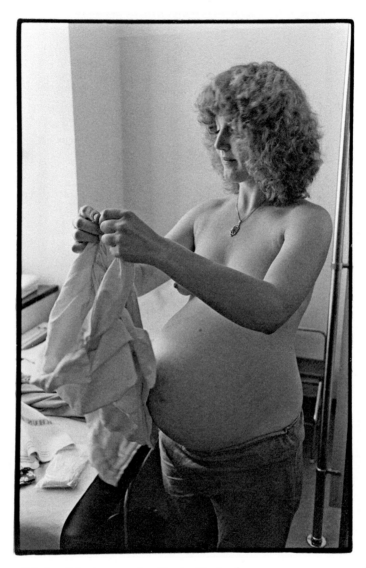

Figure I.2. Swedish photographer Monica Englund was one among many artists during feminism's second wave who thematized pregnancy and motherhood in their work. In the 1970s and 1980s, Englund documented twelve births, resulting in two books. This picture was published in *En födelse* (A birth, 1982), which followed a woman in labor and her partner from their arrival to the hospital until the birth of their child. Courtesy of Monica Englund. Reproduction: Moderna Museet.

example of this is the response to a 2021 medical illustration of a Black fetus in a Black pregnant body created by the Nigerian medical illustrator and student Chidiebere Ibe, who aimed to stimulate diversity and inclusion in medical textbooks. The picture went viral, and many commented that they had never seen an image of a Black fetus before.[9] And indeed, in many respects the contents of this volume lay bare this truth: images of fetuses and pregnant bodies of color have been largely excluded from the most predominant representations in Western culture. New work is emerging to correct this erasure, and we look forward to further historical research in this field focusing on issues of race and ethnicity and on visual representations of pregnancy outside the White norm.[10] Similarly, in contemporary representations the universal fetus also signals typical human development; that is, it seldom displays visible signs of unusual anatomy. In early modern Europe however, "monstrous bodies" were often displayed as curiosities, and disability could be understood in many ways, for example as God's work.[11]

---

9   See, for example, David Limm, "The Creator of a Viral Black Fetus Medical Illustration Blends Art and Activism, " *HealthCity*, January 13, 2022, https:// healthcity.bmc.org/policy-and-industry/creator-viral-black-fetus-medical-illustration-blends-art-and-activism (last accessed March 12, 2023). See also "The Black Fetus Illustration," on Ibe's website, https://www.chidiebereibe.com/ the-black-fetus-illustration/ (last accessed March 12, 2023).

10   See the important work done by Wangui Muigai, "'Something Wasn't Clean': Black Midwifery, Birth, and Postwar Medical Education in *All My Babies*," *Bulletin of the History of Medicine* 93, no. 1 (2019): 82–113; Deirdre Cooper Owens, *Medical Bondage: Race, Gender, and the Origins of American Gynecology* (Athens: University of Georgia Press, 2017); Karen Weingarten, "From Maternal Impressions to Eugenics: Pregnancy and Inheritance in the Nineteenth-Century U.S.," *Journal of Medical Humanities* 43 (2020): 303–17. Another example within art and activism is Michelle Browder's *Mothers of Gynecology* monument from 2022, which pays tribute to Anarcha, Lucy, and Betsey, three of the enslaved women upon whom Dr. J. Marion Sims conducted his nineteenth-century surgical experiments. See Sarah Kuta, "Subjected to Painful Experiments and Forgotten, Enslaved Mothers of Gynecology are Honored with New Monument," *Smithsonian Magazine*, May 11, 2022, https://www.smithsonianmag.com/smart-news/mothers-of-gynecology-monument-honors-enslaved-women-180980064/ (last accessed March 2, 2023). See also the website dedicated to the monument, https://www.anarchalucybetsey.org/ (last accessed March 12, 2023).

11   Lorraine Daston and Katharine Park, *Wonders and the Order of Nature, 1150–1750* (New York: Zone Books, 1998). Also see Maja Bondestam, introduction to *Exceptional Bodies in Early Modern Culture: Conceptions of Monstrosity Before the Advent of the Normal*, ed. Maja Bondestam (Amsterdam: Amsterdam University Press, 2020), and Allison P. Hobgood and David Houston Wood,

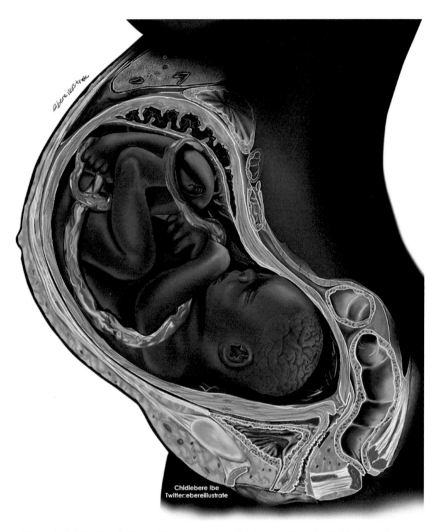

Figure I.3. The Black Fetus Illustration by Chidiebere Ibe. © Chidiebere Ibe.
Adapted from the original illustration ©QA International, 2010. https://
qa-international.com.

Second, we demonstrate that representations of fetuses and pregnant women do not carry single, transparent meanings but are dependent on specific media, material factors, and cultural and historical contexts. The view of pictures as self-explanatory is still held in many contemporary situations, not least by representatives of antiabortion groups who use prenatal ultrasound images to dissuade women from terminating their pregnancies.[12] Through our historical examples we show that visual representations of pregnancy are always mediated, shaped, and transformed through technologies and media, from wet specimen techniques in the eighteenth century to mid-twentieth-century photojournalism and early twenty-first-century remembrance photographs of fetuses that died in utero. Skilled handling of visual effects or outright manipulation of images are also taken into account, such as the case of Nilsson's early fetal photographs. In addition, several chapters highlight how film, video, and television have been powerfully linked to and reused imagery of childbirth and developing fetuses for purposes ranging from sex education to antiabortion propaganda.

Third, we highlight the multitude of actors that have been involved in the shaping of the universal, "objective fetus." Historically, nineteenth-century anatomists first established the embryological view of development, which holds that each human life begins at conception, passing through several stages before being born.[13] But as embryos and fetuses started to circulate in broader social domains, many diverse actors became engaged in the constitution of their meanings. All those involved—including antiabortion groups citing scientific "facts" to justify their views, doctors and sex educators fighting for women's health, governmental actors working to promote family planning or pronatalist agendas, feminist activists aiming to reclaim women's bodies, and advertisers wanting to sell maternity clothes or baby products—have shaped how pregnant and fetal bodies have been represented in public.[14] By following the traces of a manifold of historical actors, a more complex story of the emergence of the public fetus can be told.

However, we acknowledge that it is more difficult to find historical sources that can be used to shed light on the pregnant women who were

---

eds., *Recovering Disability in Early Modern England* (Columbus: Ohio State University, 2013.

12   This was already pointed out by Petchesky in her classic "Fetal Images."

13   Nick Hopwood, "Producing Development: The Anatomy of Human Embryos and the Norms of Wilhelm His," *Bulletin of the History of Medicine* 74, no. 1 (2000): 29–79.

14   In addition to the chapters in this volume, see Solveig Jülich, ed., *Medicine at the Borders of Life: Fetal Knowledge Production and the Emergence of Public Controversy in Sweden* (Leiden: Brill, 2024).

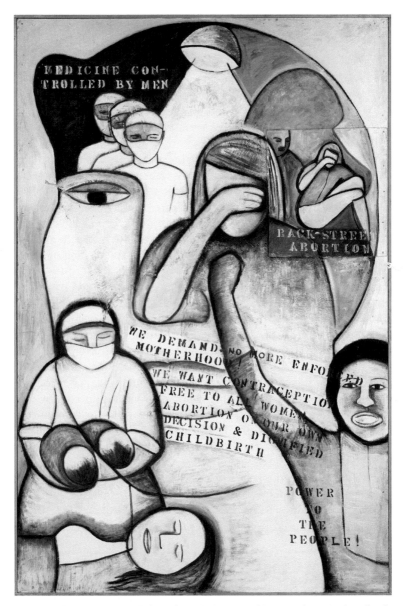

Figure I.4. Artist, activist, and ecofeminist Monica Sjöö was born in Sweden but lived most of her adult life in in the United Kingdom where she became active in women's and environmental movements and fought for minorities. Her work created a lot of controversy in the 1960s and 1970s, including the painting *Back Street Abortion: Women Seeking Freedom from Oppression* (1968), which addressed the subject of illegal abortions and took a stand for women's reproductive rights. Courtesy of the Monica Sjöö Estate. Photo: Tobias Fischer/Moderna Museet.

involved in the creation of the specimens, images, figures, machines, and models highlighted in this book. Surviving documentation suggests problematic origins and asymmetrical power relations. Many medical museums have collections of fetal specimens that were acquired in colonial contexts and used as evidence of racial differences.[15] Although some embryos and fetuses from miscarriages were willingly given by women to medical collectors, most came from poor and unmarried patients who hardly knew where the material would go or for what purposes it would be used.[16] On the other hand, women and activists have also played an active part in counteracting dominant representations of pregnancy and used visual means of expression to protest against repressive reproductive politics (see, for instance, figure I.4). The most famous example internationally is probably the book *Our Bodies, Ourselves*, published in the early 1970s by the Boston Women's Health Book Collective and translated into several languages, but there are numerous other examples.[17] More recently, pictures of pregnancy tissue from the first nine weeks of gestation, provided by the MYA Network—a group of clinicians and activists working to normalize abortion care in the United States—were published in the *Guardian* in 2022.[18]

Fourth, we demonstrate that there are national differences in how the public fetus manifests itself. Historically, national abortion legislation and debates have conditioned the making and circulation of fetal and pregnancy images. Access to aborted fetuses in 1950s Sweden was a prerequisite for Nilsson's early fetal pictures, which at the same time were used by doctors

---

15 Parry, this volume; Helena Franzén, "'Pelves of Various Nations': Race and Sex in a Mid-Nineteenth Century Obstetric Collection," in Jülich, *Medicine at the Borders of Life*.

16 Shannon Withycombe, *Lost: Miscarriage in Nineteenth-Century America* (New Brunswick, NJ: Rutgers University Press, 2019); Ray, this volume. Also see Solveig Jülich, "Embryology and the Clinic: Early to Mid-Twentieth Century Stories of Pregnancy, Abortion, and Fetal Collecting," in Jülich, *Medicine at the Borders of Life*.

17 The Boston Women's Health Book Collective, *Our Bodies, Ourselves* (New York: Simon & Schuster, 1973). This was the first commercially published version of the book. An earlier version, published in 1971, had been preceded by a course book from 1970 called "Women and Their Bodies." See Our Bodies Ourselves Today: https://ourbodiesourselves.org/about-us/our-history/ (last accessed September 2, 2022).

18 Poppy Noor, "What a Pregnancy Actually Looks Like Before 10 Weeks—in Pictures," *Guardian*, October 19, 2022, https://www.theguardian.com/world/2022/oct/18/pregnancy-weeks-abortion-tissue (last accessed January 31, 2023). See also MYA Network, "The Issue of Tissue," https://myanetwork.org/the-issue-of-tissue/ (last accessed January 31, 2023).

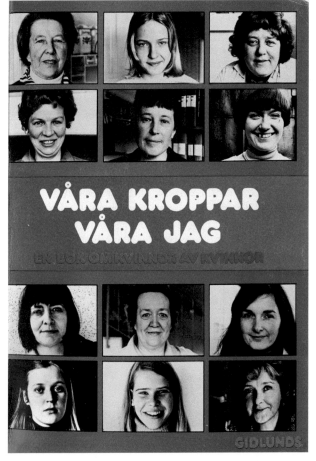

Figure I.5. Cover of the Swedish edition of *Our Bodies,
Ourselves,* published in 1975. Photographs by Monica
Englund. Published with permission from Gidlunds förlag
and Monica Englund.

opposing the relatively liberal abortion law. Later, however, they became
icons of Sweden's progressive sexual politics (figure I.7).[19] Simultaneously,
the pictures were endorsed by the censors in Franco's Spain, indicating that

19   See, for instance, Birgitta Linnér, *Sex and Society in Sweden* (New York:
Pantheon, 1967) with photographs by Lennart Nilsson. For a discussion, see
Jülich, this volume, and "Picturing Abortion Opposition: Lennart Nilsson's
Early Photographs of Embryos and Fetuses," *Social History of Medicine* 31, no.
2 (2018): 278–307.

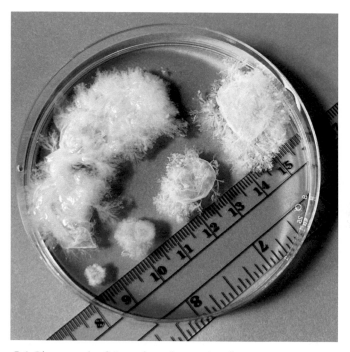

Figure I.6. Photograph of tissue from five weeks of pregnancy to nine weeks of pregnancy produced by the MYA Network in order to present information on how early abortion looks like. Courtesy of the MYA Network.

they could also be read in line with Catholic values and nationalistic goals of increasing the birth rate. And in the United States, Nilsson's images from *Life* magazine were incorporated into the visual propaganda of antiabortion groups from the 1970s onward.[20] Another example is the obstetric ultrasound, which has also been a powerful tool for antiabortion activists in the United States. This is not least obvious today, as the technology's capacity to detect early signs of embryonic cardiac activity—erroneously referred to as "fetal heartbeat" by antiabortion activists—has been used as an argument for the introduction of "heartbeat bills" in many states, aimed at banning abortion after six weeks of pregnancy. After the Supreme Court's *Dobbs v. Jackson Women's Health Organization* decision in June 2022, which overturned *Roe v. Wade* (1973), some of these laws came into effect while they were rendered

---

20   See María Jesús Santesmases's and Nick Hopwood's chapters in this volume.

moot in other states that introduced total abortion bans.[21] Meanwhile, in India ultrasound is a controversial technology, as it has been used to detect the sex of the fetus and hence has led to sex-selective abortions.[22]

In sum, we follow on from previous scholarship in arguing that there is no "universal" objective fetus. Understanding how and why fetuses have come to occupy such a powerful role in contemporary culture and society requires that we consider the longer history of visualizations of pregnant and fetal bodies. The analyses offered by the present volume give multifaceted evidence that the emergence and politics of the public fetus have involved a variety of historical actors, social categories, media forms, representational styles, and sensory capacities embedded in specific historical contexts.

The Book

The chapters in this book are organized chronologically, together spanning a period of more than three hundred years. In chapter 1, Sara Ray takes us back to the eighteenth century and Russian tsar Peter the Great's collection of hundreds of fetal bodies, which is kept at the Kunstkamera in St. Petersburg. This collection became possible through the introduction of a new technique for visualizing fetuses: wet specimen preparation, which Peter had learned in 1697 while studying under the Amsterdam physician Frederik Ruysch, whose collection of fetuses he later also purchased. In contrast to Ruysch, however, the focus of Peter's interest was "monsters"—fetuses with different kinds of malformations. In the Kunstkamera, Russia's new state museum, embryos and fetuses varying greatly in size and form were thus displayed in the same public space, and later, these "monsters" also became an important part of embryological research. In the late eighteenth century, German physiologist Caspar Friedrich Wolff used the diversity in the collection as evidence for the view that gestation was a developmental process (epigenesis). Ray also discusses the dual role of the public for these collectors. On the one hand, both Ruysch's and Peter's collections were open to the public. On the other, they were dependent on the public (women who had miscarriages, for example) for acquiring material for display.

---

21   Leslie J. Reagan, *When Abortion Was a Crime: Women, Medicine, and Law in the United States, 1867–1973* (1997; Oakland, CA: University of California Press, 2022), xxiii–xxiv. For an example of the effects of this type of legislation after *Dobbs*, see Jaime Lowe (text) and Stephanie Sinclair (photo), "What a High-Risk Pregnancy Looks Like After Dobbs," *New York Times*, September 18, 2022.

22   Dasgupta and Das Dasgupta, "The Public Fetus and the Veiled Woman," 167n13.

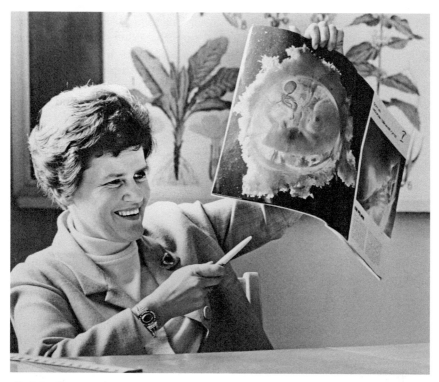

Fig I.7. Photograph by Lennart Nilsson of sex educator Maj-Briht Bergström-Walan holding up his image of the "Spaceman" at a lesson in a Stockholm school in the mid-1960s. This picture together with others showing Swedish school children and youth being educated on issues such as menstruation, contraception, abortion, and changing sex roles was included in *Sex and Society in Sweden* (1967), a book aimed at the American audience. Courtesy of Lennart Nilsson Photography/TT.

Chapter 2 stays in the eighteenth century but shifts the focus to Italy. Here, Jennifer Kosmin sheds light not only on the use of obstetrical models and machines in the instruction of male surgeons and female midwives but also on the relationship between the senses of sight and touch in this instruction. Kosmin argues that these models and machines can be placed at a shift in the ontological status of the fetus. While Catholic reformers, obstetricians, and public health experts argued for harsher legal measures regarding, for instance, abortion, and advocated the use of Cesarean section to save dying fetuses through baptism or protect them as future citizens, museums such as La Specola in Florence spread information about the female anatomy and human reproduction through the use of anatomical Venuses and other models in wax. The fetus was thus made publicly visible during this era in efforts to educate women about reproductive health. But while this observation would confirm the idea that the end of the eighteenth century was a period when sight became the dominant sense for gaining medical knowledge, Kosmin argues that obstetrical models and machines also show that touch continued to be important in medical practice.

Chapter 3 looks closely at the visual culture of medicine in the late nineteenth century and highlights representations of pregnancy in paper. Within this context, Jessica M. Dandona explores Louis-Thomas-Jérôme Auzoux's papier-mâché models of the uterus (ca. 1840s–1970s) and Gustave-Joseph-Alphonse Witkowski's printed anatomical atlas, *Progress of Gestation* (1875–78 and 1880–84). These representations appeared at a time when the groundwork for modern obstetrics was being laid, while developments in printing technology made mass production and the transnational circulation of images of pregnant bodies possible to both professional and general audiences. Through detailed analysis of these two works, Dandona argues that they represent the female body through the logic of anatomical dissection, while the fetus is represented as its intact "secret" to be discovered. Moreover, she argues that this way of representing the pregnant body occurred in parallel with the increasing use of surgical operations such as Cesarean section. Thus, they can be understood to emphasize the surgeon's way of seeing a pregnant woman.

From paper, the book moves on to sculpture. Rose Holz, in chapter 4, examines the influential *Birth Series*—a group of sculptures representing fetal development and birth created in 1939 by obstetrician-gynecologist Dr. Robert L. Dickinson and sculptor Abram Belskie on commission from the New York Maternity Center Association. These sculptures were first exhibited at the 1939–40 World's Fair in New York City and were later reproduced in different forms and distributed in sex education and other health-related contexts all over the world for several decades, reaching people across the globe. Holz argues that the *Birth Series* was a crucial part of the shift from nineteenth-century perceptions of pregnancy to late twentieth-century ones. Dickinson and Belskie were also ahead of Nilsson in picturing the unborn as alive, beautiful, and ideal, and based their sculptures on living sources (X-rays of pregnant women) to do so. This account gives new insights into the historical development of these kinds of representations, the way they were constructed, and their historical uses. Even though similar modes of depicting the unborn today are strongly associated with the modern antiabortion movement, Holz points out that Dickinson was a supporter of abortion, which affirms that interpretations of images of biological bodies are not predetermined but subjective and dependent on their historical, social, and cultural contexts.

In chapter 5, Elisabet Björklund also discusses representations used for sex education but focuses on the medium of cinema, exploring the Swedish version of the American sex hygiene film *Mom and Dad* (William Beaudine, 1944). Sex hygiene films appeared in the United States in the period around World War I, but after the war the genre was pushed to the margins by mainstream Hollywood in efforts to create respectability for the business. Consequently, when the Production Code was written in the 1930s (the self-censorship guidelines regulating the content of films made by the major studios), the purpose of cinema was defined as "wholesome entertainment," and not education. This led to the emergence of a new type of film outside the mainstream—the exploitation film. *Mom and Dad* was typical of this genre in many ways. It included information about pregnancy and explicit footage of childbirth, was made on a low budget, and was marketed and exhibited in a sensational way—for example, with fake nurses present at the screenings. However, when the film was imported to Sweden in 1949, it was adapted to the Swedish market by a medical expert at the National Board of Medicine and cut by the National Board of Film Censors, who also made demands on its marketing. Björklund examines how the edited version of the film, the censorship measures taken, and the viewing situation created for it influenced its reception as it crossed national borders, arguing that these efforts were made in order to shape its potential audience into a "public," capable of receiving its message about reproduction and venereal disease in an edifying way.

Many feminist scholars have discussed the role of Swedish photographer Lennart Nilsson's pictures of human development in the rise of the public fetus during the second part of the twentieth century. Solveig Jülich, in chapter 6, argues that however important these analyses may have been, they were often based on misunderstandings about what the pictures show and how they were produced, thereby unintentionally mythifying Nilsson's work. Jülich draws on new empirical materials to provide a fresh perspective on Nilsson's public fetus, investigating, for the first time, the relationship between the making of his images and human fetal research in 1950s and 1960s Sweden. She demonstrates that the photographer collaborated with a team of scientific and technical experts, experimenting on aborted fetuses and women scheduled for legal abortion operations. Employing both new and old techniques, he developed three different styles for visualizing human reproduction: the embryo and fetus in isolation, the fetus in bits, and the "fetoplacental unit," or, in popular terms, the fetal astronaut. In conclusion, this chapter reveals that the powerful images of embryos and fetuses that Nilsson created were anything but truthful or objective.

Chapter 7 also offers a new perspective on Lennart Nilsson's pictures, but in a different context. In María Jesús Santesmases's essay, the circulation of fetal images in Franco's Spain is explored though an examination of the translation and distribution of American science writer Geraldine Lux Flanagan's *The First Nine Months of Life* (1962) and Nilsson's *A Child Is Born* in the Spanish market. Presented as medical texts, both these works passed Spanish censorship inspection and were hence deemed acceptable to the morals of the Catholic Church and the ideology of the dictatorial regime. The books were both broadly distributed, but Santesmases also shows how the photographs were part of a larger visual culture. Some of the pictures from Flanagan's book were used in a Spanish pregnancy guide written by the Catholic activist María Salas Larrazábal in 1967. Nilsson's images were widely distributed in the catalogue advertising the book, and there were also other, competing ways of representing pregnancy in circulation. In a book by feminist cartoonist Núria Pompeia published in 1967, the fetus was absent and instead the pregnant woman's body and feelings were placed at the center. This alternative vision shifts our interpretation of the public fetus of the 1960s, as it demonstrates that the circulation of fetal images taken from a medical perspective, however dominant, occurred within a larger visual culture of reproduction in which there was also room for feminist representations.

Nick Hopwood, in chapter 8, addresses the history and circulation of Nilsson's images through an exploration of the public fetus in the United States. Hopwood takes a critical view on the public fetus by asking what was really new in the way the fetus was visualized from the 1960s onward. Combining new research with a synthesis of previous scholarship, Hopwood takes us through three decades of fetal images in the United States, beginning with examples preceding the *Life* issue of 1965, then delving deeper into Nilsson's pictures and their reception, and moving on to discuss the uses of slides, films like *The Silent Scream* (Jack Duane Dabner, 1984), and other media by antiabortion activists in the backlash against *Roe v. Wade*. Hopwood argues that Nilsson's images and the rise of photojournalism were indeed new in important ways, and that ultrasound images contributed to the widespread view of fetuses as babies. These visualizations became powerful tools for antiabortion activists. Yet, he notes, their meanings depend on context, and there are also alternative uses of visualizations. Ultrasound screening can lead to a decision to terminate a pregnancy, and seeing fetal remains after an abortion can be a way to reflect upon one's experience.

In a book focusing on public representations of pregnancy, it is fruitful to turn the perspective around and ask how bodies that do not reproduce have been represented. Camilla Mørk Røstvik addresses this question in chapter 9, where she looks at the contrasting history of public menstruation. Røstvik focuses on recent works of menstrual art by artists Rupi Kaur, Sarah Maple, Bee Hughes, and Liv Strömquist, which she historicizes in three steps, thus delineating a longer history of menstruation in public: First, the artworks are placed in the context of earlier examples of menstrual art from the 1970s onward. Second, they are considered in relation to a longer history of hiding menstruation during the twentieth century, through the growth of the menstrual product industry. And third, they are considered in light of the history of menstrual activism, also from the 1970s onward. Røstvik argues that the public menstruation shown in these recent artworks challenges the "menstrual concealment imperative," while reactions to these works reveal that making menstruation public is still controversial. Concluding the essay, Røstvik discusses similarities and differences between the visual culture of menstruation since the 1970s and the parallel rise of the public fetus.

In 2005, more than three hundred bodies of dead fetuses were discovered in the death chamber of Saint-Vincent-de-Paul Hospital in Paris, which caused a considerable scandal in France. Anne-Sophie Giraud, in chapter 10, uses this event as a starting point to discuss how the social and legal status of the unborn has shifted in France during the last thirty years. In the nineteenth century, such collections of fetuses were very common, and fetuses obtained from miscarriages or abortions were widely seen as "waste" or "specimens" that could be used in research. Over recent decades, however, a very different view has developed. In France, beginning in the 1980s, medical professionals have treated the unborn as children at earlier and earlier stages, a development that has been followed by legal changes. The limit for when a dead fetus is considered a "lifeless child" is fourteen weeks in France today, which means that many dead fetuses previously understood as "waste" are now treated as dead children—photographed, buried, and grieved in new ways. Giraud explores these practices at hospitals and among mourning parents, demonstrating that photographs of dead fetuses depict them as babies by, for instance, clothing them so that malformations cannot be seen. The photographs are often also used in remembrance ceremonies or shared on the internet, further constructing the fetuses as children and family members. These rituals are thus part of the larger development of the public fetus, Giraud argues. Yet the pictures also differ from dominant visualizations, as the fetuses are clearly represented as dead, and as individuals, rather than a universal type.

Chapter 11 ties the volume together by returning to the practice of displaying pregnant and fetal bodies in museums, also discussed by Ray. Here, Manon Parry explores reproducing bodies in contemporary medical museums. Many museums of this kind were formerly only available to medical professionals and students but during the last thirty years have been opened to the larger public. Collections of fetal remains and anatomical models displaying pregnancy and childbirth are common at these institutions, and Parry focuses specifically on wet specimen collections of fetuses ("babies in bottles") and obstetrical models in wax at museums in Vienna, Austria. She notes that while the display of human remains in general is an issue of much concern, presenting complicated ethical and legal dilemmas, collections of fetuses are understood as especially controversial—restricted, removed, and in some cases destroyed, even though there is little knowledge about visitors' reactions to these objects. Drawing on interviews and informal conversations with museum staff, Parry discusses attitudes and anxieties connected to these collections, their problematic aspects, and their potential as part of culturally authoritative institutions. She argues that while the specimens raise difficult ethical questions about, among other things, their origins and histories of display, they might also offer opportunities to, for example, reflect upon issues like pregnancy loss and abortion. Through their "de-sanitized" way of representing pregnancy and fetuses, the collections thus offer a valuable contrast to the dominant images of the public fetus.

By way of conclusion, in chapter 12, Solveig Jülich and Elisabet Björklund dive deeper into the conceptual history of the public fetus. Drawing on Mieke Bal's notion of traveling concepts within the humanities, they present a thorough reading of previous research on the visual culture of pregnancy, tracing the origins of the notion of the public fetus and following its trajectory and relevance for recent scholarship. They sum up their conclusions in four points. First, they argue that the public fetus is an interdisciplinary concept that has been used within many research fields but that an even broader interdisciplinarity could offer new perspectives on the historical phenomenon it aims to describe. Second, the concept's movement across geographical and cultural borders has been more limited. The lion's share of the scholarship has been carried out within the United States and Europe, which calls for a wider field of view in studies to follow. Third, there is also movement through history. Still a relatively young concept, the public fetus clearly sustains its relevance and continues to be used by scholars in many fields. Finally, one can observe how the concept crosses borders between the academic and nonacademic world, not least in writing at the intersection of research and activism. The authors conclude that this meta-analysis can help stimulate new research into the visual culture of pregnancy, which is vital to further deconstruct notions such as the universal fetus.

•   •   •

A note on terminology. Pregnancy, abortion, and reproductive technologies are highly politicized issues, where language use is a complex matter. Words such as "embryo," "fetus," "specimen," "life," "child," and "baby" are all politically charged and associated with different positions in contemporary abortion debates. Moreover, at what stage a "fetus" becomes an "infant," or when a "miscarriage" becomes a "stillbirth," varies legally between countries.[23] The words used and the meanings given to them have of course also changed profoundly through history. As our book has a historical focus, we find it important to use empirical concepts to avoid anachronisms and the pitfalls of attributing contemporary values to historical actors, even though this sometimes implies the use of terms that are today considered unacceptable, such as "monsters," or contested, such as "pregnant women." As editors, we have consequently allowed our authors the freedom of choosing the vocabulary they consider most appropriate for their specific cases and source materials. However, we have also been attentive to language use throughout the book and striven to employ the most neutral terms when writing more generally or theoretically about a subject, aiming for respectful discussion.[24]

---

23   For a thorough discussion of terminology related to the unborn, see Deborah Lupton, *The Social Worlds of the Unborn* (Basingstoke, UK: Palgrave Macmillan, 2013), 6–7, 26–32.

24   All translations in the chapters are by the authors if not otherwise indicated.

Chapter One

The Monsters of
Peter and Wolff

Anatomical Preparations and Embryology in
Eighteenth-Century St. Petersburg

Sara Ray

In the fall of 1776, the German physiologist Caspar Friedrich Wolff wrote to
a colleague from the Russian Academy of Sciences in St. Petersburg, saying:

> The very rich storehouse of monsters that has been collected and pre-
> served over a long series of years in the Imperial museum has now been
> handed over to me, so that I can compose a description of them and per-
> form anatomies where I decide to. In this therefore it will be necessary to
> deal once more with both the origin of monsters as well as with generation
> in general.[1]

Wolff's "storehouse of monsters" was the remarkable collection of Tsar
Peter the Great who had, in the early years of the eighteenth century, initiated a project of collecting and preserving abnormal fetuses. Collected over
several decades, the fetuses belonged to Peter's larger anatomical collection,
which became the centerpiece of his state museum—the Kunstkamera—and
its attached scientific institution, the Russian Academy of Sciences. Skilled
in anatomy and himself a towering eighty inches tall, Peter was fascinated
by bodies that seemingly defied nature. Peter collected "monsters" in hopes

---

1   Wolff's letters are reproduced in Shirley A. Roe, *Matter, Life, and Generation:
     Eighteenth-Century Embryology and the Haller-Wolff Debate* (Cambridge:
     Cambridge University Press, 1981), 170.

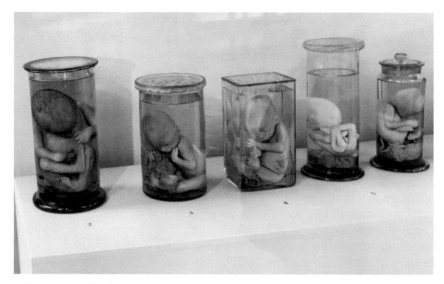

Figure 1.1. Five fetuses prepared with wax-injected placentas on display at Peter the Great's Museum of Anthropology and Ethnography (Kunstkamera). Photo by Lars Björklund.

that doing so would reveal insights into what caused them, transforming one of nature's most capricious mysteries into a scientifically rationalized phenomenon. This project of collection depended on what was, at the time, a novel innovation in visualization: wet specimen preparation, wherein the soft tissues of the body were preserved in a mixture of spirits and sometimes injected with colored wax or even mercury to accentuate certain anatomical features.

Wet specimen preparation brought the hidden processes of gestation into view for both specialist and public audiences. In her book *Disembodying Women*, historian Barbara Duden says, "Body history . . . is to a large extent a history of the unseen. Until very recently, the unborn, by definition, was one of these."[2] For Duden, the key moment in recent history was Lennart Nilsson's mid-twentieth-century photographs of the embryos and fetuses that were published in *Life* magazine. Yet Duden identifies the history of the unborn—of the fetus—as one with a longer history inextricably tied to techniques of visualization. Like Nilsson's photographs, specimens prepared

---

2   Barbara Duden, *Disembodying Women: Perspectives on Pregnancy and the Unborn*, trans. Lee Hoinacki (Cambridge, MA: Harvard University Press, 1993), 8.

in this way offered in the late seventeenth century a new technique for visualizing pregnancy: no longer hidden within the maternal body, this novel technique made gestation and its materials into tangible, observable objects. Preparations showed no single iconography of the unborn: the fetus might be shown still snugly tucked within the uterus, or with its placenta, or as an isolated body disconnected from that of its mother. Across their broad diversity in style, fetal preparations contributed to new visual narratives about pregnancy and the process of generation—what might now be called reproduction.[3]

A substantial portion of Peter's collection was purchased from the Dutch anatomist Frederik Ruysch in 1717, and this collection contained hundreds of fetuses at various gestational ages who overwhelmingly showed no anatomical abnormalities. But Peter's own project of collecting sought out "those born as monsters," and, indeed, in the first few years of the century he acquired several conjoined twins, a child with two heads, a likely case of cyclopia, and dozens of others.[4] While "monstrous births" had long been a subject of both surgical treatises and popular broadsides, wet specimen preparation also made these into material objects that could be displayed, observed, touched, verified, dissected.[5] For Peter, questions of monsters and of generation were innately bound together—in a 1718 royal *ukaz*, he rejected the idea that monsters were supernatural, claiming instead that they

---

3   Duden, *Disembodying Women;* Nick Hopwood, "The Keywords 'Generation' and 'Reproduction,'" in *Reproduction: Antiquity to the Present Day*, ed. Nick Hopwood, Rebecca Flemming, and Lauren Kassell (Cambridge: Cambridge University Press, 2018), 287–304.

4   Anthony Anemone, "The Monsters of Peter the Great: The Culture of the St. Petersburg Kunstkamera in the Eighteenth Century," *The Slavic and East European Journal* 44, no. 4 (2000): 592.

5   For more on monsters within eighteenth-century science and medicine, see Lorraine Daston and Katherine Park, *Wonders and the Order of Nature, 1150–1750* (New York: Zone Books, 2001); Katharine Park and Lorraine J. Daston, "Unnatural Conceptions: The Study of Monsters in Sixteenth- and Seventeenth-Century France and England," *Past & Present* 92, no. 1 (1981): 20–54; Michael Hagner, "Enlightened Monsters," in *The Sciences in Enlightened Europe*, ed. William Clark, Jan Golinski, and Simon Schaffer (Chicago: University of Chicago Press, 1999), 175–217; Anita Guerrini, "The Creativity of God and the Order of Nature: Anatomizing Monsters in the Early Eighteenth Century," in *Monsters & Philosophy*, ed. Charles T. Wolfe (London: College Publications, 2005), 153–68; Marie-Hélène Huet, *Monstrous Imagination* (Cambridge, MA: Harvard University Press, 1993); Palmira Fontes da Costa, *The Singular and the Making of Knowledge at the Royal Society of London in the Eighteenth Century* (Newcastle-upon-Tyne: Cambridge Scholars, 2009).

"are the result of internal damage, of fear and the thoughts of the mother during her pregnancy."[6] Wet specimen preparation brought the hidden processes of generation into view for both specialist and public audiences. Generation was a hotly contested scientific subject in the eighteenth century, and central to the subject were uncertainty and disagreements about the physical form of the fetus throughout gestation: Did it, as some believed, increase in size as if grown from an extreme miniature or, as others believed, did it emerge in successive stages? Though wet specimen preparation alone could not settle these debates, it did introduce a novel technique for investigating the questions. Because preparation transformed the body into a stable, observable, and redissectible object, it offered a new empirical tool for conceptualizing of one of the body's most hidden and mysterious processes. The ability to *collect* bodies—transformed into objects—enabled them to be more directly compared, and it was this quality that made them a crucial visual methodology in the late eighteenth century as Caspar Wolff, using Peter's collection, sought to substantiate a theory of developmental embryology.

Historians have examined the scientific, cultural, and institutional significance of the Kunstkamera's collections—the museum was a cornerstone of Peter's vision for a modernized Russia. The present chapter contributes to this rich literature by substantiating the historical connections between Peter's collecting and the later history of Wolff's embryological research. The story of Peter's travels to Amsterdam and his purchase of a remarkable anatomical cabinet has been well documented by historians of art, medicine, and Russian history;[7] Wolff's embryological research on monsters has been addressed by historians of biology and embryology who have sought to make sense of Wolff's theories and connect them to nineteenth-century

---

6   Robert Collis, *The Petrine Instauration: Religion, Esotericism and Science at the Court of Peter the Great, 1689–1725* (Leiden: Brill, 2012), 453.

7   Petros Mirilas, "The Monarch and the Master: Peter the Great and Frederik Ruysch," *Archives of Surgery* 141, no. 6 (June 1, 2006): 602; Julie V. Hansen, "Resurrecting Death: Anatomical Art in the Cabinet of Dr. Frederik Ruysch," *The Art Bulletin* 78, no. 4 (1996): 663–79; Mark Kidd and Irvin M. Modlin, "Frederik Ruysch: Master Anatomist and Depictor of the Sureality of Death," *Journal of Medical Biography* 7 (1999): 69–77; Lucas Boer, Anna B. Radziun, and Roelof-Jan Oostra, "Frederik Ruysch (1638–1731): Historical Perspective and Contemporary Analysis of His Teratological Legacy," *American Journal of Medical Genetics Part A* 173, no. 1 (January 2017): 16–41; Anemone, "The Monsters of Peter the Great"; Lindsey Hughes, *Russia in the Age of Peter the Great* (New Haven, CT: Yale University Press, 1998); Collis, *The Petrine Instauration*.

developments in the field.[8] These historical narratives are, however, firmly tied together by the Kunstkamera's fetal preparations: the fetuses within the museum's "Chamber of Curiosities" speak to the history of the "public fetus" not only because they isolated the fetal body into a novel material object but also because fetal bodies were brought together into a visual format that facilitated direct comparison. This chapter argues that fetal preparations, including especially those of "monsters," critically shaped modern conceptualizations of gestation as a developmental process by serving as "snapshots" of an unobservable physiological process and its possible pathways.

From their earliest inception, fetal preparations were not confined to the cloistered world of elite science—instead, these objects were deeply connected to the public both in their origins and in their audience. The preparations that would prove so useful to embryological science had been collected for display in museums that, while certainly catering to specialists, made public access a central part of their mission. Collected from members of the public, the museum was a space where fetal preparations might speak to narratives of obstetrical practice, parental mourning, the power of medical science, and the priorities of the state.

This chapter traces an early history of wet specimen preparation within the context of anatomical collecting. While Peter built up the Kunstkamera's collection in his own right, he relied substantially on the collection of his anatomy teacher Frederik Ruysch who, in the late seventeenth century, developed a novel technique for preserving a body part in spirits. This new technology of anatomical preparation was impactful not only to collecting practices but also to how the body could be visualized. For medical men interested in generation, the fetus was no longer relegated to anatomical drawing and description but could now be directly observed and even exchanged as objects. This, I argue, made fetal bodies deemed "monstrous" a subject of direct study that was central to eighteenth-century embryology. The collections of Ruysch and Peter emphasize the multifaceted relationship of the public as both suppliers of and audiences for fetal material displayed in museums. This chapter, then, offers insight into the human networks and

---

8   Roe, *Matter, Life, and Generation*; Janina Wellmann, *The Form of Becoming: Embryology and the Epistemology of Rhythm, 1760–1830*, trans. Kate Sturge (New York: Zone Books, 2017); L. Ya. Blyakher, *History of Embryology in Russia from the Middle of the Eighteenth to the Middle of the Nineteenth Century* (Washington DC: Al Ahram Center for Scientific Translations, 1982); A. E. Gaissinovitch, "C. F. Wolff on Variability and Heredity," *History and Philosophy of the Life Sciences* 12, no. 2 (1990): 179–201; T. A. Lukina, "Caspar Friedrich Wolff und die Petersburger Akademie der Wissenschaften," *Acta Historia Leopoldina* 9 (1975): 411–25.

scientific processes that transformed the "unborn" into something visible and even tangible well before modern embryology took shape.

The Collectors

While traveling throughout Europe in 1697, Peter the Great spent several months in Amsterdam where he worked on the docks of the Dutch East India Company and took private lessons with the famous and wealthy anatomist Frederik Ruysch.[9] Ruysch's international reputation stemmed largely from his vast and singular anatomical museum that showcased his groundbreaking method of embalming. Anatomical collections were not new, but Ruysch's method was; existing collections contained mainly osteological or dried specimens. One of Europe's most well-known anatomical collections at the time was at the University of Leiden, where Ruysch attended medical school in the seventeenth century.[10] It was while in Leiden that Ruysch, along with several classmates, devised the materials and method for the long-term preservation of a body part in spirits. The technique was exceedingly difficult, but the results were dramatic: using a combination of wax-injection and spirit preservation, Ruysch was able to create vivid, lifelike anatomical preparations from soft tissue.[11] This technique revealed minute or hidden features of the body, like glands or fine capillaries, which were difficult if not impossible to see during a traditional dissection. Preparations were also capable of showing anatomical layers, as if the viewer was privy to an ongoing dissection that had been frozen in time. Peter was captivated: he was so taken by the lifelike preservation of a young boy that, according to Ruysch, he kissed the child's face.[12]

---

9   Luuc Kooijmans, *Death Defied: The Anatomy Lessons of Frederik Ruysch* (Leiden: Brill, 2011), 244; Anemone, "Monsters of Peter the Great," 596; Blyakher, *Embryology in Russia*, 19.

10   Tim Huisman, "Resilient Collections: The Long Life of Leiden's Earliest Anatomical Collections," in *The Fate of Anatomical Collections*, ed. Rina Knoeff and Robert Zwijnenberg (Burlington VT: Ashgate, 2015), 73–92.

11   Marieke M. A. Hendriksen, *Elegant Anatomy: The Eighteenth-Century Leiden Anatomical Collections* (Leiden: Brill, 2015), 76–83.

12   Frederik Ruysch, *Alle de Ontleed-, Genees-, En Heelkundige Werken van Frederik Ruysch* (Amsterdam, 1744), 1222; Rina Knoeff, "Touching Anatomy: On the Handling of Preparations in the Anatomical Cabinets of Frederik Ruysch (1638–1731)," *Studies in History and Philosophy of Science Part C: Studies in History and Philosophy of Biological and Biomedical Sciences* 49 (February 2015): 32–33.

Ruysch's home museum was a space of both medical training and curious looking. By the 1670s, Ruysch's collection was open to the public who could pay a small fee for one of his daughters to show them around the dazzling collection: the museum quickly became an attraction both for the Dutch public and European elites traveling through Amsterdam.[13] While the artistry of Ruysch's preparations was remarkable, he understood his collection to be primarily for teaching students of anatomy, surgery, and midwifery. Among his medical colleagues, skeptics claimed Ruysch's technique ran the risk of distorting features and misguiding viewers into a false sense of objectivity.[14] Yet, Ruysch argued that preparations were valuable objects of evidence since their "truths" could be studied, verified, or contested by observers. For Ruysch's private students, like Peter, preparations were taken out of their jars and actively handled during lessons—they were often even redissected.[15] Ruysch was frustrated by the state of medical research: someone could claim to have made a discovery during a dissection but, because the body decomposed, there was no way to verify the observation outside of that researcher's own depictions and recollections. About such cases, Ruysch grumbled, "I had to leave it at that. Now I preserve everything I depict, so that I needn't resort to such stupid answers."[16] Preparations, then, introduced a new technology for extending the reach and importance of shared observations to medical research.

Roughly a third of Ruysch's collection consisted of fetal bodies collected through his supervisory work of Amsterdam's midwives.[17] Amsterdam, like many Dutch municipalities, employed a corps of midwives trained by the city physician (Ruysch, in this case) and then employed by the municipality to deliver women within a specific geographic zone. These midwives, called *stadsvroedvrouwen*, were autonomous practitioners except in cases of complicated deliveries or stillbirths, at which point they were required to call in the man midwife.[18] Ruysch both trained and supervised Amsterdam's *stadsvroedvrouwen*, and his anatomical collection sat at the intersection of these roles:

---

13   Kooijmans, *Death Defied*, 176.
14   Dániel Margócsy, "A Museum of Wonders or a Cemetery of Corpses? The Commercial Exchange of Anatomical Collections in Early Modern Netherlands," in *Silent Messengers: The Circulation of Material Objects of Knowledge in the Early Modern Low Countries*, ed. Sven Dupré and Christoph Lüthy (Berlin: Lit Verlag, 2011), 207.
15   Knoeff, "Touching Anatomy," 33.
16   Ruysch, *Alle de Werken*, 675; Kooijmans, *Death Defied*, 178.
17   Hansen, "Resurrecting Death," 672.
18   "Adviezen van de stadsdoctoren te Leiden," 1719, 0509:406, Erfgoed Leiden en Omstreken; Hilary Marland, "The '*Burgerlijke*' Midwife: The *Stadsvroedvrouw* of Eighteenth-Century Holland," in *The Art of Midwifery: Early Modern Midwives in Europe* (New York: Routledge, 1993), 199.

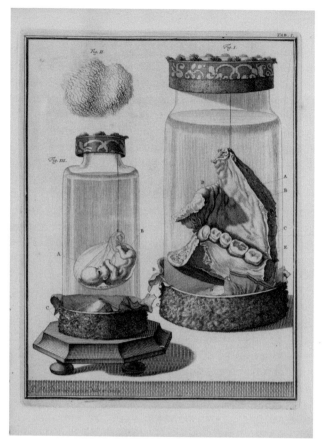

Figure 1.2. Image of two preparations by Frederik Ruysch, a fetus preserved within the amniotic sac and a section of jawbone. Ruysch often depicted his preparations in mixed arrangements that might contrast fetal or juvenile anatomy, adult anatomy, animal anatomy, and other *naturalia*, like shells. From Ruysch's *Thesaurus anatomicus* (1701). Courtesy of Rijksmuseum Boerhaave, Leiden.

he obtained fetuses for preparation through this obstetrical network, and then used the preparations to train new classes of midwives as a supplement to the dissections he performed for them.[19]

---

19   "Concept-resolutie van de burgemeesters van Leiden betreffende de opleiding van de vroedvrouwen," 1696, 0509:404, Erfgoed Leiden en Omstreken.

Fetal preparations exemplified the ability of wet preparations to bring the body's small, fleeting, and hidden components into direct sight.[20] As much as Ruysch claimed his preparations presented the body on its own terms, each preparation required decisions about visual style. Choices about how much of the maternal body to include in the preparation depended on what the preparer sought to emphasize: these choices might produce a preparation of a fetus within the womb with arteries and veins injected to highlight circulatory connections between maternal and fetal bodies, or a fetus within the delicate amniotic sac, or a fetus with its placenta still attached, or an early fetus prepared alone to demonstrate its tiny perfection. This flexibility in visual style meant fetuses could be incorporated into myriad narratives about anatomy, nature, and the body: whether skeletonized or preserved in spirits, Ruysch frequently used fetal bodies in preparations conveying moralistic messages about, for instance, the fleetingness of life or the sins of sexual promiscuity.[21] For midwives, these objects could be used to show, and thus prepare for, obstetrical emergencies like wrapped umbilical cords, vaginal abnormalities or injuries, or unusual fetal presentations. A fetus could only be prepared in *situ* if a pregnant woman had died prior to delivery and her body was available for dissection. But most fetal material in Ruysch's collection came from pregnancy losses and, as such, were preserved either with no remnant of the maternal body or only the placenta.[22]

Preparations reflected many of the questions that undergirded elite scientific interest in pregnancy during this period: namely, the nature and extent of the connection between maternal and fetal bodies and the form of the fetus throughout gestation. A fetus might appear as a body intimately enmeshed with that of its mother, or it might appear as a solitary entity disconnected from context. This second category—what might be thought of as an "embryological" in contrast to an "obstetrical" style—allowed for the isolated fetal body to be directly compared with others on the basis of anatomy. Because Ruysch saw his method of preparation as a way of venerating God and demonstrating the perfection of His design, his collection contained few fetal abnormalities and, instead, sought to preserve specimens exemplifying anatomical perfection.[23]

After months of private lessons with Ruysch, Peter returned to Russia animated by a love for anatomy. In Moscow, the tsar was said to carry a bag of surgical tools with him in case he was notified of an interesting surgery happening nearby. Peter also quickly embarked on his own project of creating

---

20　Duden, *Disembodying Women*, 45.

21　Knoeff, "Touching Anatomy," 40; Hansen, "Resurrecting Death," 669.

22　Knoeff, "Touching Anatomy," 36–37.

23　Hansen, "Resurrecting Death," 673.

an anatomical museum that he envisioned as a centerpiece of his new capital under construction, St. Petersburg.[24] Yet unlike his teacher who sought to preserve instances of perfection, Peter's interest was in nature's unusual products—particularly when it came to collecting bodies. In 1704, Peter issued an *ukaz* forbidding midwives from killing or concealing infants "born as monsters," instructing them instead to deliver such bodies to local clerics who, in a separate order, were told to send those bodies to Moscow's royal apothecary for preservation.[25] These preserved bodies were added to Peter's rapidly growing collection which, in addition to anatomical specimens, included coins, ethnographic material, and a wide variety of *naturalia*.

Peter moved his collection to St. Petersburg upon the city's establishment in 1714. Three years later, Peter returned to Amsterdam and bought his old teacher's entire collection—2,045 anatomical specimens and *naturalia*—for the sum of 30,000 guilders, roughly equivalent to $400,000 today.[26] In St. Petersburg, Ruysch and Peter's combined anatomical collections formed the core of the new state museum, the Kunstkamera. This made St. Petersburg home to a comprehensive embryological collection containing hundreds of fetuses preserved in jars—a kaleidoscopic view of gestation which included various bodily forms, gestational ages, and levels of connection to the maternal body.[27] Although wet specimen preparation proliferated across Europe and would become a mainstay of anatomical collections by the end of the eighteenth century, Peter was an early and fervent adopter of the technology: when Peter purchased Ruysch's collection in 1717, Ruysch's own medical school in Leiden had not yet begun earnestly building up its collection of wet specimens and would not do so until the early 1730s.[28] In addition to various human and animal "monsters," visitors to the museum in the 1720s report seeing bottles with human fetuses arranged from the smallest embryo to the mature fruit, a style of display that would only become scientifically commonplace in the early nineteenth century.[29]

---

24 Mirilas, "Monarch and the Master," 606; Michael Gordin, "The Importance of Being Earnest: The Early St. Petersburg Academy of Sciences," *Isis* 91 (2000), 4.

25 Collis, *Petrine Instauration*, 450; T.V. Stanyukovich, *The Museum of Anthropology and Ethnography Named after Peter the Great* (Leningrad: Nauka, 1970), 4.

26 Collis, *Petrine Instauration*, 439.

27 Stanyukovich, *Museum of Peter the Great*, 23.

28 Hendriksen, *Elegant Anatomy*, 9. For insight into the role of tacit knowledge in techniques for creating these preparations, see pp. 5–7.

29 Blyakher, *Embryology in Russia*, 22–23; Nick Hopwood, "Producing Development: The Anatomy of Human Embryos and the Norms of Wilhelm His," *Bulletin of the History of Medicine* 74, no. 1 (2000): 29–79; Nick

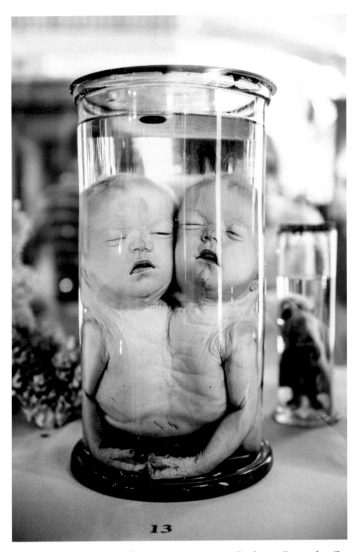

Figure 1.3. A preparation of conjoined twins on display at Peter the Great's Museum of Anthropology and Ethnography (Kunstkamera). Note the restitched incision at the neck and upper chest, indicating that the body was dissected. The anatomist here was likely interested in how the structures of the body separated. Bodies preserved in this way could be redissected, making them ideal for teaching. Photo by Annelie Drakman.

By virtue of Peter's early and aggressive collecting, St. Petersburg amassed an embryological collection that remained singular in its scale and scope for most of the century. From its earliest period, then, wet specimen preparation was used to visualize fetal bodies within multiple frameworks—obstetrically, moralistically, and embryologically. In the Kunstkamera's Chamber of Curiosities, fetuses with a wide variation of bodily forms were displayed alongside one another, which brought fetuses "born as monsters" and those considered "perfect" into a shared space and method of display. This physical merging brought together two entwined questions, both of which were of intense interest in the eighteenth century: first, the cause of "monstrosity," and, second, the physiological processes of generation. These preparations were stable objects that allowed for a wide range of audiences to share in observations of otherwise hidden or rare phenomena; as such, they were potent objects for shaping scientific narratives through their use in teaching, public display, and research.

Before this chapter turns to the role of the Kunstkamera's fetal preparations in embryological research, it first examines the dual importance of the public to the collection. Peter and Ruysch both relied upon the public to supply their museums with fetal material, although the two men employed vastly different mechanisms for doing so. The embryological collections were meant to be seen by an audience that extended far beyond scientific specialists, even if the preparations themselves were often described and understood as tools of teaching and research. If it is significant that the Kunstkamera's embryological collection was a transformative space in visualizing the fetus, it is equally significant that the collection itself was intrinsically tied to the public: this was a visual technology that brought gestation out from the body and into the halls of the museum for viewing and contemplation.

Public as Source, Public as Audience

Wet preparations were remarkably useful to medical study. This is made plain both by Ruysch's own use of the collection in his teaching and in the widespread proliferation of wet specimen preparation across European hospitals and medical schools by the end of the century. Yet from the beginning, wet preparations were appreciated not only as powerful objects for specialist study but also for public display: the public could view Ruysch's collection at his home at Bloemgracht 15 and, after moving the capital to St. Petersburg,

Hopwood, Simon Schaffer, and Jim Secord, "Seriality and Scientific Objects in the Nineteenth Century," *History of Science* 48, no. 3–4 (September 2010): 251–85.

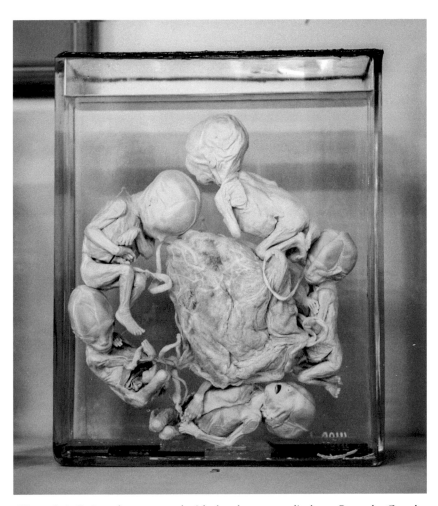

Figure 1.4. Quintuplets preserved with the placenta on display at Peter the Great's Museum of Anthropology and Ethnography (Kunstkamera). While the fetal bodies are not anatomically unusual, multiples—particularly of anything beyond twins—was another phenomenon of pregnancy whose rarity meant its physiology was poorly understood. In the same way preparation enabled the study of anatomical rarities, like conjoined twins, it also enabled physicians to observe physiological rarities, like multiples. Note also the evidence of (re)dissection in the preparation to the right. Photo by Annelie Drakman.

Peter followed his teacher's example by opening up his own collections to the public.

Fetuses are a unique object within anatomical museums with regard to their relationship to the public. Namely, fetuses had to be obtained *from* the public in a way that differed from most anatomical specimens that could be taken from hospital patients, unclaimed cadavers, criminals, or consenting adult patients. The necessity of dissection to medical education was largely accepted by European anatomists by the eighteenth century although bodies were still difficult to come by: regulations about which bodies could be anatomized differed in municipalities and countries across Europe and, even if dissection was accepted by anatomists, many in the public had reservations. Ruysch's work with Amsterdam's hospital gave him access to the bodies of some patients—hospital administration willing—and his role as the city's forensic examiner gave him access to unclaimed victims of crime.[30] Yet fetuses presented a unique challenge in that they were not isolated bodies. Instead, they were directly linked to a mother through pregnancy and, as such, the acquisition of fetal material necessitated direct contact with the parents. Elsewhere in Europe, such material might be collected from poor or unmarried women who, due to their social station, gave birth in the hospital, but because *stadsvroedvrouwen* were employed to deliver all women—regardless of income level—this was a relatively uncommon situation in Dutch municipalities; in fact, the first hospital-based maternity ward in Amsterdam wouldn't open until the turn of the nineteenth century at which point it did, indeed, become a significant site of anatomical collection.[31]

As the supervisor and trainer of Amsterdam's *stadsvroedvrouwen*, Ruysch was directly connected to the women who were attending deliveries and encountering fetal material. The regulations of this system were such that *stadsvroedvrouwen* were autonomous practitioners except in cases that either required instrumental intervention or carried a risk of maternal or fetal death; these necessitated the presence of a man-midwife. Regarding these

---

30 Kooijmans, *Death Defied*, 68, 97. For more on the acquisition of bodies for anatomical research, see Ruth Richardson, *Death, Dissection, and the Destitute* (Chicago: University of Chicago Press, 2001); Michael Sappol, *A Traffic of Dead Bodies: Anatomy and Embodied Social Identity in Ninteenth-Century America* (Princeton, NJ: Princeton University Press, 2002); Katharine Park, *Secrets of Women: Gender, Generation, and the Origins of Human Dissection* (New York: Zone Books, 2006).

31 Laurens de Rooy, "A Cabinet Departs," in *Forces of Form*, ed. Simon Knepper, Johan Kortenray, and Antoon Moorman (Amsterdam: Amsterdam University Press, 2009), 61; Justus Lodewijk Dusseau et al., *Musée Vrolik. Catalogue de La Collection d'anatomie Humaine, Comparée et Pathologique de M.M. Ger. et W. Vrolik* (Amsterdam: Impr. de W. J. de Roever Kröber, 1865), 5.

cases, Ruysch wrote in his *Works*, "I am gratified that often I was called to [miscarriages], when I found the parents very sad . . . I am in the habit of consoling them, and assuring them that perfect infants change after death in the mother's womb."[32] To these parents, Ruysch offered his method of preparation as a means of memorialization: with it, he could ameliorate the disturbing visual elements of a miscarriage and restore a fetal body to an idealized, peaceful perfection.[33] The *stadsvroedvrouwen* system in Dutch municipalities was unique in that it integrated midwives into the medical marketplace, which established a straightforward infrastructural connection between parents and elite anatomists. Thus, an enterprising anatomical collector—like Ruysch—could use this regulated medical network as a pipeline for the acquisition of fetal material from members of the public.

While Ruysch's collection consisted mostly of physically "perfect" fetuses, an account of Ruysch's negotiations with the mother of conjoined twins offers insight into these encounters. About the case, Ruysch wrote, "I myself have possession of two peoples grown together, being a birth of eight months, which I have embalmed and keep in my house on the condition that the parents are free, as often as it pleases them, to come with their friends to see the children."[34] While the father of the twins was already dead, Ruysch went on to explain his agreement with their mother that if she were to outlive Ruysch, the preparation of her children would be given back to her; if Ruysch outlived her, the twins would belong to him. Just as preparations did not provide a single iconography of the fetus, nor did they serve a uniform purpose: what Ruysch considered valuable material for teaching and research for himself, he understood as a unique and emotionally meaningful object of memorialization for parents.[35]

In contrast to Ruysch's reliance on his professional network, Peter collected fetal material using his power as an autocrat. Peter issued his 1704 *ukaz* instructing midwives to hand over the bodies of monstrous infants with the caveat that failure to do was punishable by death. Peter's interest was equated with an interest of the state, which the public was forbidden to resist. The result, however, was a similar pipeline that delivered interesting fetal material from the birthing bed to the anatomist's jar although without

32 Ruysch, *Alle de Werken*, 1022–23.
33 Knoeff, "Touching Anatomy," 43.
34 Ruysch, *Alle de Werken*, 1038.
35 For more on the relationship between anatomical collectors and mothers in the context of nineteenth-century America, see Shannon Withycombe, *Lost: Miscarriage in Nineteenth-Century America* (New Brunswick, NJ: Rutgers University Press, 2019).

the pretense of reciprocity found in Ruysch's negotiations with parents. The public's participation in Peter's project of collection was—willingly or not—their contribution to his efforts of remaking Russia into a scientific, European state.

Peter issued another *ukaz* in 1718 further detailing these acquisitions. Although the 1704 order had threatened midwives with death for failure to comply, the 1718 *ukaz* suggests that fetuses were obtained through financial incentives rather than punitive threats. The later *ukaz* set out a price list for monsters that included monstrous animals, dead fetuses, and living children with unusual bodies; this last category commanded the highest reward—one hundred roubles—and these individuals resided in the Kunstkamera as "living exhibits" who did odd jobs around the museum.[36]

From its opening in 1714, the museum was accessible to the public with low barriers to entry. The Kunstkamera was a centerpiece of the new capital of St. Petersburg, which Peter had designed according to his vision of Russia as a state aligned with European attitudes, educational standards, and institutions.[37] A key advisor was the German polymath Gottfried Wilhelm Leibniz who emphasized to Peter the chief importance of a cabinet of rarities to a modern, scientific state—Russia was, Leibniz claimed, uniquely well situated for collecting due to its massive geographic expanse.[38] Peter was adamant that his collections be open to the public, telling one resistant advisor, "It is my will and intention not only that everybody enters *gratis* but that whenever a company comes to see the cabinet, that they be offered in my name and at my expense a dish of coffee, a glass of wine, or some other refreshment in this repository of curiosities."[39]

If the Kunstkamera museum was a central piece in this broader institutional vision, the anatomical cabinet was one of its core collections. Anatomy, as a science, spoke to Peter's intentions to bring European rationalism to Russia. While dissection had become a commonplace part of medical education across Europe, it was scarcely practiced in Russia due to religious concerns and cultural beliefs, including the potential for certain bodies to become vampires; these beliefs applied most strongly to the same types of bodies that populated dissecting tables across Europe, namely criminals, suicides, and unclaimed bodies.[40] Ruysch's anatomical cabinet was one of

---

36 Collis, *Petrine Instauration*, 454; Anemone, "Monsters of Peter the Great," 592–93.

37 Mirilas, "Monarch and the Master," 603.

38 Gordin, "Importance of Being Earnest," 4.

39 Collis, *Petrine Instauration*, 443.

40 Anemone, "Monsters of Peter the Great," 588–89.

several European collections that Peter bought for his new museum, which served as an institutional link between the European scientific community and St. Petersburg society. As such, it was a powerful site for transmitting Peter's vision for Russia, and it was critical that the Kunstkamera be open to the public in order to effectively fill this role to Russian subjects. Peter strengthened the scientific messaging of the museum by joining it to the Russian Academy of Sciences when the latter was formed in 1724.[41] Thus the museum itself was a public arm of a state scientific institution—modeled directly on Berlin's academy upon Leibniz's suggestion—which signaled a new, central role of European science in Russia.

Ruysch's original collection in Amsterdam and the combined collection in St. Petersburg merged public and scientific spaces. Both museums offered the public an opportunity to observe and engage with the projects of elite science, and, in the case of St. Petersburg, they established the institutional framework for a new scientific social order. As useful to scientific research as they were, fetal preparations were objects embedded into narratives that involved the broader public, both ones intimately personal and ones of national identity. Museums are never neutral spaces: they materialize ideologies, power dynamics, and domains of knowledge.[42] In the collections of Peter and Ruysch, fetal preparations brought gestation out of the private sphere and into public view, signaling the power of medical science to reveal nature's most hidden secrets. Peter's collection of monsters, moreover, was a rejection of traditional superstition in its claim that, through collection and study, even this pernicious mystery could be brought into rational order: preserved and displayed in Peter's museum, these fetuses signaled Russia's new scientific age.

---

41 Stanyukovich, *Museum of Peter the Great*, 23.

42 Eilean Hooper-Greenhill, *Museums and the Shaping of Knowledge* (London: Routledge, 1992); George W. Stocking Jr., *Objects and Others: Essays on Museums and Material Culture* (Madison: University of Wisconsin Press, 1998); Tony Bennett, "The Exhibitionary Complex," in *Culture/Power/ History: A Reader in Contemporary Social Theory*, ed. Nicholas Dirks and Geoff Eley (Princeton, NJ: Princeton University Press, 1994), 123–54; Donna Haraway, "Teddy Bear Patriarchy," in *Primate Visions* (New York: Routledge, 1989), 22–58.

C. F. Wolff, Epigenesis, and the Storehouse of Monsters

Peter established the Russian Academy of Sciences in 1724, shortly before his death. Affiliated with the Kunstkamera, Academy physicians gained oversight of the museum's anatomical collection as well as its "living exhibits" who had come to the museum due to the *ukazi*. When possible, academy physicians attempted to gather information about the pregnancies that had produced the abnormal bodies arriving to the Kunstkamera in an attempt to discern possible causes of their bodily deviation. While Ruysch's close connection to Amsterdam's midwives gave him more direct access to parents who might answer these questions, this work was significantly more patchwork in Russia where each step of the collecting pipeline—not to mention Russia's vast geographical range—added distance between the people involved in a birth and the physicians preparing the body for display. Yet, physicians always attempted to gather as much contextual information as possible about a body given to the collection in order to discern a causal event: Had the mother experienced a fright? Did other children in the village exhibit similar abnormalities? Had the mother been ill?[43] In his 1718 *ukaz*, Peter declared, "Ignoramuses think that such monsters are born from the actions of the devil . . . monsters are [instead] caused from internal damage, also from fear and the thoughts of the mother in the time of her pregnancy."[44] With this statement, Peter aligned himself with mainstream European scientific thought and, all at once, connected his project of collecting to the dismissal of traditional beliefs and to the authority of European science to replace their explanatory power.

This belief in a connection between maternal experience and fetal body was scientifically mainstream in the early eighteenth century. The prevailing theory of generation was called "preformation," and it held that all fetuses had been fully, perfectly formed at the moment of Creation. These fully formed fetuses were stored in extremely miniature form in either the sperm or the egg until conception, which began a process of gestation that grew the fetus in size from its preformed miniature into a full-term infant.[45] Monsters were a thorny problem within this paradigm of generation. Were monsters, as some preformationists suggested, preformed by God in their imperfect state? Or were they, as others argued, the result of damage to the fetus during pregnancy?[46] The latter belief was far more widespread

---

43   Anemone, "Monsters of Peter the Great," 594.

44   Collis, *Petrine Instauration*, 453.

45   Joseph Needham, *A History of Embryology* (New York: Arno, 1975), 205–11.

46   For more on explanations of monstrosity within a preformationist framework see Maria Teresa Monti, "Epigenesis of the Monstrous Form and Preformistic

and afforded tremendous power to the maternal mind as having potentially deformative power upon an originally perfect fetal body: in addition to illness and injury, a woman's fears or psychic shocks might imprint themselves upon the growing fruit and cause her to birth not a perfectly healthy child but a monstrous one.[47] Contextual information about a pregnancy offered insight into potential causal events.

Although the academy continued to collect fetal material into the 1740s, Peter's death in 1725 began the demise of the Kunstkamera's more carnivalesque elements. Over the next half decade, the "living monsters" residing in the museum were released, while new ones were turned away with one academy physician saying, "In the Kunstkamera, we keep only dead freaks."[48] A devastating fire ripped through the museum in 1747 and, while the anatomical preparations were undamaged, most were removed from display for nearly twenty years as the museum underwent extensive renovations. These preparations comprised the "storehouse of monsters" that Caspar Friedrich Wolff referenced in his 1776 letter explaining his new research into the cause of monstrosity and, more generally, into questions of generation.

Wolff had arrived at the Russian Academy of Sciences in 1766 after being named chair of anatomy and physiology. His appointment to the Russian Academy of Sciences came after Wolff failed to obtain an academic post in Germany—a denial due, at least in part, to his controversial 1759 dissertation on generation, which had refuted the preformationist theories of one of Europe's most highly regarded scientific minds: Albrecht von Haller.[49] Wolff's was a theory of epigenesis, an ancient theory of generation positing that a body emerges through successive stages of differentiation. Though the theory of epigenesis had its roots in Aristotle, it had fallen out of favor in the mid-seventeenth century due to the philosophical and mechanistic elegance of preformation that, unlike epigenesis, required no "occult" force to explain its operation. Preformationists needed only to accept the possibility of exceptionally miniature bodies; epigenesists, however, had to explain *how*, exactly, undifferentiated matter "knew" how to differentiate and mature into the parts of a coherent animal body. Wolff's research brought epigenesis into the language and practices of eighteenth-century physiological research. He conceptualized of gestation as a developmental process characterized by rhythmic elements of repetition, regularity, and variation and driven by an

'Genetics' (Lémery-Winslow-Haller)," *Early Science and Medicine* 5, no. 1 (2000): 3–32.

47   Huet, *Monstrous Imagination*.

48   Hughes, *Russia*, 316.

49   Needham, *A History of Embryology*, 220–22. For a comprehensive account of the dispute between Wolff and Haller, see Roe, *Matter, Life, and Generation*.

immaterial organizing force inherent to organic matter itself.[50] Wolff was particularly fascinated by the phenomena of variation: How did traits within a species remain stable or undergo variation, and what variations could be passed down through generations?

Wolff saw monsters as proffering a unique line of evidence for the study of epigenesis precisely because they were dramatic physical variations.[51] Within this framework, the anatomical features of "monstrous" bodies offered insight into the stabilization or variation of traits during the shared, physiological process of development. Put another way, monsters were not singular aberrations that could be explained away by a woman's fright or sinful desire; instead, they were natural varieties within a species that did not propagate down generations due to the simple fact that most severe "monstrosities" did not survive birth, much less reach reproductive age.[52] This was a major conceptual transformation that placed variation— or "monstrosity"—at the heart of understanding both generation and the physicality of the fetal body. This transformation, however, required others: as historian of the life sciences Janina Wellmann observes, "Wolff needed pictures in order to 'see' development . . . a new conceptual framework had to be built, along with new experimental practices, new techniques of observation, and, crucially, new forms of visual representation."[53] The hundreds of fetuses in the Kunstkamera's collections—those of Ruysch, of Peter, and later academy acquisitions—offered a powerful form of visual representation that was uniquely well suited to Wolff's research: the collection contained a large number of fetuses preserved in bodily isolation— bodies spanning an enormous range of physical forms and gestational ages. Thus, Wolff could not only dissect a diversity of fetal bodies, but he could also directly compare them against one another and form a visual "map" of embryological development and its possible pathways. Wolff began his research on the fetal preparations shortly after his arrival and remained preoccupied by them until the 1780s, collecting his observations and ideas into an unpublished treatise titled *Objecta meditationum pro theoria monstrorum* that would include a description of "the whole catalog of monsters in possession of the Academy."[54] *Objecta* remained unpublished at Wolff's

50 Wellmann, *Form of Becoming*, 95; Lukina, "Caspar Friedrich Wolff Und Die Petersburger Akademie Der Wissenschaften," 416.

51 Roe, *Matter, Life, and Generation*, 126.

52 Roe, 142; C. F. Wolff, *Objecta Meditationum pro Theoria Monstrorum; Predmety Razmyshlenij v Svjazi s Teoriej Urodov*, trans. Ju. Kh. Kopelevich and T. A. Lukina (Leningrad: Izdatel'stvo, 1973), 229.

53 Wellmann, *Form of Becoming*, 16.

54 Wolff, *Pro Theoria Monstrorum*; Gaissinovitch, "C. F. Wolff on Variability and Heredity," 71.

death in 1794, and Wolff himself died a fairly marginal figure within the European scientific community.

Wolff's research, however, found two crucial champions in the German embryologists J. F. Meckel the Younger and Karl Ernst von Baer. Meckel is largely responsible for bringing Wolff to a wider European audience through his translations of Wolff's published works and for his own research. Meckel, too, was highly interested in the subject of fetal abnormality and built on Wolff's work through research and observations made from his own substantial anatomical collection in Halle.[55] While visiting St. Petersburg in 1830, von Baer encountered an archive containing the unfinished fragments of *Objecta*, and he seized upon both its novel source of evidence—the fetal preparations—and the work's utility to the field of embryology. Appealing to his fellow embryologists to collaborate on a translation of the work, von Baer stressed that Wolff's anatomical descriptions of the fetal preparations were "the most important and elaborate part,"[56] and praised the collection by saying "it is only through Peter's personal interest in such effects of nature, which attracted him through their veil of mystery, that these objects are brought together . . . [Wolff] regarded the work undertaken as a fruit of the seed of the great emperor."[57]

From the early days of the Kunstkamera's collection, the fetuses within it were understood as offering a valuable line of inquiry into scientific questions of generation. For Peter, this was directly related to his larger project of aligning Russia with European sensibilities, sensibilities that his 1718 *ukaz* on the collections set in contrast to the "ignorant superstitions" that Peter believed guided existing Russian attitudes toward unusual bodies. Yet the utility of the collection to actual embryological research in Peter's time was largely rhetorical. Because monsters were thought to be isolated aberrations whose causes were located in the experiences of the mother, an aberrant fetal body by itself demonstrated little more than the fact that such a body could, and did, exist. Building up the Kunstkamera's collections and creating an affiliated scientific institution was, for Peter, a project of statecraft, but an embryological *collection*—one large and diverse—proved to be

---

55   Owen E. Clark, "The Contributions of J. F. Meckel, the Younger, to the Science of Teratology," *Journal of the History of Medicine and Allied Sciences* 24, no. 3 (1969): 310–22.

56   Ernst von Baer, "Ueber Den Littärischen Nachlass von Caspar Friedrich Wolff, Ehemaligem Mitgliede Der Akademie Der Wissenschaften Zu St. Petersburg," *Bulletin de La Classe Physico-Mathématique de l'Académie Impériale Des Sciences de Saint-Pétersbourg* 5, no. 9–10 (1846): 159–60.

57   Von Baer, "Ueber Den Littärischen Nachlass von Caspar Friedrich Wolff," 158.

an extraordinarily useful visual methodology for a paradigm of generation that required comparison.

Conclusions:
Entwined Narratives in the Chamber of Curiosity

The development of wet specimen preparation in the late seventeenth century marks a key moment in the history of the public fetus. Referencing contemporaneous early modern advancements in microscopy and illustration, Barbara Duden says, "The technogenesis of the fetal image of embryology can be related to these instruments of visualization."[58] Wet preparations of fetuses surely belong within these consequential visual technologies. These preparations brought the fetal body into direct scientific sight both as a body dependent upon and enmeshed with that of its other, as well as a body that could be considered its own isolated being. Although the "disappearance" of the pregnant body from fetal iconography has been largely associated with the twentieth century—exemplified by Lennart Nilsson's photography for *Life*—wet specimens also allowed the fetus to be evaluated as an autonomous physical being devoid of maternal context.

The technique of anatomical preparation pioneered by Ruysch allowed fetuses to be integrated into a number of overlapping narratives: of obstetrical practice, of personal memorialization, of the power of medical science, and of the nature of gestation as a physiological process. Such narratives were never confined to cloistered halls of elite science; instead, they represent intimate entanglements between researchers and the public's perception of the scientific enterprise. For Ruysch, fetal preparations were not only useful objects of research but also demonstrated to the public the power of medical science to alleviate emotional suffering and create space for grief. For Peter, fetal preparations—particularly those of monsters—represented the centrality of European scientific methods and knowledge in the state's new transformative moment.

The anatomical collection at the Kunstkamera merged the scientific and the public into a shared space of reconceptualizing gestation. While fetuses were sometimes preserved *in situ* within the maternal body, anatomists seized upon the fact that stillborn or miscarried fetuses could be preserved, making it possible to transform relatively common obstetrical events into new scientific opportunities. This "embryological style" facilitated the comparison of fetal bodies that, in the Chamber of Curiosities, varied from the very tiny to the mature fruit, from the physically "perfect" to myriad

---

58   Duden, *Disembodying Women*, 92.

iterations of physical abnormality that had long fallen under the scientific designation of "monstrous." Wet preparations themselves would not necessarily disabuse an observer of preformationist views. The extraordinarily tiny embryos are remarkable for the way in which they do, indeed, show body parts in extreme miniature. Yet a *collection* of preserved and isolated fetal bodies proved to be a potent methodology for visualizing generation as a developmental process. Since the physiological process itself could not be directly observed, fetal preparations served as "snapshots" that collectively showed not only the stages of development but also "monsters" as its potential variations.

That the fetal body develops during gestation, its body emerging in successive stages of refinement, is so fundamental to modern embryology as to be cognitively invisible to us in the twentieth century. But we owe this conceptualization to a much earlier visual technology which today persists in anatomical collections as curious relics of the past. The embryological collections of Ruysch and Peter are still on display in the Kunstkamera in St. Petersburg, still in the original building that was completed in 1727. Although St. Petersburg was unrivaled in the scale and scope of its embryological collection, fetal preparations became ubiquitous features of anatomical collections across Europe as Ruysch's original technique was replicated and modified. Today, these preparations remain magnetic to museumgoers. Even as fetal imagery has become widespread, these bodies are still a unique, nearly tangible window into an unseen world.

Chapter Two

"What Does the Eye Have to Do with Obstetrics?"

The Fetus between Sight and Touch in Eighteenth-Century Italy

Jennifer Kosmin

During the summer of 1791, in anticipation of the opening of a midwifery school in Pavia, near Milan, Vincenzo Malacarne requested a full-sized obstetrical machine and a number of additional wax anatomical preparations from the Florentine wax workshop of Felice Fontana.[1] Fontana's wax workshop was renowned in Italy and abroad for its lifelike anatomical models.[2] Midwifery instructors like Malacarne often employed a variety of three-dimensional obstetrical representations to help students, both midwives and surgeons, coordinate their visualization of internal structures with their tactile sense of the female body and the position and movement of the fetus in utero. On models and machines, midwives, who often lacked formal training, could practice manual skills and become familiar

---

1 Parts of this chapter were previously published as "Modelling Authority: Obstetrical Machines in the Instruction of Midwives and Surgeons in Eighteenth-Century Italy," *Social History of Medicine* 34, no. 2 (2021): 509–31. With the permission of Oxford University Press.

2 A collection of documents relating to the commission and transfer of these models can be found in the Archivio di Stato di Milano (ASM), *Sanità*, Parte Antica, 273, "Ostetricia, Pavia, Macchine."

with a more scientific and standardized anatomical vocabulary.[3] Models also allowed students to develop a sophisticated understanding of gestation as a temporal process: they could see the changes the pregnant body and fetus underwent—down to the transformation of the umbilical vein and arteries— over time.[4]

Unlike inert models, obstetrical machines were intended to simulate the processes of birth and assist in student's acquisition of applied manual skills.[5] Machines ranged in their construction and complexity, though they tended to incorporate some kind of mechanization that produced effects such as the contracting and dilating of the uterus and cervix and the release of fluids.[6] This was essential, according to the Pavia machine's designer, Giuseppe

---

3   On obstetrical models made in Italy see Maurizio Armaroli, *Le cere anatomiche bolognesi del settecento* (Bologna: CLUEB, 1981); A. Zanca, *Le cere e le terrecotte ostetriche del Museo di Storia della Scienza a Firenze* (Florence: Arnaud, 1981); Francesca Vannozzi, "Fantocci, marchingegni e modelli nella didattica ostetrica senese," in Francesca Vannozzi, ed. *Nascere a Siena. Il parto e l'assistenza alla nascita dal Medioevo all'età moderna* (Siena: Nuova Immagine, 2005), 35–42; Claudia Pancino and Jean d'Yvoire, *Formato nel segreto. Nascituri e feti fra immagini e immaginario dal XVI al XXI secolo* (Rome: Carocci, 2006), 48–63; Alessandro Riva, *Cere. Le anatomie di Clemente Susini dell'Università di Cagliari* (Nuoro: Ilisso, 2007); Rebecca Messbarger, *The Lady Anatomist: The Life and Work of Anna Morandi Manzolini* (Chicago: University of Chicago Press, 2010); Lucia Dacome, *Malleable Anatomies: Models, Makers, and Material Culture in Eighteenth-Century Italy* (Oxford: Oxford University Press, 2017).

4   Pietro Sografi, *Corso Elementare dell'Arte di Raccogliere I Parti, Diviso in Lezioni* (Padova, 1788), 1–25.

5   On obstetrical machines see Pam Lieske, "'Made in Imitation of Real Women and Children': Obstetrical Machines in Eighteenth-Century Britain," in *The Female Body in Medicine and Literature*, ed. Andrew Mangham and Greta Depledge (Liverpool: Liverpool University Press, 2011), 69–88; Bonnie Blackwell, "*Tristram Shandy* and the Theater of the Mechanical Mother," *ELH* 68 (2001): 81–133; Margaret Carlyle, "Phantoms in the Classroom: Midwifery Training in Enlightenment Europe," *KNOW: A Journal on the Formation of Knowledge* 2 (2018): 111–36; Lucia Dacome, *Malleable Anatomies*, esp. chapter 5 "Blindfolding the Midwives"; Messbarger, *Lady Anatomist*, esp. chapter 3.

6   Madame du Coudray's models incorporated sponges that released dyed fluids to represent blood and amniotic fluid. On Coudray, see Carlyle, "Phantoms in the Classroom." In England, some of William Smellie's obstetrical machines may have been capable of accommodating a fluid-filled amniotic sac. Bonnie Blackwell writes that Smellie's students would often sneak into the operating room before lessons and fill the machine's bladder with beer. If a student practicing forceps delivery applied the instruments incorrectly,

Galletti, since lecturing students about the various positions a fetus might assume in utero could not accustom them to negotiating the surprising force of the uterus during labor.[7] The Pavia machine also paid particular attention to the accompanying fetal dolls, which were elastic, bendable at the joints, and contained internal structures that provided an accurate feel and sense of the resistance of fetal bone.[8] It was this attention to detail, to the lifelike recreation of human skin and bone, that made the Pavia machine unique among other eighteenth-century obstetrical machines, which tended to eschew realism in favor of instructional capacity.[9] In fact, Malacarne admitted that because the machine was "so elegant and seductively naturalistic," he felt compelled by decency to cover it with a sheet when used for instruction.[10] For Galletti, the machine mimicked the movements and feel of the human body so "splendidly . . . that it was almost as if it were produced by the secret workings of nature."[11]

This chapter argues that the Pavia commission's visually striking obstetrical machine and lifelike fetal models intended to cultivate tactile sensitivity was informed by new sensibilities toward the fetus in a period that saw the interests of the medical profession, absolutist states, and the Catholic Church projected onto the unborn in new ways. First, the models can be situated as part of an important period in the development and professionalization of the field of obstetrics. Their manufacture and use were largely contemporaneous with the emergence of formal midwifery schools and more stringent

---

it was common to puncture the bladder (a serious and life-threatening mistake). Blackwell, "*Tristram Shandy* and the Theater of the Mechanical Mother," 92–93.

7 Giuseppe Galletti, *Elementi di Ostetricia, del Dottore Gio. Giorgio Roederer, Tradotti e Corredati di Figure in Rame da Giuseppe Galletti* (Firenze: Albizziniana, 1775), xiii.

8 Galletti, *Elementi di Ostetricia*, xiv–xv.

9 In contrast to the extreme, even uncanny, verisimilitude of the anatomical wax models produced in Italy during the eighteenth century, obstetrical machines tended to eschew realism in favor of pedagogic functionality. The stuffed fabric and bone machines popularized by the renowned French midwife Madame du Coudray at midcentury suggest, for instance, utility over anatomical accuracy. Fashioning machines with durability in mind indeed made sense given that these objects were intended to be used over and over. By contrast, the Pavia machine was more delicate but seems to have been modeled with the explicit intent of erasing, or at least reducing, the conceptual boundaries between model and body.

10 ASM, *Sanità*, Parte Antica, c. 273. Letter from Vincenzo Malacarne, 9 November 1792.

11 Galletti, *Elementi di Ostetricia*, xiii.

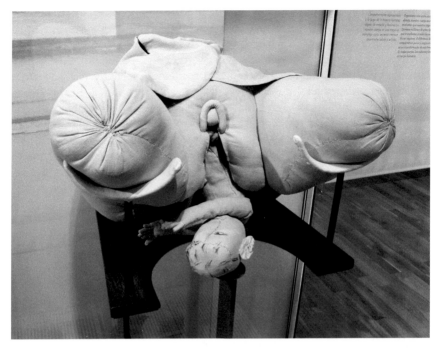

Figure 2.1. Obstetrical machine designed by Madame du Coudray, Musee Flaubert et d'Histoire de la Medecine, Rouen. Photo by Ji-Elle, courtesy of Wikimedia Commons Public Domain.

requirements for training and licensing for both midwives and surgeon-obstetricians. Extensive collections of three-dimensional obstetric models were critical components of instruction in a period when maternity wards, and thus opportunities for regular clinical training, were not widespread. Obstetrical machines like the Pavia commission also remind us that, despite scholarly emphasis on the ascendance of sight and visuality in medical practice at the end of the eighteenth century, touch continued to be a critical medical skill, particularly in obstetrics.

Second, the Pavia commission was produced in the context of a dramatic shift in thinking about the ontological status of the fetus. New research into embryonic development raised novel questions about the point of ensoulment and whether the fetus could be understood as living while still in its mother's womb. What emerged was the figure of the "unborn citizen," an imagined future component of the body politic whose life was deserving of certain legal protections even before being born. To this end, states promoted initiatives to protect infant life, while harshly criminalizing infanticide, abortion, and abandonment. In Italy, these interests were shaped by a reinvigorated Catholic concern with fetal baptism and came together most dramatically in legal requirements for surgeons and midwives to perform the Cesarean operation in cases where the life of the fetus was at risk. Such prescriptions upturned a long-standing hierarchy in which the life of the mother was valued above that of her unborn child. The result was a deontological shift on the part of medical practitioners to save the life of the fetus/child over or on par with that of the mother.

The Ontological Status of the Fetus

The Catholic Church's long-standing preoccupation with baptism was reinvigorated in the eighteenth century in response to new scientific discoveries related to embryology and the heated debates about ensoulment and animation that resulted. While some natural philosophers argued that the advanced organization that the animal embryo attained during development existed complete in some form from the time of conception (preformationism), others held that the embryo developed gradually from unorganized matter (epigenesis).[12] The argument behind preformationism that essentially an entire human being was present at conception, only waiting to be revealed over time, appealed to some theologians in that it seemed to demonstrate God's perfection and omniscience. To such thinkers, the preformation thesis also allowed for the argument that human ensoulment began at conception. Although this view aligned well with the idea of Mary's Immaculate Conception, it represented a quite drastic revision of traditional Aristotelian and Thomistic doctrine on ensoulment, which held that animation began at between thirty and forty days for males, and seventy to eighty for females. These figures, which roughly corresponded to quickening, when the mother could feel the child move in utero, had long provided the basis for both religious and secular legal codes. That is to say, abortion was typically only considered a crime (or only a severe crime) if carried out after these supposed points of animation.[13]

---

12 On the debate over preformationism in Italy, see Ivano dal Prete, "Cultures and Politics of Preformationism in Eighteenth-Century Italy," in *The Secrets of Generation: Reproduction in the Long Eighteenth Century*, ed. Raymond Stephanson and Darren N. Wagner (Toronto: University of Toronto Press, 2015), 59–78.

13 Eve Keller, *Generating Bodies and Gendered Selves: The Rhetoric of Reproduction in Early Modern England* (Seattle: University of Washington Press, 2007), 132–33.

The zealous adoption of preformationism by some Catholic reformers is best exemplified by Francesco Emmanuele Cangiamila's extraordinarily influential treatise, *Embriologia sacra: Ovvero dell'uffizio de' sacerdoti, medici e superiori circa l'eterna salute de' bambini racchiusi nell'utero* (Sacred embryology: That is, on the duty of parish priests, physicians, and officials with respect to the eternal well-being of infants still in the womb).[14] Cangiamila, a Palerman priest and jurist, was both deeply influenced by the writings of preformationists and acutely aware of existing theological debates over the fate of babies who died without baptism, an argument toward which he took a hardline approach.[15] Although nonsurgical interventions to assure baptism, such as inserting a syringe filled with holy water into the uterus during a distressed delivery, had long been discussed by theologians and clergy, by the eighteenth century the validity of such measures was increasingly being called into question.[16] Instead, it was the postmortem Cesarean operation that emerged as the resounding consensus on how to avoid what Cangiamila and his followers viewed as a massacre of innocent souls.[17]

Cangiamila, whose own pastoral work in Sicily brought him face to face with the tragedy of infant and maternal death, was deeply concerned about questions of salvation, particularly amid what he perceived as rising rates of abortion (including what today we would call miscarriage). In many cases, Cangiamila lamented, no efforts had been made to baptize these pitiful unborn children.[18] Owing to his belief that ensoulment followed closely if not immediately after conception, the priest argued that baptism should be performed on all abortions, even those that occurred in the early days of a pregnancy.[19] Most unconventionally, he advocated that the Cesarean operation be performed not only on all dead women that were suspected or known to be pregnant but also in certain cases on living women as well. This despite the fact that many medical experts in the eighteenth century argued

---

14   F. E. Cangiamila, *Embriologia Sacra, ovvero dell'Uffizio de' Sacerdoti, Medici, e Superiori, circa l'Eterna Salute de' Bambini racchiusi nell'Utero* (Milan: Giuseppe Cairoli, 1751), all quotes in this article refer to the 1751 Milanese edition, though Cangiamila's text was first published in Palermo in 1745.

15   Nadia Maria Filippini, *La Nascita Straordinaria: Tra madre e figlio la rivoluzione del taglio cesareo (sec. XVIII-XIX)* (Milan: Franco Angeli, 1995), 59–63, 81–84.

16   Adriano Prosperi, *Dare l'anima: storia di un infanticidio* (Turin: Einaudi, 2005), 215.

17   Filippini, *La Nascita Straordinaria*, 75.

18   Filippini, *La Nascita Straordinaria*, 60.

19   On ideas about ensoulment in this period see Adriano Prosperi, *Dare l'anima*, esp. 218–99.

it was extremely unlikely that the mother would survive such an operation.[20] Indeed, most jurists and public health writers questioned the logic of undertaking a procedure that was almost surely guaranteed to kill the mother when the child's likelihood of survival was itself extremely low. Cangiamila's position thus only made sense when the baptism of the fetus was prioritized over the mother's life. As Adriano Prosperi has pointed out, "In the cesarean section . . . the priest and the physician exchanged roles, and the life of the soul was the prize gained with the physical death of the mother and fetus."[21]

In Italy, obstetric writers were also deeply interested in the Cesarean section, which they approached with a combination of religious and professional interest. Subtle shifts in the surgeon's understanding of the relationship between mother and fetus were thus also underway.[22] Florentine professor of surgery Pietro Paolo Tanaron, for instance, wrote stridently in favor of performing the Cesarean section if there was any hope of saving the fetus's life. If the birth was hopelessly obstructed, were there men, he wondered, "so barbarous, and so deprived of humanity, that they could plunge a knife into the breast of a poor, little infant (*creatura*) and cut it to pieces . . . so that it could be pulled out?"[23] For Tanaron, the Cesarean section was the more humane option when compared to the horrors of embryotomy, even when the operation might put the mother's life at risk. In fact, Tanaron went so far as to argue that the learned practitioner who failed to perform the Cesarean operation in a situation where it could be of aid should be judged in line with any other murderer:

> Princes, and Magistrates judge to be the offenders those prostitutes, and other women, known to have caused the deaths of their children, either through a procured Abortion, or an Infanticide; so why not punish similarly those, who because of fault, or negligence, cause to perish within the womb those unfortunate infants . . . even though they could have saved them with the application of their profession? Since this question concerns [the loss of] the physical life, no less than the spiritual one, and as there should be equal consideration for the one as for the other crime, then any

---

20   Renate Blumenfeld-Kosinski, *Not of Woman Born: Representations of Caesarean Birth in Medieval and Renaissance Culture* (Ithaca, NY: Cornell University Press, 1991), esp. chap. 1.

21   Prosperi, *Dare l'anima*, 216.

22   Prosperi, *Dare l'anima*, 252–65.

23   Pietro Paolo Tanaron, *Il Chirurgo-Raccoglitore Moderno, che assiste le Donne nei parti* (Bassano: 1774), Bk. III, 26. At the time, apart from the Cesarean section, the only sure method for delivering an obstructed fetus was to perform a craniotomy or embryotomy and pull the baby out in pieces, a procedure typically performed by a surgeon. This was seen as the safest procedure for the mother.

Practitioner who out of negligence, or, even more if out of politics, or maliciousness omits [to perform] the Cesarean Operation he should receive a severe penalty, as grave as that for the perpetrator of Homicide.[24]

Although there were obviously differences in how eighteenth-century theologians and medical practitioners wrote about the Cesarean operation, there was an increasing consensus on its utility, at the very least in postmortem cases. Surgery and theology had combined in this instance to reimagine the nature of the relationship between mother and fetus. The Cesarean operation thus signaled something much more consequential than the development of a novel medical intervention. As Nadia Maria Filippini has argued, the new sensibilities toward the fetus gestured to a "profound rupture of tradition, one that disrupted the hierarchy of moral, professional, and social ethics."[25] For the first time, the life/soul of the fetus was considered equally, if not paramount, to that of the mother.

The Emergence of the Unborn Citizen

Public health experts like Johann Peter Frank also wrote in this period with a new sensibility about the nature of the being contained in the womb. In his widely read and translated *Sistema completo di polizia medica* (Complete system of medical police), Frank asked, "Are not the citizens still enclosed in their mother's wombs nonetheless members of the state?"[26] When considering whether a state should prescribe different punishments for deliberate abortions procured during different stages of pregnancy, Frank wrote that "there is no reason why I should deny a living creature . . . endowed with human shape, the title of human being, merely because it is connected to the mother by the umbilical cord."[27] Although he conceded that laws tended to distinguish between abortion and infanticide, and therefore recognized a qualitative legal division between the born and unborn child, Frank wrote that distinctions made on the basis of a fetus's gestational age were senseless: "The prevalent general conviction of all physicians . . . [is]

---

24   Tanaron, *Il Chirurgo-Raccoglitore Moderno*, Bk. III, Ch. III, 95.

25   Filippini, *La nascita straordinaria*, 13.

26   Frank, *Sistema completo di polizia medica*, Vol. II (Milan: Pirotta e Maspero, 1807), 166.

27   Johann Peter Frank, *A System of Complete Medical Police: Selections from Johann Peter Frank*, ed. Erna Lesky (Baltimore: Johns Hopkins University Press, 1976), 104.

that a child is just as much a living creature before half the pregnancy is over, as it is after the first half."[28]

Influenced more by the political arithmetic of populationism and new conceptions of the state's responsibility for public health as he was by the spiritual concerns of religious writers like Cangiamila, Frank nonetheless drew similar conclusions regarding the value of the life contained within the womb. For Frank, the unborn fetus was deserving of the protection of the state through laws and institutional responses.[29] Frank's treatise on medical police thus details a variety of measures a society should undertake both to protect pregnant women and to punish harshly those who would threaten the unborn fetus in some way. The Cesarean operation was therefore just one yardstick by which new attitudes regarding the responsibility of mothers toward the "future citizens" in their wombs might be measured. By investing the fetus with a greater worth than ever before, the changed ontological outlook of the eighteenth century brought pregnant women under greater scrutiny and legal supervision. According to Prosperi, the prospect of the Cesarean operation had dramatically "changed the social condition" of the *creatura* that existed in its mother's womb; it had "become the object of great investment by powers and disciplines of all kinds, just as a special system of surveillance had been put into place over unmarried mothers."[30] Frank, for instance, called for the maintenance of lists of all women who were pregnant, in the interest of caring

> for the safety of the not yet born posterity, and to give this class a guardian who could safeguard the right of such human beings and give them our most tender protection, and put a limit to the wantonness and malice of presumptuous and irresponsible mothers.[31]

This new revaluation of the ontological status of the fetus, combined with the Catholic Church's long-standing condemnation of illegitimacy, resulted in an intense web of institutional and legal efforts to curb abortion and infanticide. Women caught in such a web of suspicion and surveillance were doubly burdened in cases of illegitimacy where shame forced many to abandon their infants at one of Italy's many foundling homes.[32]

---

28   Frank, *System of Complete Medical Police*, 104.
29   Filippini, *La nascita straordinaria*, 117–21; Prosperi, *Dare l'anima*, 216–17.
30   Prosperi, *Dare l'anima*, 217.
31   Frank, *A System of Complete Medical Police*, 75–77.
32   See David I. Kertzer, *Sacrificed for Honor: Italian Infant Abandonment and the Politics of Reproductive Control* (Boston: Beacon, 1995).

Making the Fetus Public

In addition to institutional and legal responses aimed at protecting fetal life, Frank also wrote about the responsibility a society had to educate its daughters so that they could best manage their own reproductive health. Women needed to be aware of the behaviors that might either harm or enhance their fertility; when pregnant, they were duty bound to avoid activities— like excessive drinking or exercise—that might compromise the health of the child within their wombs. This was especially true for elite city women, softened by the comforts of advanced civilization, whose labors, according to the conventional wisdom of the day, were more difficult than those of either rural women or Indigenous women outside of Europe.[33] Moreover, other members of a society needed to direct the proper "veneration and all possible consideration" to women during their pregnancies, including by protecting such women from marital abuse or long hours laboring in fields or factories.[34] In other words, pregnancy was a condition of such significance for the long-term prosperity of a state that it required an informed attentiveness on the part of all community members, especially pregnant women themselves.

In Italy, a number of novel social spaces were intended to provide the necessary framework for cultivating just this kind of sensibility toward pregnancy and public health. New scientific institutions such as the Institute of Sciences in Bologna (established in 1714) and the Royal Museum of Physics and Natural History (known as "La Specola" for its observatory) in Florence (opened in 1775) were viewed as critical organs through which to promote the civic values and intellectual prestige of their home cities, both domestically and abroad. Anatomical wax models, which contemporaries agreed particularly embodied the Enlightenment project of deriving wonder, edification, and knowledge from nature, often held a position of pride in such museums.[35] They possessed a particular valence for viewers who marveled at the talent and ingenuity of those who could use science to imitate life with such exactitude. Felice Fontana, La Specola's director, related upon the

---

33   Frank, *A System of Complete Medical Police*, 64–65, 83.

34   Frank, *A System of Complete Medical Police*, 70–74.

35   Anna Maerker, *Model Experts: Wax Anatomies and Enlightenment in Florence and Vienna, 1775–1815* (Manchester: Manchester University Press, 2011); Rebecca Messbarger, *The Lady Anatomist: The Life and Work of Anna Morandi Manzolini* (Chicago and London: University of Chicago Press, 2010), 28–29.

museum's opening in 1775 that the aim of the museum was no less than to "enlighten the people and to make them happy by making them civilized."[36]

What became the true centerpieces of museums like La Specola and the Institute of Sciences were lifelike models of reproductive women. Often referred to as anatomical Venuses,[37] these full-length wax models evoked the artistic Venuses of Titian and Botticelli, and the Medici Venus, the Hellenistic marble statue said to display perfect female proportions.[38] They may also have been the inspiration for Galletti's fully embodied obstetrical machine with its striking natural beauty. Displayed in a museum setting, the anatomical Venuses were intended to merge the aesthetic pleasure of classical art works with scientific and public utility. Although the Venuses lacked the obvious signs of pregnancy that were emphasized in obstetrical machines like the one commissioned for Pavia—these women's stomachs are decidedly flat and their seductiveness rooted in a feigned virginal modesty—under scrutiny they, too, revealed the wonders of reproduction. Not dissimilar to the anatomical flapbooks and fugitive sheets of the sixteenth and seventeenth centuries,[39] the wax Venuses could be dissected part by part, always to reveal in the end a developing fetus in utero.

As both men and women viewed the models, the intention of Fontana and others seems to have been one of *nosce te ipsum*, "know thyself," and

---

36   Felice Fontana, *Saggio del Real Gabinetto di Fisica, e di storia naturale di Firenze* (Rome, 1775), 4, quoted in Anna Maerker, "'Turpentine Hides Everything': Autonomy and Organization in Anatomical Model Production for the State in Late Eighteenth-Century Florence," *History of Science* 45 (2007): 258.

37   On the Anatomical Venuses, see Roberto Carli and Elisa Mazzella, "Ophelia at the Museum: Venuses and Anatomical Models in the Teaching of Obstetrics between the XVIIth and XVIIIth Centuries," *History of Education and Children's Literature* 3 (2008): 61, 80; Roberta Ballestriero, "Anatomical Models and Wax Venuses: Art Masterpieces or Scientific Craft Works?," *Journal of Anatomy* (2010): 223–34; Elizabeth Stephens, "Venus in the Archive: Anatomical Waxworks of the Pregnant Body," *Australian Feminist Studies* 25 (2010): 133–45; Rebecca Messbarger, "The Re-Birth of Venus in Florence's Royal Museum of Physics and Natural History," *Journal of the History of Collections* 25, no. 2 (2013): 195–215; Joanna Ebenstein, "Ode to an Anatomical Venus," *Women's Studies Quarterly* 40 (2012): 346–52; Corinna Wagner, "Replicating Venus: Art, Anatomy, Wax Models, and Automata," *19: Interdisciplinary Studies in the Long Nineteenth Century* 24 (2017): 1–27.

38   Wagner, "Replicating Venus," 13.

39   Andrea Carlino, *Paper Bodies: A Catalogue of Anatomical Fugitive Sheets 1538–1687*, trans. Noga Arikha, (London: Wellcome Institute for the History of Medicine, 1999).

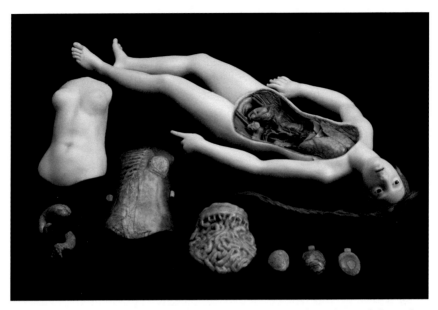

Figure 2.2. Anatomical Venus (late eighteenth century) from the workshop of
Clemente Susini, displayed at La Specola, Florence. Image courtesy of the Science
Museum, London and Wellcome Trust.

through that knowledge to assume personal responsibility for one's health.[40]
For young women who visited the displays, that meant to be initiated into
matters of reproductive and sexual health. The *Encyclopédie* author Denis
Diderot, for instance, sent his daughter, Marie Angelique, to view anatomical models on display in France prior to her marriage in order to gain a better
understanding of male and female sexual anatomy.[41] In addition to seeing
laid bare the successive layers of the anatomical Venuses, visitors might
compare female and male reproductive anatomy, or observe the organization of arteries and glands that allowed maternal breasts to produce milk.

40 On the connection between anatomical models and public health, see Anna
Maerker, "Anatomizing the Trade: Designing and Marketing Anatomical
Models as Medical Technologies, ca. 1700–1900," *Technology and Culture* 54,
no. 3 (2013): 531–62, 545–46.

41 Margaret Carlyle, "Artisans, Patrons, and Enlightenment: The Circulation
of Anatomical Knowledge in Paris, St. Petersburg, and London," in *Bodies
Beyond Borders: Moving Anatomies 1750–1950*, ed. Kaat Wils, Raf de Bont, and
Sokhieng Au (Leuven: Leuven University Press, 2017), 38.

Such waxworks sometimes weighed in on contemporary debates about the processes of generation and were intended to impart an understanding of human reproduction as a biological imperative encoded within the organs themselves.[42] Far from lewd exposure, defenders of such public displays argued that bodily knowledge acquired from anatomically accurate models was consistent with the development of both public virtue and sexual modesty.[43]

In addition to the anatomical Venuses, young men and women might view detailed anatomical waxes of fetuses in utero. In Bologna in 1757, for instance, the scientifically minded Pope Benedict XIV purchased the obstetrician Giovanni Antonio Galli's entire obstetrical collection for the Institute of Sciences.[44] In this way, the models, which numbered over 170 clay and wax representations of placentas, fetuses in utero, and other aspects of female reproductive anatomy, might continue to be used for instructional purposes while also becoming a part of the museum's permanent collection. As Lyle Massey has pointed out in relation to William Hunter's and William Smellie's obstetrical atlases, on which many three dimensional fetal models were based, such representations encoded a "highly refined pictorial link between dissection and the practices of midwifery" that fashioned "pregnancy as an illness" in need of the management of expert practitioners.[45] To lay audiences, the lesson of such models was not the cultivation of obstetrical skills needed to handle birth complications but the notion that childbirth was a dangerous medical event that required the assistance of skilled midwives and/or surgeons. Responsible citizens were duty bound to prepare appropriately for childbirth and to call for a trained professional well before a birth became difficult. Ultimately, enlightened rulers like Florence's Pietro Leopoldo and Pope Benedict XIV intended both the wax Venuses and fetal models to convey the potential of anatomical knowledge to empower laymen and women to produce and protect new life.

Obstetrical Machines and the Instruction of Touch

As instructional tools, obstetrical models were prized for their capacity to demonstrate comparative anatomy and to depict temporal change in a single space. Midwives long familiar with judging changes in breast size,

---

42   Messbarger, *Lady Anatomist*, 144–57.

43   Carlyle, "Artisans, Patrons, and Enlightenment," 38.

44   Messbarger, *Lady Anatomist*, 82.

45   Lyle Massey, "Pregnancy and Pathology: Picturing Childbirth in Eighteenth-Century Obstetric Atlases," *The Art Bulletin* 87, no. 1 (2005): 73.

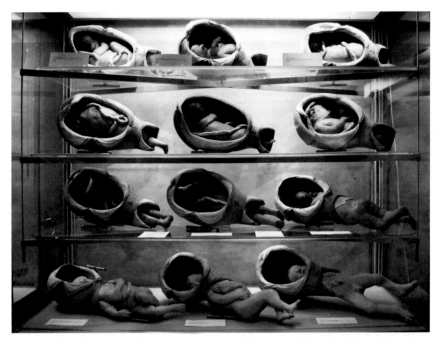

Figure 2.3. Obstetrical Models, Palazzo Poggi, Bologna. Photo by Elena Manente, courtesy of Wikimedia Commons Public Domain.

vaginal wetness, or the dilation of a cervix could easily grasp the usefulness of seeing and comparing such transformations side by side. Models also allowed students to observe and compare different types of potential complications. Students could simultaneously see and feel the ways in which various kinds of abnormalities—a pelvis distorted by rickets, a fetus with an enlarged head—might obstruct a labor. Galli's collection, for instance, included a series of twelve models representing breech births at progressive stages of delivery, and at least three models depicting various ways the placenta might mis-attach to the fundus, a complication about which Galli was especially concerned.[46] His collection also included examples of errors that practitioners might commit, including the perforation of the uterus during a manual extraction of the placenta, highlighting the disastrous impact of an unskilful touch.[47]

---

46   Messbarger, *Lady Anatomist*, 83.
47   Owen, *Simulation in Healthcare Education*, 119.

Indeed, the widespread use of obstetrical models and machines in eighteenth-century Italy reminds us that touch was and continued to be considered an essential, embodied skill in medical practice, despite claims that
this period saw the emergence of an epistemic "regime of visuality."[48]
Eighteenth-century midwifery instructors did, however, face certain unique
challenges in their efforts to define touch as a legitimate medical technique
and source of scientific knowledge. In addition to the inherent difficulties of
verbalizing the sense of touch,[49] instructors had to work against at least two
opposing tendencies. First, critiques of both midwives and man-midwives
in this period often constructed such practitioners' touch as dangerous and
harmful.[50] Women's touch was uneducated and impatient. Man-midwives'
and surgeons' touch was aggressive, sexually charged, and clumsy, made
especially perilous by the incorporation of unwieldy surgical instruments. In
both cases, touch was destructive and threatening; hands delivered babies
that were misshapen, broken, or scarred. Second, the early modern period
increasingly saw touch, long associated with eroticism and carnality, "subordinated to the senses that support a greater distance between bodies," that
is, to sight and hearing.[51] In *The Birth of the Clinic*, for instance, Foucault
suggests that eighteenth-century visual representations of pathological anatomy functioned to redirect the sensory knowledge derived from touch and
smell into a multisensory gaze in which sight is the predominant mode of
knowing.[52] Obstetrical models resisted these impulses and provided a controlled space for both male and female practitioners to cultivate touching as

---

48   On visuality and modernity see, for instance, Charlotte Epstein, *Birth of the
      State: The Place of the Body in Creating Modern Politics* (Oxford: Oxford
      University Press, 2020), 260–61.

49   Susan C. Lawrence, "Educating the Senses: Students, Teachers and Medical
      Rhetoric in Eighteenth-Century London", in *Medicine and the Five Senses*, ed.
      W. F. Bynum and Roy Porter (Cambridge: Cambridge University Press, 1993),
      154.

50   Eve Keller, "The Subject of Touch: Medical Authority in Early Modern
      Midwifery," in *Sensible Flesh: On Touch in Early Modern Culture*, ed. Elizabeth
      D. Harvey (Philadelphia: University of Pennsylvania Press, 2003), 64–65.

51   Elizabeth D. Harvey, "'The 'Sense of All Senses,'" *Sensible Flesh: On Touch in
      Early Modern Culture*, ed. Elizabeth D. Harvey (Philadelphia: University of
      Pennsylvania Press, 2003), 1–21, 8. Harvey is following Norbert Elias here;
      Mark M. Smith, *Sensing the Past: Seeing, Hearing, Smelling, Tasting, and
      Touching in History* (Berkeley and Los Angeles: University of California Press,
      2007), 93–116.

52   Michel Foucault, *The Birth of the Clinic: An Archaeology of Medical Perception*
      (Abingdon, UK: Routledge, 1989), 202–04.

a legitimate and scientifically rational mode of knowing the body that was as important as seeing, if not more so.

In addition to wax and clay fetal models, midwifery instructors like Malacarne and Galli also incorporated obstetrical *machines* in their teaching.[53] Distinct from models, which tended to be limited to disembodied wombs, obstetrical machines were intended to simulate childbirth and allow trainees to practice manipulating fetal dolls placed in a variety of positions. Galli's machine, comprising simply a torso with legs cut abruptly at the upper thigh, performed a kind of maternal erasure that was a prominent feature of obstetrical illustration in a period that saw the professionalization of the male obstetrician.[54] The machine's pelvis was composed of wood, while its uterus, sized to a full-term pregnancy, featured a glass womb. This most distinctive feature of Galli's machine allowed for students to view a fetal doll in various positions in the womb and observe as Galli performed the proper procedures to manage each situation. In time, the students themselves would practice these manoeuvres as Galli observed and corrected.

As Lucia Dacome has described, the most spectacular aspect of Galli's obstetrical instruction was his practice of testing midwives on the machine blindfolded. These moments, Dacome writes, "combined training and surveillance with a striking performance. By blindfolding the midwives, Galli could downplay their visual skills and, at the same time, subordinate their tactual expertise to his own visual control."[55] In this way, the use of the obstetrical machine validated touch as essential to obstetrical practice, yet maintained a (gendered) hierarchy that placed sight at the pinnacle of the senses. Galli was also re-creating the drama of birth with new protagonists. While the mother herself had been subordinated and silenced—reduced to nothing more than a torso—the midwife became the figure under scrutiny, acting strictly by touch and memory, the professor the protagonist guiding events to their successful conclusion.

The fame of Galli's obstetrical machine was such that obstetrics professors from across the Italian peninsula traveled to Bologna in hopes of a firsthand demonstration.[56] In fact, a visit to Galli's obstetrical collection was the inspiration for Giuseppe Galletti to finance a similar collection in Florence. Jacopo Bartolommei, professor of obstetrics in Siena, also sought out Galli, meeting

---

53 Giambattista Fabbri mentions two machines, though it is possible that one was designed but never actually realized. See Dacome, *Malleable Anatomies*, 174.

54 Massey, "Pregnancy and Pathology"; Nora Doyle, *Maternal Bodies: Redefining Motherhood in Early America* (Chapel Hill: University of North Carolina Press, 2018), chap. 1.

55 Dacome, *Malleable Anatomies*, 174.

56 Francesca Vannozzi, "Fantocci, marchingegni e modelli nella didattica ostetrica senese," in *Nascere a Siena: Il parto e l'assistenza alla nascita dal Medioevo all'età moderna*, ed. Francesca Vannozzi (Siena: Nuova Immagine, 2005), 37.

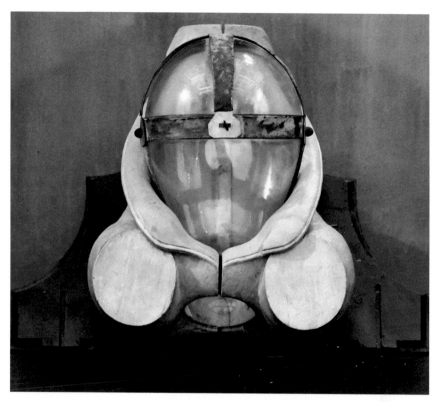

Figure 2.4. Giovanni Antonio Galli's glass womb obstetrical machine, Palazzo Poggi, Bologna. Courtesy of Alma Mater Studiorum University of Bologna—Sistema Museale di Ateneo.

him in Bologna in May of 1762 in order to observe how he trained students on his obstetrical machine. The demonstration apparently proved impressive, as Bartolommei soon ordered some forty terracotta models of his own and a duplicate of Galli's obstetrical machine. Six years later, Bartolommei featured the latter in a speech he delivered to Siena's *Accademia delle Scienze dette dei Fisiocratici* (Academy of sciences). During the talk, the professor demonstrated how a crystal uterus (like Galli's), or one modeled from cowhide with the top opened, could be used to instruct blindfolded surgical and midwifery students as they maneuvered the fetus within the womb into a more favourable position for birth.[57] Again, the glass obstetric machine provided for a spectacular demonstration of scientific ingenuity and mastery over the

---

57   Vannozzi, "Fantocci," 38.

reproductive body, embodied in the person of the obstetrics professor who oversaw the entire drama.

Midwifery professors like Galli, Jacopo Bartolommei, and Vincenzo Malacarne all viewed obstetrical machines as critical instructional aides for several reasons. First, female midwifery students often had only basic literacy, meaning extensive verbal or textual instruction would be of limited use. Second, opportunities for consistent clinical instruction were still rare in eighteenth-century Italy, where public maternity wards served only a minute fraction of the childbearing population. Third, given the general disapproval of male practitioners in childbirth in Italy, most surgeons could claim only very limited practical experience with obstetrics.[58] Given these limitations, many midwifery instructors argued that machines were necessary for the repeated and regular exercise of skills that it would be either impossible or inhumane to practice on live patients.[59] The Milanese surgeon, Giovanni Battista Monteggia, further argued that simulated training was particularly important for male surgeons because they were called almost exclusively to difficult labors, which were chaotic and required haste. It was almost impossible under such circumstances, Monteggia wrote, for a practitioner "to reason scientifically on individual cases and operate composedly behind the true principles of the art, without rushing to deliver the woman as quickly as possible with a blind touch."[60] On machines, by contrast, a professor could unhurriedly "exercise the hand[s] of the students to know" the shape and contours of the gravid uterus and the placement of the fetus within. Students could reflect on their progress calmly, "far from the commotion caused by the screaming of the pregnant patient and the consternation of onlookers."[61]

In Pavia, Vincenzo Malacarne similarly aimed to cultivate in his students a scientifically informed tactility. Touch conceived of systematically entailed subdividing tactile sensations into conceptual categories like shape, texture, resistance, and wetness, from which expectations and norms could be defined.[62] A skilled touch of this kind provided a knowledge that could not

---

58 ASM, *Sanità*, Parte Antica, c. 268, "Riflessioni di Bernardino Moscati intorno allo stabilimento della nuova Scuola pe' Parti," 1767.

59 In fact, the government in Milan had consulted Galli during the planning stages of the midwifery school. ASM, *Sanità*, Parte Antica, c. 268, "Riflessioni di Bernardino Moscati intorno allo stabilimento della nuova Scuola pe' Parti," 1767.

60 G. B. Monteggia, "Osservazioni Preliminari," in *Arte Ostetricia di G.G. Stein*, vol. 1, trans, G. B. Monteggia (Venice: 1800), 5–6.

61 Monteggia, "Osservazioni Preliminari," 6.

62 ASM, *Sanità*, Parte Antica, c. 273, "Istituzione della Scuola Pratica d'Ostetricia nella Regia Università di Pavia al Leano,'" October 3, 1792.

simply be conveyed through lectures or textbooks.[63] Indeed, it may have been Malacarne's conviction in the importance of touch that compelled him to request an obstetrical machine rather unlike those of any of his contemporaries. Distinct from the obstetrical machine used by Galli and his followers, which, while life-sized, reproduced the pregnant woman only from the mid-thigh to the lower torso, the Pavia obstetrical machine featured a wholly embodied woman.[64] Interior devices mimicked the resistance the uterus might exert at its opening or around the fetus.[65] Most dramatically, the machine included eyes that responded to pressure applied to the genital area.[66] Although this feature clearly rendered the machine a potentially sexual and sexualized object—one that Malacarne felt compelled to cover in the name of modesty—it also reconnected the ostensibly mechanical processes of birth to the rational, embodied subject of the mother. In this way, the Pavia machine counteracted a dominant tendency in obstetrical representation in the eighteenth and nineteenth centuries, which had the effect of erasing the maternal body (including any suggestion of female desire) and focusing instead on the womb as a disembodied, and sometimes almost autonomous, structure.[67]

The accompanying fetal dolls were likewise constructed so as to mimic nature as closely as artificial means would allow. Rather than the simple leather dolls often used with obstetrical machines, Galletti's artificial fetuses were elastic, with bendable joints and an internal frame that realistically reproduced the resistance and fragility of fetal bone and tissue. According to Galletti, the fetal head included "membranous spaces, the interstices of

---

63   G. B. Monteggia, "Osservazioni Preliminari," 29–30.

64   The closest examples to the Pavia machine may be a series of eight obstetrical models produced by the Roman anatomist and wax sculptor, Giovanni Battista Manfredini, who was active in Bologna in the 1770s. The models, produced in colored terracotta for instructional use at the midwifery school in Modena, feature full-size women from the head to mid-thigh, such that seated on a table they appear standing. The models move from an intact full-term pregnant belly to greater and greater penetration into the womb, often with the woman holding open her own skin (as was a familiar convention in Renaissance anatomical drawing). These models are not, however, machines. They have no internal mechanisms and were not intended to be practiced upon. On Manfredini, see Owen, *Simulation in Healthcare Education*, 125; Thomas Schnalke, *Diseases in Wax: History of the Medical Moulage*, trans. Kathy Spatschek (Carol Stream, IL: Quintessence Publishing, 1995), 38–39.

65   Galletti, *Elementi di Ostetricia*, xiii.

66   ASM, *Sanità, Parte Antica*, c. 273. Letter from Vincenzo Malacarne, November 9, 1792.

67   See Doyle, *Maternal Bodies*, chap. 1.

the skull, and [was] suceptible to enlongation and compression."[68] Indeed, obstetrical writers often wrote of horrific mistakes where practitioners used too much force while maneuvering the child's head during delivery.[69] It was essential that practitioners had a learned sense of just how much pressure could be applied, particularly when there was a malpresentation or obstruction. Thus, the obsterical machine in Pavia did not encourage haste or excessive force as some scholars have argued was the case with British obstetrical machines;[70] instead, it cultivated a touch that was sensitive to the natural feel of the fetus and aware of the delicacy of newborn skin and bone.

Critiques of Simulation

The use of obstetrical machines was widespread in Italy by the end of the eighteenth century. As Johann Peter Frank and others noted, in Italy in particular a combination of entrenched custom and female modesty meant that male professors were limited in their opportunities to instruct students at the bedside of living patients. Even at the largest public maternity homes, frequented mainly by the most desperately poor and/or unmarried women, the number of live births per year would fail to support a robust instructional program. Models and machines could fill in the gaps and, in areas without public maternity hospitals, might comprise the majority of practical instruction.[71] Yet, while they deemed models necessary, Frank and others also warned practitioners of their limitations.

Frank himself favored training on live patients and cadavers where possible.[72] Though Frank conceded the need for obstetrical models to assist

---

68 Galletti, *Elementi di Ostetricia*, xiv–xv.

69 Keller, "Subject of Touch," 65; The Turin surgeon and midwifery professor Ambrogio Bertrandi warned that too much force applied to a fetal head wedged against the mother's pelvis would lead to the head "tearing and ripping away from the chest." Ambrogio Bertrandi, *Opere Anatomiche, e Cerusiche di Ambrogio Bertrandi: Arte Ostetricia*, vol. VIII (Torino: Fratelli Reycends, 1790), 165.

70 For such critiques, see Pam Lieske, "'Made in Imitation of Real Women and Children'"; Blackwell, "*Tristram Shandy* and the Theater of the Mechanical Mother."

71 Johann Peter Frank, *Sistema Completo di Polizia Medica di G.P. Frank traduzione dal Tedesco del Dottor Gio. Pozzi*, vol. 15 (Milan: Giovanni Perotta, 1827), 293–94.

72 Frank was nonetheless acutely aware of the detriments and moral dubiety of subjecting pregnant women, poor and/or unmarried, in public hospitals to the endless ministrations of unskilled surgeons and students. According to Frank,

training, he also argued that it was difficult for students to gain an accurate sense of the feel of the fetus in utero with bulky dolls. Nor was it possible for surgical students to practice procedures like embryotomy on cloth or leather dolls. He advocated instead for the use of recently deceased fetal cadavers with obstetrical machines.[73] In Macerata around 1770, the professor of surgery and obstetrics, Antonio Santimorsi, developed an obstetrical machine with just this kind of instruction in mind. Santimorsi's machine featured a stuffed leather uterine cavity lined with waxed silk to make it waterproof. In this way, students could practice on fetal cadavers, including performing embryotomies, without damaging or staining the machine itself.[74] Contending that it was largely a waste playing around with padded dolls and pelvises, the Milanese surgeon Monteggia went one step further. In 1800, he outlined his own method for preparing maternal and fetal cadavers for practical training. Monteggia noted that initially the progress of the fetus might be blocked by the prolapse of any remaining parts of the female cadaver's peritoneum, vagina, or intestine, which would act as a strong bridle on the fetus' head, though this would resolve with additional "deliveries" as the tissues stretched.[75] These authors generally do not indicate either moral or legal concerns over the acquisition of such maternal and fetal remains. In this way, they were like many of the male obstetrical practitioners across Europe and North America in this period whose careers were made by training and experimentation on the bodies of desperately poor and marginalized women, those who took recourse to public maternity wards to be delivered and/or to hide the evidence of illegitimacy.[76]

five, ten, or fifteen students practicing the "exploration" of a pregnant woman would cause the poor woman not only shame and fear but also negative physical effects, such as inflammation. In fact, he warned against turning pregnant patients into veritable "rope dancers" (*ballerina da corda*), particularly in cases where a professor was paid per student instructed. Frank, *Sistema Completo*, 15:271–72.

73 Frank, *Sistema Completo*, 15:292.

74 Giambattista Fabbri, "Antico Museo Ostetrico di Giovanni Antonio Galli, restauro fatto alle sue preparazioni in plastica e nuova conferma della suprema importanza dell'ostetricia sperimentale," in *Memorie dell'Accademia delle Scienze dell'Istituto di Bologna*, serie III, tomo II (Bologna: Gamberini e Parmeggiani, 1872), 143; Giovanni Calderini, "Come si deve imparare a fare le diagnosi e le operazioni ostetriche," *La Clinica Moderna: Repertorio delle Cliniche Italiane*, 1895, 7, 185–87.

75 G. B. Monteggia, "Osservazioni Preliminari," 7–9.

76 See, for example, Dierdre Cooper Owens work on the importance of enslaved and poor Irish women's bodies to the professionalization of obstetrics and

Frank's position on simulated training came from his firm belief in the primacy of touch for the practice of midwifery and obstetrics. "What does the eye have to do with obstetrics?" he asked rhetorically, referring to the tendency of some professors and man-midwives to demonstrate techniques and point out reproductive structures to rooms filled with young surgeons. How could one expect students to comprehend what a professor was doing with his hands while they were moving *inside* the uterus? Or understand how to maneuver forceps from watching at a distance? It was learning by touch, Frank argued, "that should be the only pursuit that has a place in obstetrics."[77] Recalling his own experiences with obstetrical training, Frank cautioned that performing operations only on immobile models poorly prepared him for the actual sensation of turning the fetus in the face of uterine contractions.[78] Despite its potential for visual theatrics, Galli's glass simulator was thus arguably of less value than Malacarne's obstetrical machine, the mechanisms of which allowed for simulated contractions and resistance to the practitioner's touch. Neither, however, could perfectly re-create the sensations of the fetus in utero and the impressive force of a contraction might yield.

Looking back on the development of theoretical and practical obstetrics from the nineteenth century, the Ferrarese physician Augusto Ferro articulated just this kind of distaste for mechanical aids. At a speech delivered at the *Accademia Medico-Chirurgica* in Ferrara in 1852, Ferro spoke passionately on the subject. Obstetrics, he argued, is learned

> in the dark, [and] he who is a practitioner must have eyes on his fingers, and fingers exercised on parts that resist, and that move with their own force; and not from some mechanical impulse they receive from shapeless dolls, placentas made of rags, stuffed pelvises, and uteruses of wire!!!!! Oh, tragic blinding of the mind! Oh, most disastrous hardening of the heart!![79]

This impassioned plea may reflect changing understandings after 1800 of what animated living beings. Although mechanistic understandings of the body had already been challenged during the eighteenth century, vitalist conceptions of nature had strengthened by the end of the century and became prevalent in the next. Vitalism, "the theory that life is generated and

gynecology in America. Owens, *Medical Bondage: Race, Gender, and the Origins of American Gynecology* (Athens: University of Georgia Press, 2017).

77 Frank, *Sistema Completo*, 15:267–68.
78 Frank, *Sistema Completo*, 15:274–75.
79 Augusto Ferro, "Sulle Presenti Condizioni dell'Insegnamento Teorico Pratico di Ostetricia in tutte le Università e Ginnasi Comunali del Nostro Stato," speech read at the Accademia Medico-Chirurgico di Ferrara, 15 October and 19 November, 1852.

sustained through some form of non-mechanical force or power specific to and located in living bodies," opposed the notion that living beings could be defined by mechanical laws.[80] Enlightenment discussions about vitalism had particular relevance for the field of embryology, as a range of interested parties, from medical practitioners to theologians to jurists, debated what the precise mechanisms were that prompted fetal development and growth in utero.[81] Ferro's objection to the possibility that mechanical devices could ever re-create the intrinsic force that animated pregnant bodies and fetuses suggests a rejection of mechanical thinking about the body. In this view, obstetrical machines would never sufficiently simulate childbirth precisely because they lacked the unique vital forces that constitute living things but that are absent from inert ones. Although obstetrical machines continued to be used in the nineteenth century, it is clear that some practitioners had begun to question whether wax and wood bodies, even those as ingeniously constructed as Galletti's obstetrical machine, could truly instill students with the human compassion and manual sensitivity required to attend real women.

Conclusions

During the eighteenth century, the ontological status of the fetus emerged as a question for jurists, reformers, medical practitioners, and theologians in compelling and novel ways. As scientific investigations revealed more about the nature of fetal growth and development, the combination of dissection and artistic wax modeling allowed for technologies that made visible in new ways what had before been hidden. New social spaces allowed a wide range of Europeans, including ample numbers of women, to experience such models and to know their own bodies in a categorically different way, from the inside out. The proponents and patrons of new natural history museums saw the potential for expert knowledge about the natural world to be harnessed for state interests, including bolstering procreativity. At the same time, the Catholic Church found in new scientific theories of generation and embryological development a justification for aggressive medical intervention on

---

80   Catherine Packham, *Eighteenth-Century Vitalism: Bodies, Culture, Politics* (New York: Palgrave Macmillan, 2012), 1. See also Peter Hanns Reill, *Vitalizing Nature in the Enlightenment* (Berkeley: University of California Press, 2005).

81   On the debates between preformationists and epigenesists, see Shirley A. Roe, *Matter, Life, and Generation: Eighteenth-Century Embryology and the Haller-Wolff Debate* (Cambridge: Cambridge University Press, 1981).

behalf of the fetus in the womb. Theology and scientific theory converged to upset long-standing hierarchies in which medical practitioners had traditionally placed the value of the living mother above that of her unborn child. Obstetrical models and machines, such as those Vincenzo Malacarne commissioned for his obstetrical instruction, embodied both the reimagined status of the unborn child and the increasingly expansive public health interests of eighteenth-century states.

Chapter Three

Paper Pregnancies

Visualizing the Maternal Body, 1870–1900

Jessica M. Dandona

At the end of the nineteenth century, rapidly increasing immigration to the United States, France's humiliating defeat in the Franco-Prussian War, and the controversial impact of evolutionary theory on British science provoked intense public debate around the perceived fitness, vitality, and reproductive potential of these nations' citizenry.[1] Influenced by the emerging discourse of eugenics and contemporary theories of "degeneration,"[2] public health officials, reformers, and physicians sought to harness the power of science to ensure a strong and abundant population by dramatically reducing infant mortality and promoting the health and safety of mothers and children.[3] During the same period, the groundwork was being laid for modern

---

1   For a discussion of the French context, see Fae Brauer, "Eroticizing Lamarckian Eugenics: The Body Stripped Bare during French Sexual Neoregulation," in *Art, Sex and Eugenics: Corpus Delecti*, ed. Fae Brauer and Anthea Callen (Aldershot: Ashgate, 2008), 97–136 and Tamar Garb, *Bodies of Modernity: Figure and Flesh in Fin-de-Siècle France* (London: Thames and Hudson, 1998). For the British context, see Anthea Callen, *Looking at Men: Anatomy, Masculinity and the Modern Male Body* (New Haven, CT: Yale University Press, 2018).

2   For a discussion of the concept of "degeneration" in a European context, see Daniel Pick, *Faces of Degeneration: A European Disorder, c. 1848–c. 1918* (Cambridge: Cambridge University Press, 1989) and Robert A. Nye, *Crime, Madness, & Politics in Modern France: The Medical Concept of National Decline* (Princeton, NJ: Princeton University Press, 1984).

3   For more on this, see Rima D. Apple, *Mothers and Medicine: A Social History of Infant Feeding, 1890–1950* (Madison: University of Wisconsin Press, 1987);

obstetrics. By 1900, physicians would attend over half of births in the United States,[4] although less than 5 percent of all births took place in a hospital. Meanwhile, increasingly stringent regulations governing the practice of midwifery led to changes in how birth attendants in Britain and France were trained and their profession regulated. The medicalization of childbirth and the increasing use of instrumental and surgical interventions marked the culmination of an evolution away from midwife care that began in the sixteenth century and greatly accelerated in the eighteenth and nineteenth.[5] Sara Dubow has noted the crucial importance of this period in the history of reproduction: by 1900, "embryology became a modern science, obstetrics became a profession, abortion became a crime, birth control became a movement, eugenics became a cause, and prenatal care became a policy."[6]

Central to these efforts were visual representations produced in a wide array of forms, including anatomical atlases, clinical pamphlets, and obstetrical models, as well as abundantly illustrated studies in medical journals. With few exceptions, such works define the female anatomical form as youthful and above all productive: the ideal body is, in these images, a pregnant body.[7] Such depictions circulated not only in professional contexts but also in popular medical treatises, public anatomy lectures, and childcare guides,

---

Deborah Dwork, *War Is Good for Babies & Other Young Children: A History of the Infant and Child Welfare Movement in England 1898–1950* (London: Tavistock, 1987); and Elisa Carniscioli, "Producing Citizens, Reproducing the 'French Race': Immigration, Demography, and Pronatalism in Early Twentieth-Century France," *Gender and History* 13 (2001): 593–621.

4　Judith Walzer Leavitt, "'Science' Enters the Birthing Room: Obstetrics in America since the Eighteenth Century," *Journal of American History* 70 (1983): 281–304, here 295.

5　Ornella Moscucci, *The Science of Woman: Gynæcology and Gender in England, 1800–1929* (Cambridge: Cambridge University Press, 1990), 10. For more on this transition from midwife-assisted to physician-managed childbirth, see Deborah Kuhn McGregor, *From Midwives to Medicine: The Birth of American Gynecology* (New Brunswick, NJ: Rutgers University Press, 1998); Judith Leavitt, *Brought to Bed: Childbearing in America 1750 to 1950* (New York: Oxford University Press, 1986); and Adrian Wilson, *The Making of Man-Midwifery: Childbirth in England, 1660–1770* (Cambridge, MA: Harvard University Press, 1995).

6　Sara Dubow, *Ourselves Unborn: A History of the Fetus in Modern America* (Oxford: Oxford University Press, 2011), 7.

7　For an example of widely circulated late nineteenth-century representations that depict the female anatomical body as pregnant, see *Vinton's Anatomical Model of the Human Body (Female): Student's Edition* (London: Millikin & Lawley, ca. 1900); W. S. Furneaux, *Philips' Anatomical Model of the Female Human Body* (London: George Philip & Son, ca. 1900); and W. S. Furneaux,

familiarizing lay audiences with the basic precepts and visual language of anatomical science. In this period, medical texts, images, and objects also traversed national borders at an increasingly rapid pace, often appearing nearly simultaneously in European and American collections. The rapidity of this circulation, as well as the number and variety of images available to viewers of all socioeconomic levels, was unprecedented in the history of medicine.

Yet, relatively little scholarly interest has been paid to the material dimensions of medical visualization in this period. Scholars such as Anna Maerker, Margaret Carlyle, and Lucia Dacome have explored in detail the ambivalent status of obstetrical models as "medical technologies," their role in the training of midwives and *accoucheurs*, and the gendered associations of materials such as wax. Yet these scholars' accounts focus more on handcrafted seventeenth- and eighteenth-century models than on mass-produced nineteenth-century works.[8] Similarly, much of the work done on early obstetrical images, including the incisive analyses of Lyle Massey, Rebecca Whiteley, and Lianne McTavish, centers on the properties of luxuriously produced copperplate engravings and large-format anatomical atlases—not their proliferating, late nineteenth-century progeny.[9] By contrast, scholars writing on twentieth-century obstetrical images have more often concentrated their analysis on the impact of technological modes of visualization such as ultrasound and MRI scans, while failing to fully consider the origin of their visual codes in nineteenth-century anatomical depictions of the pregnant body.[10]

Dr. Minder's Anatomical Manikin of the Female Body (New York: American Thermo-Ware Company, ca. 1900).

8   Lucia Dacome, "Women, Wax and Anatomy in the 'Century of Things,'" *Renaissance Studies* 21, no. 4 (September 2007): 522–50; Margaret Carlyle. "Phantoms in the Classroom: Midwifery Training in Enlightenment Europe." *Know* 2, no. 1 (Spring 2018): 111–32; Anna Maerker, "Anatomizing the Trade: Designing and Marketing Anatomical Models as Medical Technologies, ca. 1700–1900," *Technology and Culture* 54, no. 3 (July 2013): 531–62.

9   See Lyle Massey, "Pregnancy and Pathology: Picturing Childbirth in Eighteenth-Century Obstetric Atlases," *Art Bulletin* 87, no. 1 (March 2005): 73–91; Rebecca Whiteley, *Birth Figures: Early Modern Prints and the Pregnant Body* (Chicago: University of Chicago Press, 2023); and Lianne McTavish, *Childbirth and the Display of Authority in Early Modern France* (Aldershot, UK: Ashgate, 2005).

10   See Kelly A. Joyce, *Magnetic Appeal: MRI and the Myth of Transparency* (Ithaca, NY and London: Cornell University Press, 2008); Lisa Cartwright, *Screening the Body: Tracing Medicine's Visual Culture* (Minneapolis: University of Minnesota Press, 1995); and José Van Dijck, *The Transparent Body: A Cultural Analysis of Medical Imaging* (Seattle and London: University of Washington Press, 2005).

This privileging of craft and technology, I would argue, elides the transition from one dominant visual mode to the other and ignores the crucial role of late nineteenth-century physicians and anatomists in defining the concept of scientific objectivity. Between the wax model and the ultrasound scan, in other words, lies a wealth of mechanically reproduced images and objects that map the territory of the female reproductive body in an increasingly detailed and direct manner. This chapter thus takes as its case study two such depictions of the pregnant body that circulated widely in Europe and the United States: Louis-Thomas-Jérôme Auzoux's papier-mâché models of the uterus (ca. 1840s–1970s) and Gustave-Joseph-Alphonse Witkowski's printed *Progress of Gestation*, from his series of anatomical atlases, *Human Anatomy and Physiology* (1875–1878 and 1880–1884). Both works crossed national borders, foregrounded the relationship between the pregnant body and the fetus, and circulated in both professional and popular contexts, helping to establish a shared understanding of the reproductive body defined through its anatomical structure. Despite their disparate formats, moreover, both Auzoux's three-dimensional models and Witkowski's printed atlas make paper, as a material at once inexpensive, industrial, and ubiquitous in nineteenth-century visual culture, central to their representation of the body.

These works, like many others produced in this era, offer a dramatic contrast between their depiction of the pregnant body and their representation of the fetus. Both allow the viewer to imaginatively peer inside the womb in order to reveal its reproductive "secrets," a privileged metaphor for the acquisition of anatomical knowledge since at least the Middle Ages.[11] This process ends abruptly at the limits of the fetal form, however. While the pregnant body is represented as an anatomical specimen or dissected cadaver, associating the pregnant woman's anatomy with the specter of death, in both works the fetus appears as if living, intact, and whole. Close study of these works therefore provides new insight into the historical origins of a phenomenon more often associated with the twentieth century—namely, the tendency to picture a pregnant woman and her fetus as potentially distinct, autonomous beings.[12] At the same time, it also reveals the growing authority of medical discourse in this period, as efforts to professionalize the field of obstetrics increasingly cast pregnancy and childbirth as inherently dangerous conditions requiring treatment by trained physicians.

---

11   See Katharine Park, *Secrets of Women: Gender, Generation, and the Origins of Human Dissection* (Cambridge, MA: MIT Press, 2006).

12   For more on this history, see Karen Newman, *Fetal Positions: Individualism, Science, Visuality* (Stanford, CA: Stanford University Press, 1996).

Popular Displays of the Pregnant Body

Although depictions of the female reproductive body proliferated in the visual culture of late nineteenth-century medicine, members of the public also encountered fetal and pregnant bodies in both institutional and domestic settings—as illustrations in popular medical treatises, at the bedside of friends and relatives during childbirth, and in the form of specimens and models displayed in popular anatomy museums. As Samuel Alberti has argued, "Bodies, living and dead, were to be found in all corners of the nineteenth century exhibitionary complex, not only in fairgrounds and freak shows, but also in private cabinets and grand museums, great exhibitions, and shilling anatomy shows."[13]

Popular exhibitions included Pierre Spitzner's *Grand Musée Anatomique et Ethnologique,* which opened in Paris in 1856, and similar museums in New York, Philadelphia, London, and other cities. In many cases, the very same objects and images employed to teach students in medical schools also appeared in displays for popular audiences, similarly inscribed as "pedagogical" in purpose. In 1893, for example, Friedrich Ziegler's series of wax models depicting embryological and fetal development appeared at the World's Columbian Exposition in Chicago, where they earned their maker the fair's top prize.[14] Similar works by Ziegler can today be found in the historical collections of many university anatomy museums, including those of Harvard, Oxford, and Edinburgh, suggesting that such works routinely traversed the boundaries separating "popular" and "professional" audiences.

Popular anatomy museums often exhibited a disproportionately large number of objects linked to human reproduction, including wax and papier-mâché models as well as fetal and pathological specimens. A "Florentine Venus, Dissected" features prominently in advertisements for Drs. Jordan & Davieson's Gallery of Anatomy in Philadelphia,[15] for example, while the New York Museum of Anatomy promised visitors daily lectures on "the functions and derangements of the generative organs."[16] The catalogue for Dr. Kahn's

---

13   Samuel J. M. M. Alberti, *Morbid Curiosities: Medical Museums in Nineteenth-Century Britain* (Oxford: Oxford University Press, 2011), 3.

14   Nick Hopwood, *Embryos in Wax: Models from the Ziegler Studio* (Cambridge: Whipple Museum of the History of Science, 2002), 1.

15   Samuel Davieson and Henry J. Jordan, *Grand Anatomical Museum, 807 Chestnut Street, c.* 1872, handbill, collection of the Library Company of Philadelphia. For an image of this figure, see *Startling Additions at Drs. Jordan & Davieson's Gallery of Anatomy and Museum of Science and Art, c.* 1872–73, handbill, collection of the Library Company of Philadelphia.

16   Drs. Jordan and Beck, *Catalogue of the New-York Museum of Anatomy* (New York: Charles F. Bloom, 1865).

Museum of Anatomy and Medical Science, also located in New York, similarly lists numerous obstetrical "dissections"—most likely in the form of wax models—as well as a series of eight models "illustrating the development of the fœtus in the Womb," which may have been made by Auzoux.[17]

Indeed, the catalogue of Dr. Kahn's Museum foregrounds the museum's role in educating the public regarding matters of human reproduction. Writing of "the science of Anatomy and Physiology," the author asserts,

> This knowledge is beyond all question of the utmost importance, [yet] there are few who possess even a smattering of such information, more especially as regards the last point, how we have our being; a false sense of propriety has not only prevented the discussion of this subject, but rendered it most difficult to obtain reliable information.[18]

Such efforts, however, were not entirely disinterested: popular anatomy museums often exhibited highly illusionistic wax models depicting the symptoms of venereal disease, helping to drive demand for the spurious "remedies" sold by the museums' enterprising proprietors.[19] Given that many of these museums were open to women at select times, displays on human reproduction may also have reflected visitors' curiosity regarding methods of preventing conception and their fears regarding illegitimate pregnancy at a time before reliable pregnancy tests were available.

By the end of the nineteenth century, many of these museums had fallen prey to accusations that they displayed "obscenities" and, one by one, closed their doors. Their contents were gradually integrated into university and hospital collections that offered only limited access to members of the public. For both popular and professional audiences, then, paper in all of its various forms came to be a prime route through which images of human reproduction circulated, allowing for their use in the home as well as in the lecture theater.

Touch and Sight: Modes of "Seeing" the Pregnant Body

For late nineteenth-century medical students, obstetrical training entailed applying knowledge gained from a wide variety of sources—written commentary, lectures, study of anatomical models and specimens, and printed images—to the examination and treatment of living bodies. Access to

---

17   L. J. Kahn, *Hand Book and Descriptive Catalogue of Dr. Kahn's Museum of Anatomy and Natural Science* (1875), pamphlet, collection of the Library Company of Philadelphia, 17 and 27.

18   Kahn, *Hand Book*, 3.

19   A. W. Bates, "'Indecent and Demoralising Representations': Public Anatomy Museums in mid-Victorian England," *Medical History* 52 (2008): 12.

patients in labor was often quite limited,[20] especially prior to the establishment of clinical training as a standard element of medical education,[21] and students rarely had the opportunity to engage in the dissection of women who died during pregnancy or childbirth. For women medical students and midwives, who were often denied access to both clinical training and dissection, the problem was even more acute.

Indeed, access to an adequate supply of bodies for dissection remained an ongoing issue, even after the passage of laws requiring unclaimed bodies from hospitals, workhouses, and asylums to be turned over to local medical schools in Britain and the United States.[22] A number of anatomical models and printed works produced at the end of the nineteenth century, therefore, were introduced to supplement direct observation of the female reproductive body. In many cases, these works claimed to replicate the logic and visual forms of anatomical dissection, which continued to occupy a central place in medical education.[23]

The second half of the nineteenth century, as Jonathan Crary and other scholars have noted,[24] was marked by a growing emphasis on visuality. In medical discourse, this took the form of an intensification of visual practices associated with the diagnosis, study, and representation of the patient body. While physicians increasingly relied on printed charts, diagrams, and even early radiographs in their clinical practice, medical publishers turned to efficient and economical methods of mechanical reproduction such as chromolithography and half-tone printing to create works richly illustrated not only with line drawings but also with photographs and even full-color images. This growing emphasis on visuality functioned in tandem, however, with other modes of studying the body, including haptic and auditory forms

---

20 Abraham Flexner, *Medical Education in the United States and Canada: A Report to the Carnegie Foundation for the Advancement of Teaching* (Boston: The Carnegie Foundation for the Advancement of Teaching, 1910), 117–18.

21 Thomas Neville Bonner, *Becoming a Physician: Medical Education in Britain, France, Germany, and the United States, 1750–1945* (New York and Oxford: Oxford University Press, 1995), 268–78.

22 For more on this history in an American context, see Michael Sappol, *A Traffic of Dead Bodies* (Princeton, NJ: Princeton University Press, 2002).

23 For more on the history of dissection, see Helen MacDonald, *Human Remains: Dissection and its Histories* (New Haven, CT: Yale University Press, 2006); Ruth Richardson, *Death, Dissection and the Destitute*, 2nd ed. (Chicago: University of Chicago Press, 2000); and Sappol, *A Traffic*.

24 See, for example, Jonathan Crary, *Techniques of the Observer: On Vision and Modernity in the Nineteenth Century* (Cambridge, MA: MIT Press, 1990); Nicholas Mirzoeff, "On Visuality," *Journal of Visual Culture* 51 (2006): 53–79; and Hal Foster, ed., *Vision and Visuality* (Seattle, WA: Bay Press, 1988).

of patient assessment such as palpation and auscultation and with increasingly instrumentalized forms of examination.[25] The works discussed in the pages that follow likewise served as a bridge between the body and its representation by inviting viewers to explore a simulacrum of the corporeal form through both touch *and* sight—by turning flaps, taking apart models and putting them back together again, and even reenacting the processes of childbirth itself. In these works, the visual text becomes a substitute for the body at the same time that flesh becomes a text, its "truths" legible through both visual inspection and tactile exploration.

Auzoux's Paper Dissections

According to French manufacturer Louis-Thomas-Jérôme Auzoux, his life-sized papier-mâché anatomical models permitted students to transform the lecture hall into a virtual dissecting room. Manufactured by hand between 1827 and the 1980s, the models can be found in large numbers in historical medical collections in the United States, Britain, France, and other countries.[26] Auzoux termed his models *anatomie clastique*, a term he invented based on the Greek word "to break," as each model could be taken apart, studied, and reassembled using a special tool. While the models continue to be used for study even today in many medical schools, in the nineteenth century they also served to illustrate popular anatomy lectures, including those given by Auzoux himself.

Produced in a factory employing dozens of specially trained workers, Auzoux's models represent a blending of artisanal and industrial modes of production. Models were made from papier-mâché shaped in metal molds and then painstakingly finished by hand—first coated with plaster, then elaborated with applied details such as nerves and veins, and finally, painted with a high degree of naturalism. While some visual conventions were employed, such as the use of red and blue to signify arteries and veins, by and large Auzoux's models sought to replicate closely the structures they represented. Small paper labels indicated the proper order in which to assemble

25 Elizabeth Hallam, *Anatomy Museum: Death and the Body Displayed* (London: Reaktion, 2016), 278.

26 Auzoux's models also appeared in collections in Australia, Asia, and Africa. For a discussion of the models' use in Egypt, for example, see Anna Maerker, "Papier-Mâché Anatomical Models: The Making of Reform and Empire in Nineteenth-Century France and Beyond," in *Working with Paper: Gendered Practices in the History of Knowledge*, ed. Carla Bittel, Elaine Leong, and Christine von Oertzen (Pittsburgh: University of Pittsburgh Press, 2019), 177–92.

and disassemble each model and directed users to an accompanying book-
let describing the structures depicted, thus inscribing the language of anatomical science directly onto the bodily forms represented and providing an
interpretive framework for viewing the work.[27]

Auzoux first began manufacturing a series of models depicting the stages
of fetal development in the early nineteenth century, advertising a life-size
figure of a woman complete with a detachable pelvis and 14 uteri representing the stages of pregnancy.[28] It seems demand for such figures was high:
by the 1840s, Auzoux was producing at least four works devoted to human
reproduction, including the aforementioned life-sized figure, two series of
uteri, and two different models of the female pelvis, one depicting the external organs and one with three uteri.[29] The series considered here, which
consists of six models showing the progressive development of the fetus
inside the womb and two models representing extrauterine pregnancies, was
likely produced in the twentieth century but is essentially identical to similar
models produced as early as the 1870s or 1880s.[30]

I focus here on the largest work in the series, which depicts a full-term
fetus (figure 3.1). The model represents the uterus as an isolated yet undamaged organ, visually and surgically severed from the rest of the pregnant
body. The anterior portion of the uterus lifts off as a single piece, allowing
users to re-create the spectacle of revealing its mysterious contents (figure
3.2). The painted detail of the uterine wall in cross-section reveals the surgical procedures entailed in opening the womb, but the cut depicted here is
bloodless and crisp—an idealized incision into an impossibly intact organ.
It should be noted that despite their intense naturalism, models such as this
proffer an abstracted view of the human body—one free of the fluids, fat,
and fascia that so frustrated the anatomist. The sectioning employed here
thus corresponds to neither surgical practice nor the procedures utilized in

27 Examples of these booklets, few of which have survived, can be found in the
    collection of the Bibliothèque nationale, in Paris.
28 191 *Catalogue of Preparations of Artificial Anatomy by Dr. Auzoux, of Paris*
    (Albany: Henry Rawls & Co., 1841), 3–4.
29 The earliest mention of the set that I have found is in an American catalogue
    published in 1844 where it is described as "No. 9. UTERI, with the fœtus
    and its membranes, at different periods of gestation." *Catalogue of Anatomical
    Models, Made by Dr. Auzoux, and For Sale by George Dexter* (Albany: Stone &
    Henly, 1844), 4.
30 B. W. J. Grob dates the series to around 1858 based on a catalogue published
    by Auzoux in that year. B. W. J. Grob, "The Anatomical Models of Dr. Louis
    Auzoux: A Descriptive Catalogue," *Museum Boerhaave Communication* 305
    (2004): 121.

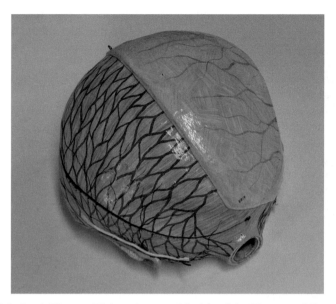

Figure 3.1. Louis-Thomas-Jérôme Auzoux, Models of the Uterus and Fetus: Ninth Month, n.d. Papier-mâché. Collection of University of Dundee Museums.

anatomical dissection,[31] but rather serves to provide users with the greatest possible degree of visual and physical access to the uterus.

In her study of images of childbirth in theory, literature, and science, Alice Adams argues,

> Since the advent of ultrasound, representations of the womb in medical literature have shifted from "black box" images, in which the womb was viewed as an opaque, almost impermeable barrier between the fetus and the outside world, to images of the womb as a penetrable "window'" onto the fetus.[32]

While Adams is right, I think, to point to the transformation wrought by the use of twentieth-century imaging technologies, the example of Auzoux's

---

31 It was common practice in this period to divide the anterior wall of the uterus vertically. See, for example, Christopher Heath, *Practical Anatomy: A Manual of Dissections* (London: Churchill, 1881), 286.

32 Alice E. Adams, *Reproducing the Womb: Images of Childbirth in Science, Feminist Theory, and Literature* (Ithaca, NY: Cornell University Press, 1994), 155–56.

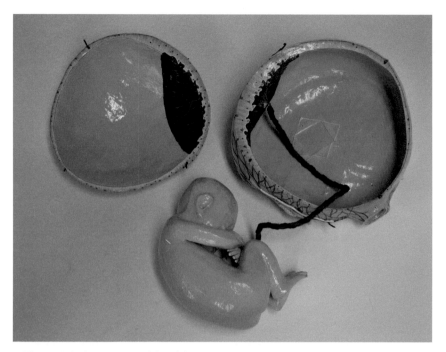

Figure 3.2. Auzoux, Models of the Uterus and Fetus: Ninth Month, n.d. Papier-
mâché. Collection of University of Dundee Museums.

models demonstrates that in some ways the ultrasound scan is the technological realization of an incursion that first found expression in the realm
of visual representation. In the model, we see a desire to render the womb
accessible to both sight and touch. A thin layer of parchment covering the
opening of the cervix and a square of paper peeled back to represent the
membranes of the amniotic sac, for example, suggest the fragility of human
tissues and evoke themes of layering and transparency as the body is progressively opened to the view.

    This penetration of the corporeal form is paired with a play between the
body's exterior and its interior, as the uterus itself, in isolation, comes to
represent the "outside" of the pregnant form with the fetus as its "inside."
Whereas users of eighteenth- and early nineteenth-century "Anatomical
Venuses" lifted off the torso of the wax model to reveal its hidden fetus,
those using Auzoux's model instead remove the anterior surface of the
womb itself. The model thus allows for a double breach of corporeal boundaries, revealing both the internal organs of the female body *and* the secrets

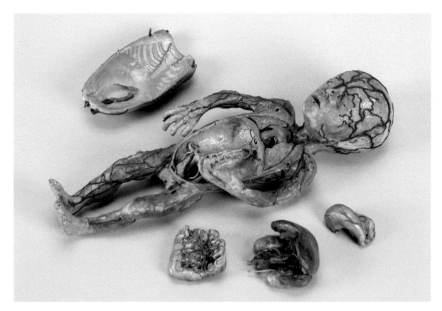

Figure 3.3. Auzoux, Model of Fetus, 1867 or earlier. Papier-mâché. Warren
Anatomical Museum collection, Center for the History of Medicine in the Francis
A. Countway Library of Medicine, Harvard University.

contained therein. In her discussion of anatomical wax models, Ludmilla
Jordanova likens this act of penetration to an unveiling that is at once sexual
and intellectual, suggesting its highly gendered dimensions in the history of
anatomical discourse.[33]

This exploration ends abruptly, however, when the viewer encounters
the fetus. While Auzoux manufactured a model of a full-term fetus that
could be disassembled (figure 3.3), in this series the body of the fetus is
whole, undamaged, and inviolate: a convention so well-established that it
appears even in contemporary illustrations depicting frozen slices of a pregnant female cadaver, as seen in A. H. F. Barbour's well-known treatise *The
Anatomy of Labour* (1889) (figure 3.4).[34] The implicit logic here is simple:

33 Ludmilla Jordanova, *Sexual Visions: Images of Gender in Science and Medicine
between the Eighteenth and Twentieth Centuries* (Madison: University of
Wisconsin Press, 1989), 55 and 99.

34 A. H. F. Barbour, *The Anatomy of Labour, Including That of Full-Term
Pregnancy and the First Days of the Puerperium Exhibited in Frozen Sections
Reproduced Ad Naturam,* 2nd ed. (Edinburgh and London: W. & A. K.
Johnston, 1889), frontispiece.

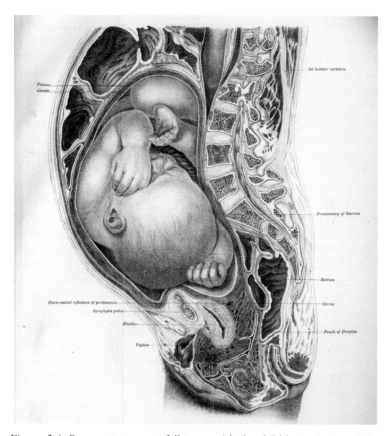

Figure 3.4. Pregnant uterus at full term, with the child lying right occipito anterior, from A. H. F. Barbour, *The Anatomy of Labour, Including That of Full-Term Pregnancy and the First Days of the Puerperium Exhibited in Frozen Sections Reproduced Ad Naturam*, 2nd ed. (Edinburgh and London: W. & A. K. Johnston, 1889), Figure 1. Collection of University of Dundee Library.

the pregnant body serves as a frame for the fetus within. "Life," it is suggested, requires the woman's progressive disassembly in order to preserve the self-contained unity of the unborn.

Unlike twentieth-century images of a seemingly autonomous, free-floating fetus,[35] in Auzoux's model the unborn infant remains connected to the

---

35 Rosalind Pollack Petchesky, "Fetal Images: The Power of Visual Culture in the Politics of Reproduction," *Feminist Studies* 13 (1987): 264.

pregnant body via a red and blue umbilical cord and painted depiction of the placenta. The fetus can be removed from its protective shell, however, by lifting it out of the model uterus and unhooking the umbilical cord from the uterine wall. The radical simplicity of this format is especially striking given that most models manufactured by Auzoux include dozens and, in some cases, even hundreds of separate parts. The only "use" to which the model uterus can be put, in other words, is a kind of symbolic birth, as the user "delivers" the fetus by removing it from the womb.

It is clear from nineteenth-century accounts that Auzoux's models were employed primarily for demonstration purposes, in the context of a large audience, rather than for use in practicing hands-on obstetrical techniques.[36] In this way, they served as illustrations for a verbal description of the various anatomical structures progressively revealed by their disassembly. References to the models as "specimens" confirm both the tendency to conflate them with the structures they depicted and their function as objects of display.[37] Unlike the so-called obstetrical machines commonly employed in midwifery courses, then, Auzoux's model uterus does not allow the user to pass the fetus through an opening in the pelvis. Indeed, the pelvis itself is absent from the model. Nor does the model reproduce the surgical procedures employed in birth by Cesarean section, which in this period typically involved a midline incision along the *linea alba* rather than the dramatic surgical cut depicted here.[38] This bloodless and lifeless "birth," then, is not one experienced by living mothers: the radical disassembling of the model in effect evokes a postmortem *dissection*, not the act of parturition.

---

36 For example, "A complete set of abnormal pelves, Auzoux models of the uterus and contents of the various periods of gestation and charts are employed for demonstration." *Catalogue: Sixty-Fifth Report of the Curators to the Governor of the State, 1906–1907, Columbia Missouri Bulletin of the University of Missouri* VIII, no. 5 (May 1907): 245. Similar references appear in many university catalogues of the time. Auzoux's models were likewise used in the context of presentations before professional societies. For an example, see Dr. Sawyer. "Proceedings of The Dublin Obstetrical Society. Twenty-Ninth Annual Session," *The Dublin Quarterly of Medical Science* XLIV (August and November 1867): 451.

37 "Review of a Lecture upon Clastic Anatomical Models, Delivered before the Baltimore College of Dental Surgery, by F. G. Lemercier, Co-operator of Dr. Auzoux and Professor of the Polytechnic Association of Paris," *American Journal of Dental Science* 3, no. 1 (May 1869): 3.

38 The transverse and Pfannenstiel incisions commonly employed today were developed slightly later, around 1900. Samuel Lurie and Marek Glezerman, "The History of Cesarean Technique," *American Journal of Obstetrics and Gynecology* 189, no. 6 (December 2003): 1804.

Indeed, comments comparing Auzoux's models with the products and processes of anatomical dissection appear frequently in nineteenth-century accounts. Contemporaries underscored the models' exquisite detail and "anatomical accuracy," for example, suggesting that they illustrated difficult-to-see processes, such as the progress of gestation, "in a way no dissection could possibly do."[39] Some also commented on the way in which Auzoux's models fixed and rendered legible the form of soft, "movable" and thus difficult-to-study structures such as the uterus.[40] Even though commentators underscored the differences between Auzoux's papier-mâché forms and the cadaver, they nonetheless described the models as representing not only the human body, but also the *practice* of dissection. Auzoux himself described his models as works "which can easily be assembled and disassembled, with parts removed one by one, as in a real dissection."[41] In restaging the process of childbirth through the progressive dismantling of the pregnant body, then, Auzoux's model of the uterus in the ninth month of gestation imagines an *anatomized* birth, one accomplished through dismemberment, and here presented as necessary to the safe delivery of the fetus. In the process, the pregnant body is bifurcated, to use Janelle Taylor's term, into not one but two subjects: mother and fetus.[42]

Paper-Thin: Witkowski's *Progress of Gestation*

Auzoux's models of fetal development made touch, as well as sight, central to the way they introduced users to the pregnant body. The same is true of another medium of anatomical representation that found widespread popularity at the end of the nineteenth century: the flap anatomy. Like Auzoux's models, flap anatomies sought to emulate the temporal, tactile, and visual dimensions of anatomical dissection, transforming the body into thin, superimposed layers that allowed users to penetrate the secret recesses of the body as if turning the pages of a book. In the late nineteenth century, these layers

39 "Review of a Lecture," 2; "The various stages of development of the gravid uterus and evolution of the embryo and fœtus are illustrated by two series of beautiful models, which are most life-like and true to nature." *Twenty-Fifth Annual Announcement of the Medical College of Georgia, Augusta* (Augusta, GA: James McCafferty, 1856), 8–9.

40 W. Symington Brown, "Chronic Cystitis in Women," *Transactions of the Gynaecological Society of Boston* 1 (1889): 105.

41 Louis Auzoux, *Anatomie clastique du Docteur Auzoux, Catalogue de 1869* (Paris: Imprimerie Adolphe Lainé, 1869), frontispiece.

42 Janelle S. Taylor, "The Public Fetus and the Family Car: From Abortion Politics to a Volvo Advertisement," *Public Culture* 4 (1992): 78.

were produced using chromolithography, an early, labor-intensive method of color printing that employs a succession of lithography stones to print colors one by one, resulting in vivid, highly saturated images.[43] Such flap anatomies often decorated the pages of home medical treatises and anatomical atlases but also appeared as large folding displays and even life-size figures intended for professional use.

Perhaps the best known of the nineteenth-century flap anatomies are the works produced by the French physician and medical popularizer Gustave-Joseph-Alphonse Witkowski, whose series of eleven full-color anatomical atlases appeared in visually identical form as *Anatomie iconoclastique* in France (1875–1878 and 1880–1884), *Human Anatomy and Physiology* in Britain (*c.*1878–1888), and *A Pictorial Manikin, or, Movable Atlas* in the US (*c.*1880s).[44] The set includes a work dedicated to the *Progress of Gestation*, first published in French in 1884, with the text of both English language editions translated by an obstetrician from Edinburgh, R. Milne Murray (figure 3.5). The same image of a pregnant woman and fetus, scaled down, also appears in some editions of Witkowski's volume *La génération humaine* (1880), a popular medical treatise published just four years earlier.[45]

Well known as the author of highly diverting and heavily illustrated texts on topics such as birth at the French court, famous midwives, and the female breast, Witkowski crafted an atlas that was no doubt as appealing to curious collectors as it was to physicians, nurses, and midwives in training. The work presents the figure of a pregnant woman standing in profile and unclothed except for the drapery around her shoulders, which serves to obscure the less palatable aspects of anatomical investigation while also lending her the air of

---

43   For more on this process and flap anatomies, see Meg Brown. "Flip, Flap, and Crack: The Conservation and Exhibition of 400+ Years of Flap Anatomies," *Book and Paper Group Annual* 32 (2013): 6–14.

44   G.-J. Witkowski, *Anatomie iconoclastique* (Paris: H. Lauwereyns, 1875–78 and 1880–84); G.-J. Witkowski, *Human Anatomy and Physiology* (London: Baillière, Tindall & Cox, 1878–88); G.-J. Witkowski, *A Pictorial Manikin, or, Movable Atlas* (New York: Joseph Cristadoro, 1880–?). The British edition lists the printers as Lemale et Cie, Havre, suggesting that the chromolithographed plates were printed in France and shipped to publishers in the United States and Britain. Witkowski's *Atlas* was also reprinted in Japan, possibly in the form of a pirated edition. Masatane Ando, *Zenkei kaibo dzukai* [A movable atlas of the human body, reproduced from G. J. Witkowski.], 3 vols. (Tokyo, 1884–86).

45   Gustave-Joseph Witkowski, *La génération humaine* (Paris: H. Lauwereyns, 1880). The flap anatomy of "*Grossesse à terme,*" with Witkowski credited as the draughtsman and Léveillé as the lithographer, appeared at least as early as the sixth edition, published in 1886, and as late as 1927.

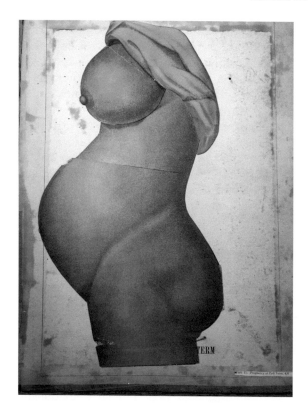

Figure 3.5. G.-J. Witkowski, *Human Anatomy and Physiology Part XI: A Movable Atlas Showing the Progress of Gestation by Means of Superposed Coloured Plates* (London: Baillière, Tindall and Cox, 1879–88). Courtesy of Thomas Jefferson University Archives.

a fragmentary but idealized classical sculpture. In this context, the connotations of purity, beauty, physical vitality, and racialized Whiteness associated with Greek art in this period reinforce the suggestion that the figure represents at once an anatomical, racial, and maternal ideal.[46] Like the figures in William Hunter's famous eighteenth-century engravings of the gravid uterus, this pregnant woman is amputated at mid-thigh and just above her breast, which lifts up to reveal the mammary glands, reducing the corporeal form to its reproductive function. The absence of limbs transforms the individual, living model into a universal and idealized depiction of pregnancy but also invites viewers to imaginatively reconstruct the missing details according to their own preferences.

Witkowski depicts the figure naturalistically, using careful tonal modeling to suggest the roundness of her swelling, fertile body. The use of a strict profile view, however, quickly begins to compartmentalize and fragment

---

46   For more on this topic, see Callen, *Looking at Men*.

what is otherwise illusionistically depicted as a fully rounded form. This view foreshadows the layering that will take place as successive cross-sections of the pregnant figure's body are revealed by turning the flaps. In each case, a curious doubling of the figure results, an overly literal sectioning that produces two similar but unequal halves. The use of a profile view, meanwhile, strongly recalls the conventions of display employed in ethnographic, criminological, and natural history discourses,[47] defining the female reproductive form as the object of the clinical gaze. It is worth noting that the effect of mastery thus produced is reinforced by the securing of the figure to the inside cover of the atlas with red string, evoking at once the line of a surgical incision, the laces of a corset, and the ropes used to position cadavers for dissection.

By folding the topmost flap of paper (the figure's "skin") to the left, the viewer unveils a series of thin layers, some translucent, that must in turn be peeled back. Meant to evoke the body of the uterus, its internal surface, the decidua, the chorion, and the amnion, these layers intensify the drama of anatomical and temporal unfolding that takes place and provide tantalizing glimpses of what lies beneath. The attentive viewer can easily perceive the ghostly fetus through the translucent paper representing the amnion, for example, as well as the placenta (figure 3.6). Witkowski thus considerably simplifies the complex tissues of the human form, taking inspiration from the layered membranes of the pregnant body itself to render impossibly precise and improbably intact paper-thin strata. He similarly omits any reference to the amniotic fluid, creating an image that transposes complex three-dimensional volume into crisp two-dimensional form.

Contemporary responses to Witkowski's work noted the limitations of this approach. A review of the volume in the *Glasgow Medical Journal*, published in 1888, thus describes the work:

> This is a series of chromo-lithographic plates of pregnancy at full term, so arranged as, when lifted the one from above the other, to show the uterus in position, the placenta, membranes, and fœtus. The drawing is fairly correct, and will give a student a good idea of the disposition of parts and their relation to each other, but further than this it can hardly go in the way of instruction.[48]

Despite the temporal dimensions of its use, the reviewer's critique points to the fact that Witkowski's atlas depicts not the *stages* of childbirth, nor even the "progress of gestation" as promised, but rather the anatomy of a

---

47 Sandra Matthews and Laura Wexler, *Pregnant Pictures* (London: Routledge, 2000), 112.

48 "*A Movable Atlas, showing the Progress of Gestation by Means of Superposed Coloured Plates,*" *Glasgow Medical Journal* XXX, no. 3 (September 1888): 255.

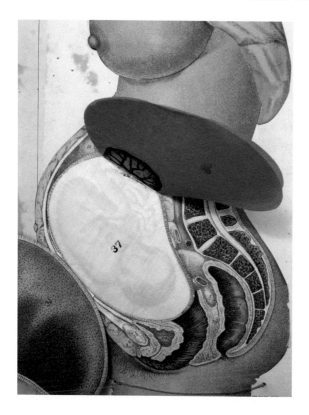

Figure 3.6. Witkowski, detail of *Human Anatomy and Physiology Part XI: A Movable Atlas Showing the Progress of Gestation by Means of Superposed Coloured Plates* (London: Baillière, Tindall and Cox, 1879–88). Courtesy of Thomas Jefferson University Archives.

woman at a single moment in her pregnancy. The image would therefore have been of limited usefulness for those training to be obstetricians, as it fails to depict the various malpresentations or other conditions that might necessitate medical intervention. Nor does it depict the process of childbirth itself; instead, the atlas serves primarily to map the relation of various organs and anatomical structures to the whole. Witkowski's *Progress of Gestation* thus constructs an idealized version of pregnancy, one depicted primarily in anatomical rather than physiological terms.

While Witkowski's flaps are viewed in succession, moreover, the individual images themselves are static. Their successive revelation marks not the passage of *time*, as suggested by the work's title, but the progressive elimination of impediments to our visual access to the fetus. As the flaps are folded to the side, the pregnant body itself is flayed, layer by layer, in order to reveal its hidden "secret"—the fetus dwelling within, at the heart of its colorful paper petals.

Like Auzoux's models, commentators often compared movable flap anatomies such as Witkowski's to an anatomical dissection. Even though the atlas's flaps remain attached during viewing, for example, reviews of the work describe how "successive layers may be removed."[49] Witkowski's American publisher likewise praised the series' ability to present "an exact counterpart of each organ," so that "the necessary knowledge of its anatomy and physiology [is] acquired almost as readily as from actual dissections."[50] The process of creating the atlas thus relied upon the *pictorial* dissection of the female body by the viewer as much as it did upon close observation of an actual anatomical dissection by the artist.

The word "iconoclasm," derived from the Greek *eikonoklastes*, refers to the breaking or destroying of images. The title of the French edition of Witkowski's work, *Anatomie iconoclastique* (Iconoclastic anatomy), thus connotes the symbolic violence entailed in this act of pictorial dismemberment, even as it invokes Auzoux's *anatomie clastique*, perhaps in an effort to emulate the latter's success. Indeed, Witkowski acknowledged his debt to Auzoux, writing, "It was in view of the magnificent anatomy models of Dr. Auzoux that we conceived the idea of doing on paper what this skillful anatomist did with a special paste."[51]

The printer's proofs for *The Progress of Gestation* reveal that in order to produce its layered flaps and create its narrative of discovery, the artist and lithographer, J.-B. Léveillé, first had to disassemble the pregnant body into its component parts (figure 3.7). While the fetus is here shown as whole and untouched, as in Auzoux's model, the pregnant figure's body is depicted in cross-section. In the finished work, the shift from picturing the left leg in the first image to showing the right leg in subsequent layers bisects the figure neatly, and yet the fetus pictorially appears to project outward from the pregnant uterus, seemingly spared the knife. From this perspective, the pregnant figure in Witkowski's atlas does not produce a fetus so much as reveal it through her own gradual elimination.

The bifurcation of the female figure into unequal halves, one bearing the rounded uterus and the other a concave emptiness, also strongly recalls the process of symphysiotomy, or separation of the cartilage connecting the pelvic bones, a surgical procedure employed in cases of obstructed labor.

49   "A Movable Atlas, Showing the Progress of Gestation, by Means of Superposed Colored Plates," *The American Journal of the Medical Sciences* 46 (1888): 64.

50   G.-J. Witkowski, *A Pictorial Manikin, or, Movable Atlas Showing the Mechanism of the Organs of Hearing and Mastication* (New York: Joseph Cristadoro, 1880).

51   G.-J. Witkowski, *Le Corps humain*, 2nd ed. (Paris: Librairie H. Lauwereyns, 1882), III.

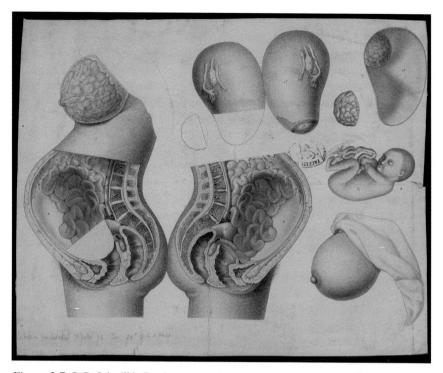

Figure 3.7. J.-B. Léveillé, *Dessins anatomiques et épreuves d'imprimerie* [*Anatomie de la grossesse*], *c.*1878. Collection of BIU Santé, Paris.

Indeed, the visually severed pubic symphysis joint can be seen just in front of the bladder. Considered less risky than Cesarean section, in the 1880s and 1890s, symphysiotomy was widely discussed in contemporary medical literature and popularized by renowned obstetricians such as Adolphe Pinard (1844–1934).[52]

In this way, practices first employed in anatomical dissection to divide the body, physically, into its component parts found their way into both visual representation and the material practice of medicine. It should be noted, however, that there are significant differences between the procedures employed in conventional anatomical illustration and those entailed in *The Progress of Gestation*. While Witkowski's illustrations depict a sagittal section of the pelvis, a view commonly found in contemporary textbooks and dissection manuals, it includes not only the now-standard view of the pelvic organs

---

52   Leavitt, *Brought to Bed*, 56.

in profile, with viscera removed, but also successive perspectives showing organs *in situ* before their removal. Thus, certain structures—including the vertebral column and bones of the pelvis—appear in full cross-section, while other details, such as the intestines, are illusionistically rendered to suggest their three-dimensionality. By layering subsequent views of the body in cross-section, yet depicting some areas in depth, Witkowski calls to mind anatomical dissection's process of gradually penetrating the body *and* its goal of thereby revealing previously hidden structures. Anatomist and illustrator thus follow similar conventions, portioning the body into its constituent parts and working from the outside in to penetrate its depths, while in the process casting the body's surface, its skin, as an impediment to sight, touch, and thus knowledge.

The flatness and discretely bounded character of the images in Witkowski's atlas are also significant in this regard. The carefully delimited, crisp-edged paper die-cuts of forms such as the uterus, each of which was stamped out using a brass die before being painstakingly glued into position by the printers, parallel anatomy's efforts to describe, delineate, and name discrete bodily structures. They also recall contemporary efforts to standardize the techniques employed in surgical procedures to remove internal organs, such as hysterectomy, successfully performed and subsequently described by Italian obstetrician Eduardo Porro in 1876.

The paper-thin layers composing Witkowski's figure eliminate volume from the body, collapsing its structures as if they were slices of tissue examined on a microscope slide. The female form here functions, symbolically, as a mere echo of the messy physicality of living bodies. The flattened figures of the pregnant woman and fetus can thus not only be manipulated at will but are also safely secured within the cardboard covers of the atlas, itself stored inside a hinged wooden box, signaling their status as collected objects, simulated specimens, and intensely private portals to a largely invisible world.[53]

Indeed, the voyeurism thematized in Witkowski's work is clear on multiple levels. The figures of pregnant woman and fetus are depicted from both the front and the back and can be removed from the atlas for closer inspection, giving the viewer full and unimpeded visual access to the figures' exterior and, in the case of the pregnant female form, interior as well. The female figure's sinuous shape and amputated arms, legs, and head focus attention on the sexualized aspects of her anatomy. The depiction of drapery, meanwhile, evokes classical antecedents praised for their beauty and eroticism,

---

53 A surviving example of this box can be found in the archives of the Wellcome Collection, London.

such as the *Venus de Milo*, as well as the marriage bed in which both conception and childbirth often took place. The small scale and minute detail of the work, moreover, lends itself to an intimate viewing experience rather than to display in the lecture theater.

The use of paper flaps, meanwhile, allows the viewer to imaginatively "undress" the figure, a process also employed in numerous erotic postcards produced in this era. The atlas's understated and utilitarian cardboard cover brings to mind similarly presented folios of erotic engravings. Readers would also have been familiar with two other, much more detailed works in the same series, which depict the male and female "organs of generation" in an unprecedentedly graphic manner (figure 3.8). The erotic component of Witkowski's pregnant creation is nonetheless safely contained within the parameters of medical discourse, for the drapery's resemblance to hospital sheets also conveys the figure's status as an obstetrical patient.

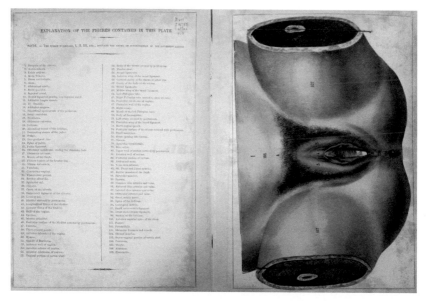

Figure 3.8. Witkowski, detail of *Human Anatomy and Physiology Part III: A Movable Atlas Showing the Positions of the Female Organs of Generation and Reproduction by Means of Superposed Coloured Plates* (London: Baillière, Tindall and Cox, *c.*1879). Collection of the Wangansteen Historical Library of Biology and Medicine, University of Minnesota, Minneapolis.

Anatomizing Pregnancy: Pictorial and Surgical Dissections

In these two widely circulated works, we have seen physicians and artists repeatedly invoke the idea of penetrating and even disassembling the pregnant body in order to reveal its "secrets." This logic of fragmentation and bodily incursion clearly evokes the power and authority of the anatomist. It also, however, betokens the growing influence of another medical professional: the surgeon. By the turn of the century, the gradual shift away from procedures such as craniotomy, increasingly viewed as outmoded and even barbaric, and toward surgical Cesarean sections in cases of obstructed or difficult labor helped to consolidate the medical authority of obstetrician and surgeon alike.

It should be noted that in surgical procedures, the techniques employed—physically separating joints, removing organs, and piercing the body through surgical incision—parallel both anatomical practice and the *visual* strategies employed in obstetrical illustration. An anatomical structure defined and delimited is one that can be severed from surrounding tissues. A body pierced by sight is one that can be penetrated by the hand. I would argue that in a very powerful way, anatomical images of the pregnant body produced in this era thus helped to lay the conceptual framework for modern medical practice, even as physicians employed visual illustrations to record, publicize, and promote the surgical and clinical innovations they helped to pioneer.[54]

In their numbered and labeled representations of bodily structures, Auzoux and Witkowski unite the naturalism of the fine art tradition with the increasingly standardized conventions of anatomical illustration, creating hybrid works that offer evidence of a transitional moment in medical visualization. Grounded in the practice of close observation, their works nonetheless anticipate the indexical yet highly conceptual pictorial language of modern scanning methods. Both Auzoux and Witkowski created works that blend realism with abstraction, Auzoux by substituting a singular and seemingly self-contained organ for the complex pregnant body, and Witkowski by rendering the pregnant form in a series of crisply delineated leaves of paper. In the process, they reflect anatomy's ongoing struggle to define the universal through study of the particular but also look forward to new, technologically mediated methods of representing the body's interior.

In time, a new palette of black, white, and gray—the visual language of the X-ray and the ultrasound scan—would replace the richly descriptive color and carefully modeled forms of Auzoux's models and Witkowski's atlas,

54   For an example, see Frederic Shepard Dennis and John S. Billings, *System of Surgery*, 4 vols. (Philadelphia: Lea Brothers, 1895).

just as the machine would replace the hand of the artist. By mobilizing and widely disseminating the material and visual practices of anatomical science, Auzoux and Witkowski's depictions of the pregnant body lay the ground-work for this transformation, confirming the discursive power of anatomy and its privileged role in shaping our understanding of the human body. As nineteenth-century physicians, obstetricians, and surgeons united the authority of this anatomical discourse with increasingly "objective" methods for generating images of the body, they began to fundamentally redefine the ways in which we understand the pregnant body and, in the process, created a new medical subject: the fetus.

Chapter Four

Biological Bodies, Unfettered Imaginations

The 1939 Dickinson-Belskie *Birth Series* Sculptures and the Unexpected Origins of Modern Antiabortion Imagery

Rose Holz

Although only briefly touched upon by scholars, *The Birth Series*—a series of sculptures that depicted in utero development from fertilization through delivery—was a monumental scientific and artistic achievement.[1] Commissioned by the New York Maternity Center Association for an exhibit on women's health and reproduction and created by Dr. Robert L. Dickinson and Abram Belskie, the sculptures went on display at the 1939–1940 World's Fair in New York City where they were seen by hundreds of thousands of people. Wildly successful and much in demand in the decades

---

1   Parts of this chapter appeared in Rose Holz, "The 1939 Dickinson-Belskie Birth Series Sculptures: The Rise of Modern Visions of Pregnancy, the Roots of Modern Pro-Life Imagery, and Dr. Dickinson's Religious Case for Abortion," *Journal of Social History* 51, no. 4 (June 2018): 980–1022 and are reprinted here with permission. Also in Rose Holz, "'Art in the Service of Medical Education:' The 1939 Dickinson-Belskie Birth Series and the Use of Sculpture to Teach the Process of Human Development from Fertilization Through Delivery," in *Visualizing the Body in Art, Anatomy and Medicine Since 1800: Models and Modeling*, ed. Andrew Graciano (New York: Routledge, 2019), 129–56, reproduced with permission of the licensor through PLSclear.

thereafter, the sculptures were reproduced in a variety of forms and sent out to medical teaching institutions and health museums across the nation and overseas. And this was just the beginning. For several decades after their debut, *The Birth Series* made its way into sex education materials in classes for expectant parents as well as high school and university students. Local businesses, global philanthropic organizations, authors of books on childbirth, and makers of movies and television programs found use for its imagery. Even the military was intrigued. But then, as quickly as they appeared they disappeared, swept aside by the latest innovations in pregnancy imaging technology that had emerged by the 1970s. Left behind as a result was a significant historical gap in our knowledge about the rise of modern visions of pregnancy that we are only now able to fill.

As this chapter will demonstrate, *The Birth Series* sculptures participated in the shift from nineteenth-century conceptualizations of pregnancy to those that had emerged by the latter third of the twentieth. As Leslie Reagan demonstrated, the nineteenth-century notion of quickening as the start of life still held sway well into the early twentieth century, despite the medical profession's efforts to convince women otherwise. Likewise, the experience of pregnancy was still largely regarded as a woman's experience with what grew inside her womb, not of two separate identities that existed from the moment of conception forward.[2] However, by the latter third of the twentieth century both notions had eroded dramatically. As Sara Dubow noted in describing the rise of fetal medicine in the 1970s: no longer did pregnancy care involve merely two people (doctor and woman); a third (the fetus) had entered the equation, dramatically affecting the choices women had in their pregnancies and the care they received.[3]

This chapter further reveals how *The Birth Series* changed the visual narratives that were in place by the 1930s, decades before Lennart Nilsson's much-heralded photographs in *Life* magazine in the 1960s.[4] There was already a long history of representing and displaying the contents of a pregnant womb. While Karen Newman traced this phenomenon back to religious/anatomical art of the ninth century, Nick Hopwood described the

---

2   Leslie J. Reagan, *When Abortion Was a Crime: Women, Medicine, and Law in the United States, 1867–1973* (Berkeley: University of California Press, 1997), 8–14 and chapter 3.

3   Sara Dubow, *Ourselves Unborn: A History of the Fetus in Modern America* (Oxford: Oxford University Press, 2011), chapter 4.

4   For the impact of Nilsson's photos and other contemporary visual imagery of in utero development, see the historiographic discussion in chapter 12.

rise of wax and marble embryonic models in the nineteenth.[5] By the early twentieth century, moreover, lay and medical audiences were increasingly familiar with mass-produced papier-mâché uteruses and anatomical gestational atlases (as described by Jessica M. Dandona in the present volume) in addition to displays of *real* embryos and fetuses in public exhibits and medical teaching institutions, as discussed by Lynn Morgan and Catherine Cole.[6] But *The Birth Series* introduced something new—the product of Dr. Robert L. Dickinson's desire to marry eighteenth-century obstetrical art with twentieth-century science and technology.

Indeed, *The Birth Series* ushered in a dramatic new narrative about in utero human development. In the generations preceding the sculptures' 1939 debut, depictions of this process embodied a tone of dispassionate science or grotesque morbidity as they were often modeled after dissected cadavers. This was not so, however, with *The Birth Series* sculptures. Instead, they represented a crucial shift in visualization of the process, from depicting figures modeled on the inert and dead, to ones modeled after alert and alive subjects, producing a compelling new story about human development that audiences loved. Part of the appeal was the practical story the series told about the mechanics of reproduction. Combining art with the latest in scientific knowledge and technology, Dr. Dickinson and sculptor Abram Belskie gave audiences a view of something with which most were familiar but had not seen in quite this way: what happens inside a pregnant woman's body from the moment of fertilization through delivery. However, there was something else buried within the aesthetic of *The Birth Series* that drew audiences in. With these sculptures, the story of in utero development became a tale of creative perfection, with an idealized fetus whose story began at the moment of conception and culminated in the birth of a sweet and innocent child. Thus, not only did Dickinson and Belskie shape modern gynecological education for aspiring practitioners while educating ordinary Americans in matters of public health and pregnancy, but they also inadvertently articulated over three decades in advance the imagery that would become the

---

5   Karen Newman, *Fetal Positions: Individualism, Science, Visuality* (Stanford: Stanford University Press, 1996); Nick Hopwood, *Embryos in Wax: Models from the Ziegler Studio* (Cambridge: Whipple Museum of the History of Science, 2002); and Nick Hopwood, "A Marble Embryo: Meanings of a Portrait from 1900," *History Workshop Journal* 73 (Spring 2012): 5–36.

6   Lynn M. Morgan, *Icons of Life: A Cultural History of Human Embryos* (Berkeley: University of California Press, 2009) and Catherine Cole, "Sex and Death on Display: Women, Reproduction, and Fetuses at Chicago's Museum of Science and Industry," *Drama Review* 37, no. 1 (1993): 43–60.

hallmarks of the modern antiabortion movement, even though Dickinson himself was an ardent supporter of abortion.

The Birth Series as Visual Meditation

While space does not allow for the reproduction of all twenty-four of the original sculptures, the nine that appear here give a good impression of what the series looked like and the impact it may have on both past and present viewers. Questions to consider when looking at them include: What do you see? What don't you see? What else do they conjure up?

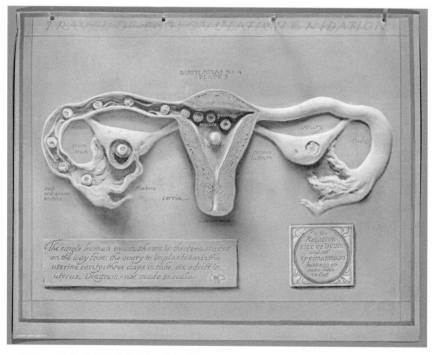

Figure. 4.1. *Birth Atlas* (1940), plate 3. Birth Atlas © National Partnership for Women & Families. All images used with permission.

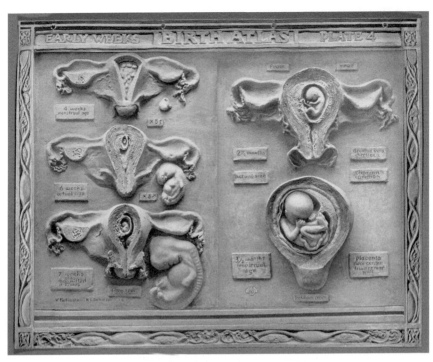

Figure 4.2. *Birth Atlas* (1940), plate 4.

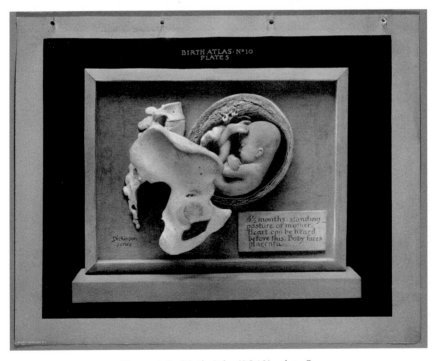

Figure 4.3. *Birth Atlas* (1940), plate 5.

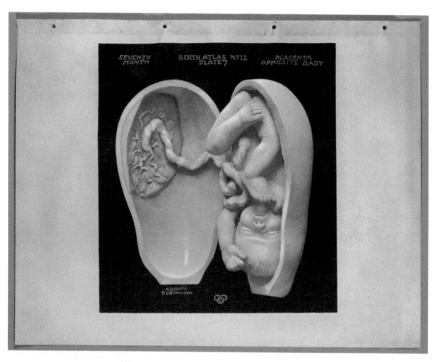

Figure 4.4. *Birth Atlas* (1940), plate 7.

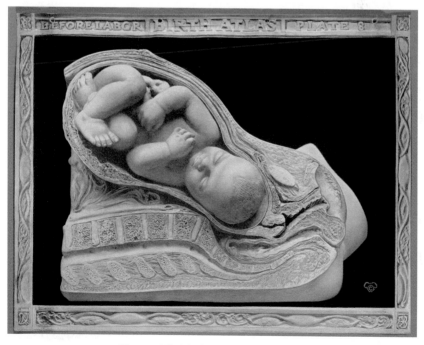

Figure 4.5. *Birth Atlas* (1940), plate 8.

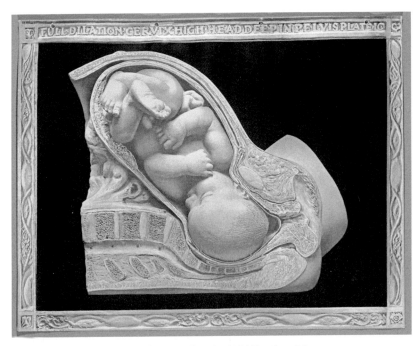

Figure 4.6. *Birth Atlas* (1940), plate 10.

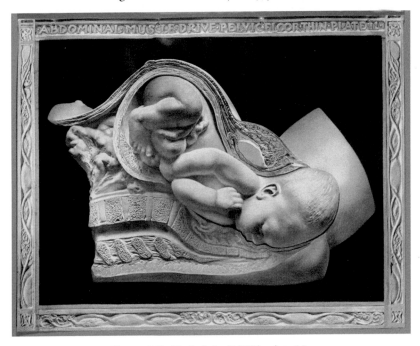

Figure 4.7. *Birth Atlas* (1940), plate 11.

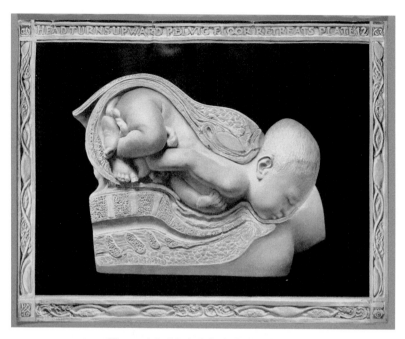

Figure 4.8. *Birth Atlas* (1940), plate 12.

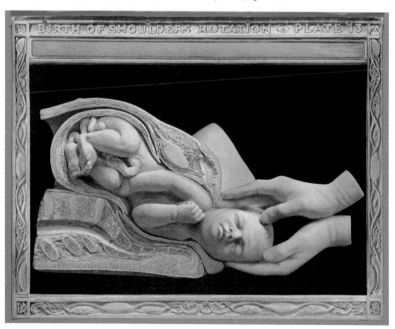

Figure 4.9. *Birth Atlas* (1940), plate 13.

The Birth of *The Birth Series*

The Birth Series came about as a result of the convergence of Dr. Robert L. Dickinson, Abram Belskie, the Maternity Center Association, and two World's Fairs. Dr. Dickinson was a prominent and well-published American gynecologist, obstetrician, and sexologist, who practiced from the late nineteenth through the early twentieth centuries. Although most known for his involvement in the early twentieth century birth control movement (in the organization now known as Planned Parenthood), he laid the foundation for prominent sexologists—Alfred Kinsey and Masters and Johnson—who followed in his wake. Significantly, Dickinson was also a prolific artist, driven to create both for personal pleasure as well as to engage in medical and scientific practice. In fact, by the 1930s, he had committed himself to bridging the worlds of art and science to improve the practice of medicine throughout the profession. Forty-six years his junior was the sculptor Abram Belskie. Born in England but raised in Scotland, Belskie came to New York City in the 1920s to make his mark. There he met the noted sculptor Malvina Hoffman who would later put him in touch with Dickinson who was in desperate need of assistance to finish his massive sculptural undertaking in time for the April opening of the 1939 New York City World's Fair. The two hit it off and went on to collaborate for the next decade until Dickinson's death in 1950.[7]

But it was the Maternity Center Association that first served as the spark to set the whole process in motion. Indeed, during the 1930s, just when Dickinson began to proselytize the educational power of science and art, the Maternity Center Association (MCA) stepped up its efforts to educate the public about women's health and reproduction. According to historians Laura E. Ettinger and Ziv Eisenberg, the MCA was a classic product of the Progressive Era movement for infant and maternal welfare reform. Founded in 1918 by obstetricians, social reformers, and public-health nurses in New York City, its purpose was to provide maternity care education in the hopes of reducing the high infant and maternal mortality rates that plagued the nation. Its work had consisted of classes for expectant mothers, but by the 1920s the MCA began to publish maternity care handbooks. By the 1930s, it established a nurse-midwifery clinic and school and broadened its public educational efforts by setting up exhibits at two World's Fairs—Chicago in 1933 and New York City in 1939–1940.[8]

---

7   Holz, "The 1939 Dickinson-Belskie Birth Series Sculptures" and Holz, "'Art in the Service of Medical Education."

8   Laura E. Ettinger, *Nurse-Midwifery: The Birth of a New American Profession* (Columbus: Ohio State University Press, 2006), chapter 3; Ziv Eisenberg, "The Whole Nine Months: Women, Men, and the Making of Modern Pregnancy in America" (PhD diss., Yale University, 2013).

The MCA's first display at the 1933 World's Fair was designed to educate the public about what it called "the entire maternity period"—from the moment a woman was aware of her pregnancy through six weeks after she delivered. The goal was to encourage medical supervision throughout the pregnancy and not merely at the moment of delivery. As an illustration of the mindset the MCA hoped to change, the organization repeated a common refrain in its 1933 report, "My mother had eight children and never saw a doctor until the baby came." The exhibit, in turn, used visual aids to publicize just how much happens inside a woman's body before birth takes place. To that end, it featured a series of eighteen pictures demonstrating proper maternity care techniques and a quaintly decorated nursery complete with white organdy curtains, stenciled ducks, and a cabinet and bath table constructed from cardboard boxes. Declaring the installation a great success, the organization pronounced it "made a decided impression" on those "who are still whispering 'she's going to have a baby.'"[9] However, while earnest in its message, the Chicago exhibit offered little in the way of explanation for the mechanics of reproduction. Indeed, it would be Dickinson's desire to depict "how babies come" that later stole the show at the 1939–1940 World's Fair in New York City.[10]

Whether he realized it or not, Dickinson had been working toward such a sculptural display for years, as is revealed in the extensive sourcebooks he meticulously kept for decades of his scientific research. Housed in the Rare Book Room of the New York Academy of Medicine, they vividly demonstrate Dickinson's fascination with embryonic development, in addition to his interests in contraception and human reproductive anatomy.[11] In these

---

9   Sarah Ward Gould, "Exhibits at Fairs: A Medium of Educating the People in Matters Pertaining to Maternal Health," folder 2, box 39, Maternity Center Association Records, Archives & Special Collections, Health Sciences Library, Columbia University, New York City, NY (hereafter cited as MCA Records—CU). Quotes on 3 and 1, respectively.

10   Quote from a conversation Dickinson had with a grandson over Christmas, folder 13, box 10, Robert Latou Dickinson Papers, 1881–1972 (inclusive), 1883–1950 (bulk), B MS c72, Boston Medical Library, Francis A. Countway Library of Medicine, Boston, Mass. (hereafter cited as Dickinson Papers—CLM).

11   The general name of this collection is Medical Illustrations of Human Sex Anatomy, With Some Text, and Many Original Drawings (New York 1924–1940), New York Academy of Medicine Library, New York, New York (hereafter cited as NYAML). The specific folios I relied upon include: The Living Vagina, Outlines and Case Records, Parts I and II; Topographical Anatomy of the Uterus, Tubes and Ovary, Parts I and II; Location of Embryo, Size of Fetus, Parts I and II; Shape and Size of Uterus and Its Cavity, Parts I and II; Topographical Anatomy of the Uterus, Tubes and Ovary, Parts I and II;

sourcebooks, Dickinson supplemented the clinical data derived from his private practice patients with clipped articles from medical journals and notes taken on the images and information he found. He also drew extensively, sketching contraceptive devices, women's and men's sexual and reproductive anatomies, as well as countless versions of in utero development. Tracing, and in particular tracing over X-rays, was an important method in his scientific/artistic process, for it facilitated clear linear drawings, useful for illustrations and sculptural models of messy anatomical interiors.[12]

Notably, Dickinson's creative and scientific vision also reflected his appreciation for earlier representations of in utero development, in particular those from eighteenth-century Europe. He spoke glowingly of the British midwives William Smellie and William Hunter who were among the first to publish pictorial medical atlases to illustrate pregnancy and birth.[13] Likewise, the similarity his sculptures bore to the Italian wax and clay obstetrical models used in Bologna, Italy's School of Obstetrics is unmistakable.[14] Yet the imagery of both was rooted in the science that existed before the nineteenth-century rise of embryology. Thus, in including embryonic development, Dickinson was adding a new chapter to these eighteenth-century stories.

Vaginal Pessaries; and Medical Illustrations of Female Human and Monkey Genitourary Organs.

12 For mention of tracing, see Dickinson to Hazel Corbin, July 13, 1945, folder 3, box 26, MCA Records—CU. For earlier uses of tracing technique, see Dickinson to Dr. E.V. Schubert, November 6, 1929, in Medical Illustrations of Human Sex Anatomy, Topographical Anatomy of the Uterus, Tubes and Ovary, Part II.

13 Robert L. Dickinson, "What Medical Authors Need to Know About Illustrating," *The Proceedings of the Charaka Club* 8 (1935): 141–48 and Lyle Massey, "Pregnancy and Pathology: Picturing Childbirth in Eighteenth-Century Obstetric Atlases, *The Art Bulletin* 87, no. 1 (2005): 73–91.

14 For eighteenth-century obstetrical models and their use in midwifery education, see guide to the Museo di Palazzo Poggi, "The School of Obstetrics" (Room 5), https://anatomiaitaliana.com/wp-content/uploads/2013/05/Poggi_Obstetrics.pdf (last accessed May 27, 2023) and Jennifer F. Kosmin, *Authority, Gender, and Midwifery in Early Modern Italy: Contested Deliveries* (Abingdon, UK: Routledge, 2021), chapter 4. For the histories of wax anatomical models and their makers more generally, see Anna Maerker, *Model Experts: Wax Anatomies and Enlightenment in Florence and Vienna, 1775–1815* (Manchester: Manchester University Press, 2011); Rebecca Messbarger, *The Lady Anatomist: The Life and Work of Anna Morandi Manzolini* (Chicago: University of Chicago Press, 2010); and Roberta Panzanelli, ed. *Ephemeral Bodies: Wax Sculpture and the Human Figure* (Los Angeles: Getty Research Institute, 2008).

Consequently, when Dickinson was asked to serve on the planning committee for the MCA's exhibit at the 1939–1940 World's Fair in New York City, he was well poised to make his dramatic sculptural contribution.[15] A massive undertaking, however, this task was not something Dickinson could complete alone. He made the first five sculptures mostly on his own, but with assistance from another physician/medical artist, Dr. Vladimir Fortunato, whose name appears on the fourth of these early figures. Done in bas relief, they begin with a visual representation of a woman's reproductive anatomy and then move on to illustrate the process of fertilization and early embryonic/fetal development through the first four-and-a-half months. It was at this point, though, that Dickinson sought additional help. This was in part because Fortunato unexpectedly passed away in 1938.[16] But it was certainly also true that Dickinson's grand vision was beginning to outmatch his own artistic ability and physical endurance. Not only did he lack formal training in sculpture, but the work is physically demanding and Dickinson was nearly 80.[17] Thus, the sixth sculpture marks the arrival of the sculptor Abram Belskie's talented, young hand. The next few months then saw Dickinson and Belskie—along with two other medical artists who assisted with sketching (Emily Freret and Frances Elwyn)—working feverishly to have the full series ready for the April 30 opening of the 1939 World's Fair.[18] They almost succeeded. By May 19, eighteen had been delivered and on display, three

---

15   Planning committee meeting minutes in folder 3, box 39, MCA Records—CU.

16   Keith C. Mages and Sebastian C. Galbo, "Dr. Vladimir Fortunato (1885–1938), Once Lauded but Now Obscure Russian-American Medical Model Sculptor," *Journal of Medical Biography* (2022): 1–7.

17   Belskie also mentioned that when they first met, Dickinson was "too tired to tackle the project himself." In Robert J. Demarest, "Abram Belskie, Sculptor . . . and the Famous American Sculptors with Whom He Worked," *Journal of Biocommunication* 35 (2009): e58–e66.

18   Hoffman declined Dickinson's request for assistance, but she put him in touch with Belskie. For letter of introduction between Belskie and Dickinson, see Hoffman to Dickinson, January 12, 1939, folder 80, box 1, Dickinson Papers—CLM. For more on Hoffman's life and work, see Linda Nochlin, "Malvina Hoffman: A Life in Sculpture," *Arts Magazine* 59 (September–December 1984): 106–10; Marianne Kinkel, *Races of Mankind: The Sculptures of Malvina Hoffman* (Urbana: University of Illinois Press, 2011); and Jennifer Schuessler, "'Races of Mankind' Sculptures, Long Exiled, Return to Display at Chicago's Field Museum," *New York Times*, January 20, 2016, https://www.nytimes.com/2016/01/21/arts/design/races-of-mankind-sculptures-long-exiled-return-to-display-at-chicagos-field-museum.html (last accessed May 27, 2023). As far as the other artists' work, in the months leading up to the 1939 World's Fair: Emily Freret had logged in 91 days, Frances Elwyn 29, and Belskie 48. After the Fair opened, Belskie continued to work on additional

more were ready, and four "nearly finished," as Dickinson reported with characteristic exactitude to the MCA's director, Hazel Corbin.[19] With the arrival of Abram Belskie, *The Birth Series* had finally quickened.

However, while Dickinson relied heavily on Belskie's skills as a sculptor to carry out his artistic vision, Dickinson also made direct use of the latest technology, using X-rays to capture another essential feature to which five of *The Birth Series* sculptures were devoted, the active stages of delivery. As Dickinson well understood, previous knowledge about in utero development had been derived from the dead—pregnant cadavers as well as the embryonic and fetal remains of miscarriages, abortions, and hysterectomies.[20] Prompted by the suggestion made by the MCA's Hazel Corbin to include a birth sequence in the series, he found it necessary to replace the cadaverous sources with what he called "*the alert upstanding tensions of the living.*" He then enlisted the help of his colleagues at prominent hospitals (Johns Hopkins, Sloane, Bronx, Harlem, and New Haven), who gave him access to thousands of X-rays of pregnant women perhaps during their pregnancies, but certainly as they delivered their babies.[21] Of course, it is difficult to imagine today, but periodic X-rays of pregnant women were routine at the time, and it was not until 1956 that Dr. Alice Stewart sounded the alarm about their potentially ill effect on in utero development.[22]

Notably, information about these women is elusive. Whether they were asked for permission is not clear. The records do not appear to say. Their

models. See "Modeling Account" time sheets, unprocessed Abram Belskie Papers, Belskie Museum of Art and Science, Closter, NJ.

19   Dickinson to Corbin, May 19, 1939, folder 8, box 39, MCA Records—CU. See Dickinson's attached list entitled, "List of Teaching Models Loaned to Maternity Center Association by R. L. Dickinson for Exhibit at World's Fair."

20   See "Some Dickinson Claims for Priority," January 1947, folder 2, box 59, Planned Parenthood Federation of America Records I—SC (hereafter cited as PPFA Records I—SC). See also Nick Hopwood, "Producing Development: The Anatomy of Human Embryos and the Norms of Wilhelm His," *Bulletin of the History of Medicine* 74 (Spring 2000): 29–79; Morgan, *Icons of Life*; and Shannon K. Withycombe, "From Women's Expectations to Scientific Specimens: The Fate of Miscarriage Materials in Nineteenth-Century America," *Social History of Medicine* 28, no. 2 (2015): 245–62.

21   Dickinson, "The Application of Sculpture to Practical Teaching in Obstetrics," *American Journal of Obstetrics and Gynecology* 40 (October 1940): 662–70. Quote on 662. Italics in original. See also the introduction to the *Birth Atlas*, 2nd ed. (1943). For Corbin's suggestion, see Anne A. Stevens to Dickinson, November 27, 1946, folder 8, box 39, MCA Records—CU.

22   José van Dijck, *The Transparent Body: A Cultural Analysis of Medical Imaging* (Seattle: University of Washington Press, 2005), 102.

backgrounds are equally difficult to pin down. 1938 and 1939 Hospital Annual Reports for Johns Hopkins, Sloane, and New Haven indicate that "ward" patients vastly outnumbered "private" and "semi-private," suggesting a significant patient population of modest means.[23] In addition, Harlem Hospital likely served predominantly Black women. Yet, we still do not know for certain the backgrounds of the women whose bodies were X-rayed—with one notable exception. Buried in one of Dickinson's sourcebooks are six of their names, all of whom attended Sloane Hospital for their deliveries. In this case at least, German heritage and/or German marriage seems to be a common theme.[24]

Likewise, for all the beauty to be found in *The Birth Series*, it would be wrong not to acknowledge other troubling aspects, particularly concerning race and eugenics, embedded in these and the other sculptures Dickinson and Belskie made together. Indeed, it is the particular kind of beauty embodied by the sculptures that poses the problems. Compelling critiques have already been made by historians Anna G. Creadick and Julian B. Carter about the 1945 Dickinson-Belskie *Norma* and *Normman* sculptures. As their none-too-subtle names suggest, *Norma* and *Normman* were intended to represent the average American male and average American female. However, as Creadick and Carter demonstrated, the normality they suggest is deeply problematic. Not only do the sculptures present Whiteness and White sexuality as normal or even divine, but such representations were also hardly born of naiveté nor innocence. Rather, as Creadick noted, "The Aryan look and eugenicist overtones of Norm and Norma were not aberrations, but signs of a midcentury obsession. Their boldly European features,

---

23   *The Johns Hopkins Hospital Forty-Ninth Report of the Director, 1938*, 5 and *The Johns Hopkins Hospital Fiftieth Report of the Director, 1939*, 6. Both in The Alan Masey Chesney Archives, Baltimore, MD. "Report of the Sloane Hospital for Women," in the *Seventieth Annual Report for The Presbyterian Hospital in the City of New York, The Sloane Hospital for Women, and Vanderbilt Clinic* (December 31, 1938), 51–52 and "Report of the Sloane Hospital for Women," in the *Seventy-First Annual Report for The Presbyterian Hospital in the City of New York, The Sloane Hospital for Women, Vanderbilt Clinic, and Neurological Institute of New York* (December 31, 1939), 51. In Digital Collections: Columbia University Medical Center Affiliated Hospitals, Health Sciences Library, Columbia University, New York City NY. *Annual Report of the General Hospital Society of Connecticut and the New Haven Dispensary, 1938–1939* (New Haven, CT, 1939), 10. Obtained through Yale University Library's "EliScholar." I was unable to track down comparable information for Harlem Hospital. Thanks to archivist Stephen Novak for help tracking this hospital information down.

24   Medical Illustrations of Female Human and Monkey Genitourary Organs.

their alabaster whiteness, their youthful, able bodies reveal what 'normality' had been designed to include and exclude."[25]

Moreover, if we were to combine such overtones with the MCA's habit of dismissing the knowledge of Black midwives—whose "only training comes from 'de Lawd,'" as one MCA president pronounced in a 1941 issue of *Baby Magazine*—then a rather complex story about the intersection of race and *The Birth Series* quickly bubbles to the surface.[26] Suffice to say, learning more about the women whose X-rayed bodies guided the depiction of *The Birth Series'* delivery sequence as well as using the lens of race to unpack more of the sculptures' imagery, medical use, and popular reception are important threads that deserve further investigation, especially in the wake of medical illustrator Chidiebere Ibe's drawing of a Black pregnant body that went viral in 2021 and sparked conversations about the lack of representation in medical texts.[27]

Such crucial considerations for the moment aside, the sculptures were produced in a moment of creative artistic inspiration—one born of many minds and carried out by many bodies. With X-rays in hand, tracings were made and sketches developed—whereupon *The Birth Series* sculptures were meticulously created and expertly delivered. It is little wonder that "the babies," as the sculptures were often called, looked so alive.[28]

25   Julian B. Carter, *The Heart of Whiteness: Normal Sexuality and Race in America, 1880–1940* (Durham: Duke University Press, 2007) and Creadick, *Perfectly Average*. Quote from Creadick on 16.

26   Mrs. Shepard Krech, "Saving Mothers: Tomorrow," *Baby Life* (January 1941): 27+. Quote on 27. In scrapbook 2, scrapbook box 4, MCA Records—CU. Another example of this mindset can be seen in the 1937 planning meeting minutes for the 1939–1940 New York City World's Fair. "It was agreed that the midwife, as such, should be left out of the picture. It was felt that it was wrong terminology to call most of the 30,000 mammies who practice in this country 'midwives.'" See planning meeting minutes, November 11, 1937. Quote on 2. In folder 3, box 39, MCA Records—CU.

27   David Limm, "The Creator of a Viral Black Fetus Medical Illustration Blends Art and Activism," *HealthCity*, January 13, 2022.

28   While Dickinson referred to them as such, Hoffman did so as well. See Dickinson to Hoffman, February 1, 1939, and Hoffman to Dickinson, August 3, 1939. Both in folder 80, box 1, Dickinson Papers—CLM. "The babies" is also how the curators and museum workers at the University of Nebraska State Museum for years referred to their set.

The Birth Series 1939 Debut and Their Mass Distribution in the Decades Thereafter

Much to the delight of the MCA, its exhibit at the 1939–1940 World's Fair in New York City, which now included the Dickinson-Belskie *Birth Series*, was far more successful than the one in Chicago in 1933. Housed in the "Hall of Man," it was accompanied by other exhibits, such as *The Transparent Man*, a model created in the 1920s by the world-renowned Deutsche Hygiene Museum that illustrated the workings of the human body through transparent skin and illuminated organ systems. Notably, such three-dimensional installations (including the one commissioned by the MCA) reflected the influence of the German visual health museum movement pioneered in the 1920s, which was increasingly popular among health educators and museums in 1930s America.[29] However, *The Birth Series* was, to use the MCA's words, the *pièce de résistance*. Wildly popular, the installation attracted long lines of visitors every day from ten in the morning to ten at night. Neither rain nor shine stopped the crowds from coming.[30] In fact, so well-attended was the exhibit—seven hundred thousand people had viewed it in 1939 alone—that it prompted more than a few complaints from fair organizers and fellow exhibitors who claimed that the MCA installation prevented people from visiting other exhibits.[31] When reassembled in 1940 for the second year of the New York City World's Fair, the exhibit underwent

---

29 Erin McLeary and Elizabeth Toon, "'Here Man Learns about Himself'": Visual Education and the Rise and Fall of the American Museum of Health," *American Journal of Public Health* 102 (July 2012): e27–e36. For more on the Transparent Man, see Klaus Vogel, "The Transparent Man: Some Comments on the History of a Symbol," in *Manifesting Medicine: Bodies and Machines*, ed. Robert Bud, Bernard S. Finn, and Helmuth Trischler (London: Routledge, 1999), 31–61 and José van Dijck, "Bodyworlds: The Art of Plastinated Cadavers," *Configurations* 9 (Winter 2001): 99–126.

30 "Life Begins" (1939), Maternity Center Association, folder 6, box 59, PPFA Records I—SC. Quote on 19. Italics in original. For another mention of the exhibit's popularity from opening to close, see Corbin to Sylvia Carewe, June 15, 1939, folder 5, box 39, MCA Records—CU.

31 For 1939 attendance, see the photo caption on first page of "Life Begins." See also a letter by Dickinson in which he said exhibit attendance was five thousand per day: Dickinson to Mrs. Albert D. Lasker, circa December 1941, folder 4, box 59, PPFA Records I—SC. For complaints from fair organizers, see Homer N. Calvert to Corbin, May 29, 1939, folder 5, box 39. For complaints from fellow exhibitors, see Bryan Gray to the MCA, October 23, 1939, and Corbin to Bryan Gray, October 24, 1939, folder 6, box 39. All in MCA Records—CU.

several changes. However, *The Birth Series* sculptures (of which there were now two sets) remained the star attraction.[32]

The reaction from the fair-going crowds, moreover, was overwhelmingly favorable—much to the relief of the MCA. "It was not without qualms that we decided to display the sculptures," noted the organization. The MCA had good cause to be concerned. The New York State Board of Regents had recently banned the showing of the film *The Birth of a Baby* (Al Christie, 1938), deeming it "indecent, immoral, and tending to corrupt public morals," a decision that was upheld by the courts. But not so with the 1939–1940 New York City World's Fair exhibit that featured *The Birth Series*. As the MCA further remarked, while parents were pleased to have something that explained "their children's questions about babies," doctors and nurses told their students, ministers their parishioners, and many others recommended the exhibit to family members.[33]

Similar enthusiasm was expressed when the sculptures were later exhibited elsewhere. For example, in 1941 Ruth Perkins Kuehn (Dean of the University of Pittsburgh's School of Nursing) noted how husbands and wives (expectant and otherwise), high schoolers, college students, student nurses, practical nurses, doctors, teachers, clubwomen, and ministers had come to see the sculptures in the university's "Dawn of Life" exhibit. She then described the many positive comments they had received. "Many women who have had babies were very much interested," she wrote. To which she added, "They could not understand how they could have had children without knowing how the process took place." Indeed, their many questions were decidedly practical. Among the questions that were frequently asked were, "What is the bag of water? Why is the baby's head out of shape when it is born? Why do the feet come first sometimes? Does the doctor shape the baby's head after birth? How do twins grow in the mother's body? How long is the cord? Why can some women not have babies? Does the baby change its position during the nine months before birth?"[34]

32 Corbin to Bruno Gebhard, March 4, 1940, folder 6, box 39, MCA Records—CU. See also Dickinson's remark in March 1940 that there would be "twice as many (sculptures) as last year." Dickinson to Dr. Wilcox, March 14, 1940, Unprocessed Dickinson Papers—NYAML.

33 "Life Begins." Quote on 20. Fair organizers were so concerned about the exhibit that they forbade the MCA from including the fair logo on the leaflets the organization distributed. See "RLD: An Appreciation," *Briefs: Official Publication of the Maternity Center Association* 14 (Winter 1950–1951): 1–5. Story recounted on 5.

34 Ruth Perkins Kuehn to Dickinson, June 14, 1941, folder 8, box 39, MCA Records—CU.

There were, of course, the few who disapproved. As Kuehn described, one woman "thought it was terrible to embarrass young girls who might wander into the exhibit with their boyfriends," only to find they were not embarrassed, thus prompting her to announce they "had no 'shame.'" Kuehn also recounted how another female teacher worked hard to keep the several dozen teenage girls she had brought to the museum from seeing the models and repeatedly "reprimanded" them. However, most appreciated what they saw and were deeply grateful for what they had learned.[35]

Hence, the purpose of *The Birth Series* sculptures once the 1939–1940 World's Fair was over: to be mass reproduced in a variety of forms to educate the lay public and medical professionals across the United States and the globe about the mechanics of human reproduction. Demand was great and orders placed in abundance. The sculptures themselves were much desired. During the winter months of the fair's offseason, the set displayed at the fair was exhibited at New York City's Museum of Natural History. Another set made its way to the offices of the MCA.[36] More sets went to medical and public health institutions across the country—in Flint (MI), Madison (WI), Cleveland (OH), and Chicago (IL).[37] By the 1950s still another set made its way to the University of Nebraska State Museum.[38] Even commercial interests saw use for *The Birth Series* sculptures.[39] So great was the demand for copies of *The Birth Series* sculptures (along with what was becoming the massive Dickinson-Belskie *Sculptured Teaching Models* collection) that the MCA handed the entire collection over to the Cleveland Health Museum to whom Dickinson had in 1945 granted all rights to reproduce and sell the sculptures, which it did for decades.[40]

However, most people's knowledge about and use of the sculptural imagery came through the *Birth Atlas*, a 22 x 17 1/2–inch manual put out by the MCA that depicted the entire *Birth Series* using photography and line plate

35 Kuehn to Dickinson.

36 "A Report of 'The First Year of Life:' An Exhibit at the New York World's Fair" (1939), folder 5, box 39, MCA Records—CU.

37 Dickinson to Corbin, November 14, 1940, folder 8, box 39, MCA Records—CU.

38 The University of Nebraska State Museum in Lincoln is where I first encountered them.

39 See Harper L. Schimpff to Horace Hughes, September 14, 1955, and Perry N. Zang to Horace Hughes, December 28, 1951. Both in folder 9, box 68, MCA Records—CU.

40 "The Dickinson-Belskie Collection . . . and Facilities for Its Multiple Reproduction," *Medical Times* (September 1945): 23. See also Bruno Gebhard, "The Birth Models: R. L. Dickinson's Monument," *Journal of Social Hygiene* 37 (April 1951): 169–74.

drawings.[41] Immensely popular, the *Birth Atlas* ultimately went through six editions (with many reprints of each) from 1940 through the 1960s.[42] In 1957, the MCA put out a smaller, updated follow-up, *A Baby Is Born: The Picture Story of Everyman's Beginning*, the central feature of which remained the photos of *The Birth Series*.[43]

In other words, whatever their form, *The Birth Series* sculptures were used seemingly everywhere—in medical schools, nurse-midwifery programs, nursing schools, museums, university classrooms, high schools, and elementary schools (public and parochial), marriage education classes, classes for expectant mothers and fathers, and classes for parents and children to learn about the process of reproduction together. They even made their way into an Amish community in Ohio.[44] Government agencies (including the US Navy) were also interested in them, as were such organizations as the American Red Cross, which brailled its copy of the *Birth Atlas* for use in the parenting classes for the blind. And this was in the United States alone; requests for information about and orders for *The Birth Series* in all its forms rolled in from countries across the globe—China, England, Canada, Japan, Mexico, Bolivia, Israel, New Zealand, South Africa, Switzerland, and India, to name just a few.[45] Because of the overwhelming interest from Central and South America, by the mid-1940s the MCA was working on a

41 Maternity Center Association, Robert L. Dickinson, and Abram Belskie, *Birth Atlas* (New York, 1940).
42 Editions, according to OCLC Worldcat, can be found at http://www.worldcat.org/title/birth-atlas/oclc/6034148/editions?sdasc&refererdi&seyr&editionsViewtrue&fq (last accessed May 27, 2023). For an overview of editions and reprints through 1958, see "Birth Atlas," folder 9, box 68, MCA Records—CU.
43 Maternity Center Association, *A Baby Is Born: The Picture Story of Everyman's Beginning* (New York, 1957). Later published as *A Baby Is Born: The Picture Story of a Baby from Conception through Birth* (London, 1966), it went through eleven editions, the last of which came out in 1978. It also includes a breech series not found in the *Birth Atlas*.
44 See Gebhard, "The Birth Models;" Allan C. Barnes, "The Use of the Dickinson Models in Obstetric and Gynecologic Education," *Journal of the American Association of Medical Colleges* 22 (April 1947): 261–62; David B. Treat, "Reproduction Education," *The Family Life Coordinator* 8 (September 1959): 3–8; and "RLD: An Appreciation." Mention of Amish community in Gebhard, "The Birth Models," 173.
45 Requests in folders 7–10, box 68, MCA Records—CU. For the braille version, see Gertrude Geiger Struble to the MCA, March 23, 1948, folder 8, box 68, MCA Records—CU.

Spanish-language version of the *Birth Atlas*.[46] Even the global philanthropic organization UNICEF bought "increasingly larger quantities" over the years.[47] As late as the 1980s, orders for the *Birth Atlas* still came in to the MCA.[48]

Thus the convergence of one organization, two men, two World's Fairs, the bodies of many pregnant women, and a host of other contributors set into motion a massive phenomenon that reached into big cities and small towns across America and the globe, laying the foundation for grand new ways to see—grand new ways to imagine—the process of human reproduction.

Biological Bodies, Unfettered Imaginations

As beautiful as they are as works of art and as pedagogically useful as they once were in educating lay and medical audiences about the mechanics of human reproduction, embedded within *The Birth Series* are the complexities of what it means to use art and science to reveal singular truths about biological processes. At the time of their debut, there were already other visual narratives available about in utero development. Take, for example, Friedrich Ziegler's three-dimensional wax embryos, which were displayed at the 1893 World's Fair in Chicago. While beautifully crafted and arranged in ways that captured the Victorian aesthetic of categories, balance, and order, they were not particularly humanized. That the set also included cross-sections of the embryo's inner workings further made them into modeled specimens or objects for study rather than a baby to be tenderly loved.[49] The same holds true for the increasingly common practice in the early decades of the twentieth century of displaying *real* embryos and fetuses—which showed the progression of in utero development from roughly six weeks through nine months, using either complete specimens or slices. In fact, a set of these was also on display at the 1939 New York City World's Fair, in the same building as *The Birth Series,* albeit in a different exhibit.[50]

---

46 For evidence of interest from Latin and South America, see Horace Hughes to Dr. Edward C. Ernst, October 21, 1943, folder 8, box 68, MCA Records—CU. For mention of Spanish-language version, see Hughes to Garst, March 29, 1949, folder 9. In same box.

47 Quote in Ruth Watson Lubick to Angele Petros-Barvazian, October 28, 1982, folder 10, box 161, MCA Records—CU.

48 See materials in folder 10, box 161, MCA Records—CU.

49 Hopwood, *Embryos in Wax.*

50 "Man and His Health: New York World's Fair 1939" (1939), folder 3, box 39, MCA Records—CU. On 18–19. In fact, a set had also been on display at the 1933 World's Fair in Chicago. See Cole, "Sex and Death on Display."

Audiences appreciated these sorts of exhibits as well, viewing them with much curiosity and interest.[51]

Whether wax or real, however, such displays were nonetheless derived from sources that were either inert or dead, which explains Dickinson's desire to use the latest scientific technology to capture in utero development as a dynamic and living biological process. "These are not the cadaver obstetrics of . . . textbooks," he wrote in a 1941 issue of the *American Journal of Obstetrics and Gynecology* when describing the stages of labor sequence for which X-rays played a vital part. "This is life in action, life arriving, tense and not collapsed."[52] His medical peers were equally laudatory. "In my experience, no two-dimensional teaching aids or mechanical models equal in instructional value these full-scale sculptures," noted Allan C. Barnes, associate professor of obstetrics and gynecology at The Ohio State University Medical School.[53]

The Birth Series also differed in its lack of the grotesque. The plaster sculptures' pale whiteness, for example (sometimes pale pink or creamy beige in subsequent reproductions), denied the messiness of blood and placental and other bodily fluids and excretions.[54] This was no accident; Dickinson had no interest in what one fair-goer called the "butcher shop color" found in other exhibits depicting the human body.[55] Instead, he believed in the power of "high art" to reach and move mass audiences.[56] Indeed, Dickinson was also concerned with decorum regarding the representation of the unclothed, sexual body—especially to the lay public. Decrying what he called the

---

Moreover, *The Birth Series* exhibit at the University of Nebraska State Museum also included an installation of real embryonic/fetal slices, with seven specimens ranging from six weeks to seven months.

51 For discussion of displays of fetal specimens before and after *Roe v. Wade* (1973), see Cole, "Sex and Death on Display;" Morgan, *Icons of Life*, 134–35 and 156–58 and Dubow, *Ourselves Unborn*, chapter 2. For more on the popular interest in anatomy museums, see Michael Sappol, *A Traffic of Dead Bodies: Anatomy and Embodied Social Identity in Nineteenth-Century America* (Princeton, NJ: Princeton University Press, 2002), especially chapter 9.

52 Dickinson, "Models, Manikins, and Museums for Obstetrics and Gynecology," *American Journal of Obstetrics and Gynecology* 41 (June 1941): 1075–78. Quote on 1077.

53 Barnes, "Use of the Dickinson Models." Quote on 261.

54 For various generations of the sculpture replicas, see the Dickinson-Belskie Collection, Warren Anatomical Museum, Francis A. Countway Library of Medicine, Boston, MA.

55 Dickinson, "Wall Charts and Models in Clinic Instruction" *Journal of Contraception* 4 (August–September 1939): 152–53. Quote on 153.

56 Dickinson, "Application of Sculpture." Quote on 662.

"sprawling nakedness" found in some art, he complimented figures drawn by such anatomists and medical illustrators as William Smellie, William Hunter, and Max Broedel as appropriate examples to follow.[57] In addition, across the series, the sculpted baby inside the woman's womb is the embodiment of an ideal, generalized depiction of the perfect baby, rather than directly based on any specific patient. It is never deformed, wrinkled or lumpy, mashed into weird shapes, or contorted into odd positions—not even when born breech as a later set of models would demonstrate.[58] In other words, the entire *Birth Series* represented the pregnancy process featuring an artistically idealized human developmental narrative that transpired with the union of sperm and egg. It is corrected in order to appear universal and timeless—the aspirational goal of classical sculpture.[59]

That said, Dickinson was not oblivious to the complex reality of pregnancy. Miscarriage was common among women, and he would have known from his decades in medical practice that not all conceptions yielded such perfect results.[60] Nor was he lackadaisical about the scientific-artistic process, which he knew could sometimes go awry.[61] Nonetheless, as he continued to work with Belskie, Dickinson was increasingly content to ignore the unscientific embellishments that made their way into *The Birth Series*. Chief among them were the features embedded in the sculpture of *Twinning*. Reflecting a light-hearted whimsy, each of the three sets depicted the adage of "see no evil, speak no evil, hear no evil" by using their little fetal hands to cover their little fetal eyes, mouths, and ears. Audiences, lay and medical, loved it.[62] Not even Dickinson could avoid straying from his scientist's eyes when overcome with the joy of creation—artistic or human—which as a deeply religious man he believed to be divinely inspired.

Therein lies, however, the conundrum of Dickinson's intent and the final riddle upon which this chapter ends. Although he had set out to use the tools of science and art to explain with greatest accuracy the mechanics behind the

---

57 Dickinson, "What Medical Authors Need to Know about Illustrating." Quote on 148.

58 For quick visual access to the Breech models, see *A Baby Is Born*, 53–57. The sculptures themselves are on display at the Belskie Museum of Art and Science, Closter, NJ.

59 As art historian Andrew Graciano noted in *Visualizing the Body*, this conflict between whether art should "'correct' imperfections or copy faithfully" was common among anatomists and artists. See page 151, footnote 73.

60 Lara Freidenfelds, *The Myth of the Perfect Pregnancy: A History of Miscarriage in America* (Oxford: Oxford University Press, 2020).

61 Dickinson, "What Medical Authors Need to Know about Illustrating."

62 *Birth Atlas*, 2nd ed. (1943), plate 17. For audience reactions to the twinning sculpture, see Gebhard, "Birth Models," 171.

process of human reproduction, much to his delight, the visual story he told captured so much more. As he wrote to his sculptor friend Malvina Hoffman in 1942, precisely when the mass reproduction and dissemination of *The Birth Series* was well underway:

> It is my chief and most cherished comment, the one made by a [Catholic] Sister whom I found later was the head of a large institution, to this effect. I asked "Sister, why is it that you feel your girls will want these?" and she answered, "The children always ask, 'how is a baby born,' and this is the most <u>reverent</u> way of answering that question that I have seen."[63]

Dickinson had managed to capture what he understood to be the power and glory of God and the joy found in the divine creation of human life, which unfolded with the union of sperm and egg. This visual story was later taken up, long after his death, by the modern antiabortion movement in the wake of *Roe v. Wade* (1973).

Indeed, one need not look too far to find how crucial this version of in utero imagery is to the modern antiabortion movement's educational efforts. As *NRL News Today* (the mouthpiece for the National Right to Life organization) proudly announced in a 2013 story submitted by the Minnesota Citizens for Concerned Life, after visiting its booth that featured "life-size models of unborn babies," women "canceled appointments at abortion clinics."[64] Similar stories about the power of in utero models to change people's mind about abortion abound in antiabortion publications.[65] The assumed antiabortion message in such imagery even appears in antiabortion responses to Damien Hirst's *The Miraculous Journey* (2013)—a strikingly *Birth Series*-esque series of fourteen massive bronze sculptures depicting in utero development that now stand in front of Sidra Medical Centre in Qatar.

63 Dickinson to Hoffman, December 30, 1942, folder 80, box 1, Dickinson Papers—CLM. Underline in the original. To ease the flow of reading, spelling errors have been corrected.

64 "Fetal Models Offer a Unique Glimpse at Life's Beginnings," *National Right to Life News Today* (December 12, 2013), http://www.nationalrighttolifenews. org/news/2013/12/fetal-models-offer-a-unique-glimpse-at-lifes-beginnings/#.V2GzJXrNwa4 (last accessed May 27, 2023).

65 Andrew Bair, "Abortion Advocates Go Nuts Over Pro-Lifers Distributing Fetal Models," *LifeNews.com* (July 26, 2013), http://www.lifenews. com/2013/07/26/abortion-advocates-go-nuts-over-pro-lifers-distributing-fetal-models/; Steven Ertelt, "Fetal Models Help Save Baby From Late-Term Abortion," *LifeNews.com* (June 4, 2014), https://www.lifenews. com/2014/06/04/fetal-models-help-save-baby-from-late-term-abortion/; and Kate Ewald, "Fetal Models Help Save Baby From Abortion, Mom Already Had Abortion Appointment," *LifeNews.com* (July 8, 2015), http://www. lifenews.com/2015/07/08/fetal-models-help-save-baby-from-abortion-mom-already-had-abortion-appointment/ (last accessed May 27, 2023).

As Canadian Catholic Lou Iacobelli blogged, "Consider the last piece which is a huge sculpture of the born baby. Visually it says that we cannot hide this human life away and destroy it."[66] The assumption among antiabortion activists is thus clear, only one conclusion can be drawn in the face of this imagery: that life begins at conception and that abortion is murder.[67]

However, it was never Dickinson's intent to craft a visual message that would articulate a case against abortion. On the contrary, Dickinson firmly believed in the necessity of its practice, not *despite* his religious views but *because* of them. As I describe elsewhere, it pained Dickinson deeply to see the ways in which abortion was characterized as the evil above all evils. After all, he too was a devout and religious man, and he saw quite the opposite— likely a product of his decades in gynecological practice where he listened to thousands of women's personal stories. He thus spent the 1930s also making the case for birth control and abortion, criticizing religious and medical leaders for failing to take his lead, and even providing visual instructions for how to do the abortions in fertility control manuals intended for physicians he coauthored with the public-health advocate and sexologist Louise Stevens Bryant.[68]

But the tide could not be shifted nor the die recast, not even by Dr. Robert L. Dickinson. To begin, he would be unable to deter what by the 1940s and '50s would become a massive period of legal and medical crackdown on the abortion procedure. Despite his frustration with his medical peers for failing to take up the abortion cause, the 1930s had witnessed a loosening of attitudes about the procedure, despite its illegality.[69] The frankness of his comments, not to mention his illustrated instructions, are thus a reflection of the period's more tolerant attitude. But this would quickly come to an end. In this era of renewed crackdown, all talk of abortion in

66 Quote from "14 Giant Sculptures Of Fetuses Attract Praise From Pro-Life Supporters," *Huffingtonpost.com* (October 24, 2013), http://www.huffingtonpost.com/2013/10/24/damien-hirst-fetus_n_4151500.html. See also "14 Monumental Sculptures of Unborn Babies by Controversial British artist Unveiled in Qatar," *LifeSiteNews.com* (October 8, 2013), https://www.lifesitenews.com/news/14-monumental-sculptures-of-unborn-babies-unveiled-in-qatar (both last accessed May 27, 2023).

67 Joanne Boucher made a similar observation with the antiabortion movement's use of ultrasound. See Boucher, "Ultrasound: A Window to the Womb? Obstetric Ultrasound and the Abortion Rights Debate," *Journal of Medical Humanities* 25 (Spring 2004): 7–19. See also Jennifer Holland, *Tiny You: A Western History of the Anti-Abortion Movement* (Berkeley: University of California Press, 2020).

68 Holz, "1939 Dickinson-Belskie Birth Series Sculptures."

69 Reagan, *When Abortion Was a Crime,* chapters 5 and 6.

his fertility control manuals was reduced to a handful of brief mentions, mostly to make the case that without the provision of birth control the need for abortion would increase. It was also the end of another era. In 1950 Dickinson passed away at age eighty-nine, and while Belskie would carry on, plying his trade as a sculptor until his death in 1988, this prolific and unique era of collaboration was finished.[70]

In sum, *The Birth Series* was a monumental scientific and artistic achievement. In marrying eighteenth-century obstetrical art with twentieth-century science and technology, Dickinson, Belskie, and their many collaborators gave lay and professional audiences grand new ways to see—grand new ways to imagine—the process of pregnancy, producing a visual tale of creative perfection, with an idealized fetus whose story began at the moment of conception and culminated in the birth of a sweet and innocent child. For the deeply religious Dickinson, moreover, it was a story that did not challenge his support for abortion; rather, it coalesced effortlessly alongside it. That this imagery would later be taken up by the modern antiabortion movement to make the case that abortion is murder in turn illustrates the ways in which the knowledge we create about our biological bodies are not simply singular truths to be revealed by science to justify our intellectual positions. Instead, this knowledge is far messier, complicated, and interesting—with the power, in this case, to bring together the most unlikely of people in shared curiosity and conversation: those avidly in support of abortion and those avidly against. Indeed, the riddle from which *The Birth Series* was born invites us to move beyond simple assumptions about the ideological meanings embedded in this imagery. We are thus free to dive—for one brief but beautiful moment—into the morass together. What do you see? What don't you see? What else do the sculptures conjure up?

---

70   Holz, "1939 Dickinson-Belskie Birth Series Sculptures."

Chapter Five

Creating a Public for Visualized Pregnancies

The Swedish Version of the American Sex Hygiene Film *Mom and Dad*

Elisabet Björklund

The historiography of the "public fetus" describes the increasing visibility of pregnant and fetal bodies in medicine and visual culture starting in the 1960s.[1] This development can also be observed in the history of cinema, which saw the loosening of different forms of film censorship from the 1960s onward. In the United States, for example, the self-censorship system managed by the Production Code Administration forbade the explicit depiction of pregnant bodies and childbirth in Hollywood cinema from 1930 until the late 1950s.[2] In the latter part of the twentieth century, however, this changed profoundly. Kelly Oliver has traced the transition of pregnancy "from shameful and hidden to sexy and spectacular," describing it as "exploding onto the screen" during this period.[3]

---

1   The author would like to thank Lars Gustaf Andersson and the students at the bachelor's level in film studies at Lund University for their helpful comments on a draft version of the text during a seminar in the spring of 2022. See Jülich and Björklund in this volume.

2   David A. Kirby, "Regulating Cinematic Stories about Reproduction: Pregnancy, Childbirth, Abortion and Movie Censorship in the US, 1930–1958," *The British Journal for the History of Science* 50, no. 3 (September 2017): 451–72.

3   Kelly Oliver, *Knock Me Up, Knock Me Down: Images of Pregnancy in Hollywood Films* (New York: Columbia University Press, 2012), 2, 1.

This description broadly holds true, but many scholars have shown that films visualizing the course of pregnancy and childbirth were in wide circulation much earlier in history. Different types of sex education films had been shown in various contexts in both Europe and the United States since the 1910s, and examples of childbirth scenes in films of this kind can be found at least as early as the 1920s and 1930s.[4] On the one hand, there were educational films about reproduction shown in, for example, schools and medical training. On the other, there were feature-length sex education films shown in commercial cinemas. In the United States, exploitation films—which provided content that was forbidden in mainstream cinema—often included spectacular images of birth and attracted large audiences to cinemas not belonging to the major film companies.[5] Films could also cross these social boundaries and be shown in both educational and commercial settings. This was the case with the widely successful American film *The Birth of a Baby* (Al Christie, 1938)—seen by around five million people in the United States—which triggered public debate concerning whether cinema was the proper place for education. Pictures from the film were also published in *Life* magazine, which created immense controversy.[6] Moreover, many films traveled abroad; in doing so, they sometimes also crossed over into new spaces of display, thus reaching new audiences.

Hence, films showing pregnancy and birth could be seen in various public places long before the 1960s. But as previous research has demonstrated, the content and meanings of these films could also shift depending on the context of exhibition. There were often many versions of the films in circulation, they were frequently cut by censors, and the way they were shown could vary. How viewers experienced a sex education film was thus probably

---

4   See, for example, Robert Eberwein, *Sex Ed: Film, Video, and the Framework of Desire* (New Brunswick, NJ: Rutgers University Press, 1999); Manon Parry, *Broadcasting Birth Control: Mass Media and Family Planning* (New Brunswick, NJ: Rutgers University Press, 2013); Jesse Olszynko-Gryn and Patrick Ellis, "'A Machine for Recreating Life': An Introduction to Reproduction on Film," *The British Journal for the History of Science* 50, no. 3 (September 2017): 383–409; Anja Laukötter, "Listen and Watch: The Practice of Lecturing and the Epistemological Status of Sex Education Films in Germany," *Gesnerus* 72, no. 1 (2015): 56–76; Saniya Lee Ghanoui, "Translating Sex Culture: Transnational Sex Education and the U.S.–Swedish Relationship, 1910s–1960s" (PhD diss., University of Illinois, Urbana-Champaign, 2021), 77.

5   Eric Schaefer, *"Bold! Daring! Shocking! True!" A History of Exploitation Films, 1919–1959* (Durham, NC: Duke University Press, 1999), 165–216.

6   Benjamin Strassfeld, "A Difficult Delivery: Debating the Function of the Screen and Educational Cinema through *The Birth of a Baby* (1938)," *Velvet Light Trap*, no. 72 (Fall 2013): 44–57.

dependent on how censors, film companies, and other historical actors envisioned their audiences and tried to shape them. This happened both at the textual level, through the films' address and construction of an implied audience, and in the ways in which the films' contexts of display were managed to produce certain ways of viewing.[7] Consequently, when discussing depictions of pregnancy in "public," it is important to consider what is meant by this term. It concerns the kind of public space in which the representations were made accessible, as well as how historical actors viewed and consequently constructed the people with potential access to these spaces. The films' audiences might be understood, for example, as passive consumers to attract, masses that must be controlled, or members of an ideal public who could be educated and expected to use what they learned to act as citizens.[8]

Using these points as an analytical frame, I aim to contribute to existing scholarship on the transnational circulation of sex education films and discussions of the public fetus by exploring the release of the American sex hygiene film *Mom and Dad* (William Beaudine, 1944) in Sweden.[9] This film included a film-within-the-film with animations of fetal development and explicit footage of childbirth—both a vaginal birth and a birth through Cesarean section. Clearly a "classical exploitation film," and the most successful of its kind in the United States, *Mom and Dad* presents an interesting example of such representations in a "low" form of culture.[10] Moreover, when imported to Sweden in 1949, the film was reedited and censored in such a way that it could be shown in regular cinemas. The display of pregnancy and childbirth in public, its effects on audiences, and the role of cinema were conceived differently in these contexts, and its history in the United States and Sweden makes for an interesting comparison.

---

7   Annette Kuhn, *Cinema, Censorship and Sexuality, 1909–1925* (London: Routledge, 1988), 1–8, 28–48, 126–34; Schaefer, *"Bold! Daring! Shocking! True!,"* 73–75; Laukötter, "Listen and Watch"; Elisabet Björklund, "The Most Delicate Subject: A History of Sex Education Films in Sweden" (PhD diss., Lund University, 2012).

8   For clarifying discussions of the terms "audiences" and "publics," see Sonia Livingstone, "On the Relation between Audiences and Publics," in *Audiences and Publics: When Cultural Engagement Matters for the Public Sphere*, ed. Sonia Livingstone (Bristol: Intellect, 2005), 17–41; Richard Butsch, *The Citizen Audience: Crowds, Publics, and Individuals* (New York: Routledge, 2008); and Richard Butsch, "Audiences and Publics, Media and the Public Sphere," in *The Handbook of Media Audiences*, ed. Virginia Nightingale (Malden: Wiley-Blackwell, 2011), 149–68.

9   William Beaudine, dir., *Mom and Dad* (Wilmington, OH: Hygienic Productions/Hallmark, 1944).

10   Schaefer, *"Bold! Daring! Shocking! True!,"* 197–98.

In Sweden, the United States has long been understood paradoxically as both an inspiration and a threat. On the one hand, Swedish intellectual and cultural life has been deeply influenced by developments in the United States. For instance, in the area of sexuality, Alfred C. Kinsey and his research group were very important for the Swedish debates on these matters in the decades following the end of World War II.[11] On the other hand, a fear of "Americanization" has long been prominent in Swedish public discussion, not least concerning culture and the media, and the United States has also been understood as a conservative contrast to Sweden regarding sexual values.[12] *Mom and Dad* is interesting because of what its release in Sweden reveals about these perceptions but also because it can highlight differing views about sex education and cinema audiences.

Sex education was recommended in Swedish elementary schools from 1942 and was made compulsory in 1955, which was early in international comparison. Even so, sex education films shown in cinemas were a contested genre in Sweden during the larger part of the twentieth century. During the development of the Swedish welfare state from the 1930s onward, the spreading of sexual knowledge became part of a larger aim of creating educated citizens capable of planning their futures and contributing to the "good" society that the Social Democratic government envisioned. However, it was the school that was considered the proper place for this education, and an important argument behind this was that the state needed to counteract information from the commercial market.[13] Even though they

---

11   Lena Lennerhed, *Frihet att njuta: Sexualdebatten i Sverige på 1960-talet* (Stockholm: Norstedts, 1994), 229–30.

12   See, for example, Nikolas Glover and Carl Marklund, "Arabian Nights in the Midnight Sun? Exploring the Temporal Structure of Sexual Geographies," *Historisk tidskrift* 129, no. 3 (2009): 487–510; Klara Arnberg and Carl Marklund, "Illegally Blonde: Swedish Sin and Pornography in U.S. and Swedish Imaginations 1955–1971," in *Swedish Cinema and the Sexual Revolution: Critical Essays*, ed. Elisabet Björklund and Mariah Larsson (Jefferson, NC: McFarland, 2016), 185–200; and Ghanoui, "Translating Sex Culture."

13   See, for example, Lena Lennerhed, "Taking the Middle Way: Sex Education Debates in Sweden in the Early Twentieth Century," in *Shaping Sexual Knowledge: A Cultural History of Sex Education in Twentieth Century Europe*, ed. Lutz D. H. Sauerteig and Roger Davidson (London: Routledge, 2009); Sofia Seifarth, "Från desarmering till utlösning under ansvar: Sex- och samlevnadsundervisning i skolradion 1954–1975," in *Frigörare? Moderna svenska samhällsdrömmar*, ed. Martin Kylhammar and Michael Godhe (Stockholm: Carlssons, 2005), 222–23; Birgitta Sandström, *Den välplanerade sexualiteten: Frihet och kontroll i 1970-talets svenska sexualpolitik* (Stockholm: HLS förlag 2001), 193–94.

were usually allowed to be screened, commercially produced sex education films thus became a problematic phenomenon in need of regulation.[14] This chapter argues that the efforts to adapt *Mom and Dad* to the Swedish market were attempts to shape its potential audience into a group of people capable of receiving its message in an edifying way—an audience perhaps more akin to an enlightened public than to passive cinemagoers seeking entertainment. Consequently, the chapter contributes to the investigation of the public fetus not only by detailing an early example of films showing images of pregnancy, fetuses, and childbirth, but also by highlighting that such films were shown in quite different public spaces, and that their audiences were constructed in different ways in different circumstances. Thus, the impact of public visualizations of pregnancy is not only a matter of distribution; it also depends on how the representations are made public, which, in turn, influences the ways their audiences understand themselves and relate to the images.

The Transnational Character of Sex Education Films in Sweden

Sex education films circulated internationally from an early stage in cinema history. In Sweden, films of this kind were imported from other countries beginning in the 1910s, and by the 1920s, they had become a recurring phenomenon on Swedish cinema screens. Until the end of the 1950s, when school films on the subject gradually started to replace those shown in theaters, the genre was a familiar one.[15] Many of these films were changed in various ways to fit the new market and could hence be understood as transnational, rather than simply foreign films in Sweden. Their trajectories were shaped by various factors.

First, censorship played a significant role. In Sweden, a state film censorship board—the National Board of Film Censors—had been introduced in 1911 and scrutinized all films intended for public screening, which was defined as screening in commercial cinemas. This board frequently cut parts of films that were considered harmful to viewers. In sex education films, scenes showing the effects of venereal disease on the body and scenes of childbirth were often shortened or removed. Between 1929 and 1954, the board could also require that certain films be shown only to gender-segregated audiences, or in connection with a lecture by a person trained in medicine. Earlier, distributors had often promised such measures to avoid a ban, but from 1929 the censorship board had the right to prescribe them.

---

14   For a thorough discussion of this, see Björklund, "Most Delicate Subject."
15   Björklund, "Most Delicate Subject."

The censorship board could thus both cut certain content and restrict the contexts in which films were shown.[16]

Second, while Swedish producers were aware of the limits posed by censorship and took them into account in the filmmaking process, distributors also edited imported films in order to avoid censorship. For example, they could cut films in advance and translate the intertitles in such a way that controversial content would meet Swedish requirements. One example is the American film *Where Are My Children?* (Lois Weber and Phillips Smalley, 1916). This film dealt with the controversial topics of abortion and birth control and was imported to Sweden in 1918. At this point in time, spreading information about birth control was forbidden in Sweden, but the film passed censorship inspection uncut. The version submitted to the Swedish censors had been edited and its intertitles changed in such a way that the message about birth control had been erased—thus making it acceptable.[17]

Third, Swedish sex educators could adapt the films to align better with the Swedish situation regarding, for instance, maternity care. These adjustments might be made through accompanying lectures prescribed by the censorship board. Films could also be dubbed, a Swedish voice-over could be added, and material shot in Sweden could be integrated into films. Through these methods, many foreign sex education films circulating in Sweden were reworked, translated, adapted, and reframed in efforts to control their controversial content, make them economically viable, and reach specific educational goals.

But the transnational character of sex education films was not confined to foreign films adapted to the Swedish market. Material from foreign films was also incorporated into Swedish productions. In *Möte med livet* (Encounter with life, Gösta Werner, 1952), three short films-within-the-film are shown, one about venereal disease, one about contraceptives, and one about human reproduction, which lets the viewer follow the course of fertilization, fetal development, and childbirth through animated, and some photographic, pictures. In the credits, the material is attributed to the Carnegie Institute in Washington, DC, the University of California, the United States Department of Public Health, the California State Departments of Public Health and Social Welfare, and the Ortho Pharmaceutical Corporation. Two of these scenes were also shown in the American exploitation film *Because of Eve* (Howard Bretherton, 1948), which indicates that they circulated widely. Another example is the film *Kvinnor i väntrum* (Women in waiting rooms, Gösta Folke, 1946). In an issue of the popular picture magazine *Se* (See) before the film's release, it was reported that a short film about the process of

16   Björklund, "Most Delicate Subject," 62–78.
17   Björklund, "Most Delicate Subject," 65.

fertilization, described with words such as "remarkable" and "sensational," was to be included in the feature. The film comprised material from Russian and American scientific short films, compiled by the Swedish medical doctor Sam Clason. A number of drawn and microscopic images from the film were published in the magazine, displaying, among other things, cell division, but the film-within-the-film does not seem to have been part of the version that eventually premiered.[18]

American Exploitation Cinema and *Mom and Dad*

While the term "exploitation" is often used to describe many types of low-budget "bad" films in general, American "classical exploitation film" was a genre that existed parallel to the classical Hollywood cinema and found a market by offering content that the major film studios did not allow. From the late 1910s to the late 1950s, hundreds of films on topics such as sexuality, nudity, or drugs circulated in cinemas outside the mainstream, often reaching quite substantial audiences.[19] Film scholar Eric Schaefer has demonstrated that so-called sex hygiene films played an important role in the development of this type of film. Films on sexual hygiene had appeared in the United States in the period around World War I but were suppressed by mainstream Hollywood after the war, when the studios sought to create respectability for the industry and stabilize the conventions of their product—feature-length narrative cinema.[20] This marginalization was solidified in the 1930s, when the Production Code was written. In an attempt to differentiate their films from exploitation films—which often used an educational framework as excuse to show sensational material—the mainstream industry defined the purpose of cinema as "wholesome entertainment" and not education.[21] Consequently, Hollywood cinema did not construct its audience as a public but rather as consumers of entertainment.[22]

Schaefer has carefully characterized the exploitation film's mode of production and style. Exploitation films were often made on very low budgets and dealt with topics that were forbidden according to the code. They often included a "square-up," a written statement at the beginning of the film that explained the motivation for addressing the topic. The most important stylistic element of these films was the forbidden spectacle, which in the sex

---

18   "Befruktningens mysterier," *Se*, no. 5 (1946): 6–7.
19   Schaefer, *"Bold! Daring! Shocking! True!"*
20   Schaefer, *"Bold! Daring! Shocking! True!,"* 17–41.
21   Schaefer, *"Bold! Daring! Shocking! True!,"* 154–55.
22   Butsch, "Audiences and Publics," 157.

BEFRUKTNINGENS

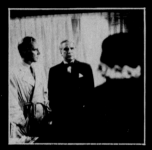

Agneta Lagerfelt spelar en ung, ogift kvinna, som blivit havande och hennes fader vill inte att hon skall föda barnet. Har ej något att invända mot ett ingrepp i fosterfördrivande syfte, läkaren, Arnold Sjöstrand, blir rasande.

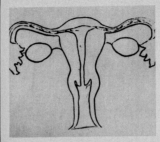

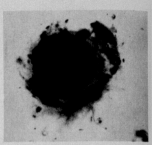

1 Befruktningen av en kvinna sker genom att de manliga spermatozoerna, sädescellerna, sammansmälter med den kvinnliga könscellen, ägget. Bilden ovan, liksom samtliga bilder i detta reportage, har hämtats dels ur en rysk medicinsk film, dels ur en amerikansk, vilka sammanställts av med. dr docenten Sam Clason. Den visar hur de manliga sädescellerna trängt upp genom sidan och livmodern och nu skall ut till äggstocken där befruktningen sker.

2 Här ses genom mikroskopisk filmupptagning det befruktade ägget omgivet av manliga sädesceller. Ägget hos en kvinna är i genomskärning ungefär 2 tiondels millimeter. Genom äggledaren hos kvinnan flyttas det befruktade ägget ned i livmoderns håldighet, där det fastnar i slemhinnan, biter sig fast och utvecklas genom den näring det håmlai av slemhinnan. På dotta sått uppstår alt normalt havandeskap, medicinskt uttryckt intrauterint havandeskap.

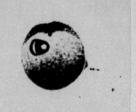

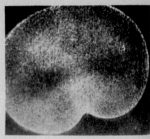

Han känner flickans fader och kallar honom upp på mottagningen, där fadern (Rudolf Wendblad) i sin dotters närvaro blir »nedklubbad» av läkaren. Han fragar bl. a. om inte han, undervisningsrådet, har några som helst moraliska begrepp.

5 Detta är befruktningsögonblicket. Sädescellen tränger in i ägget varvid på detta uppstår en mindre utbuktning. Denna spränges när spermatozoen får kontakt med äggets hinna och sädescellen tränger in i ägget — befruktningen har ägt rum.

6 Det befruktade ägget tillväxer utomordentligt hastigt och den s. k. celldelningen inträffar mycket raskt. Principen för celldelningen hos ett sjöborrägg och ägget hos en befruktad kvinna är densamma. Ovan börjar ägget ändra form.

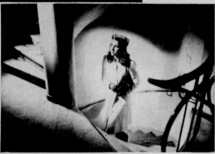

Läkaren berättar några fall ur sin praktik och visar dessutom en medicinsk film av befruktningsprocessen. Ett av »fallen» handlar om dottern till en kanslisekreterare och hennes havandeskap. Britta Holmberg spelar dottern.

En av de märkligaste kortfilmer som någonsin sammanställts presenteras snart inför svensk publik. Den handlar om befruktningsprocessen — vad som verkligen händer när en kvinna blir havande. Filmen har upptagits av dels ryska, dels amerikanska vetenskapsmän och sedan sammanställts till några minuters kortfilm av docent Sam Clason och visningen blir i samband med att Sandrew-Baumanfilms spelfilm »Kvinnor i väntrum» får sin premiär.

Den medicinska filmen ingår nämligen i stora filmen och visas där för ett undervisningsråd som inte har något emot, att hans havande ogifta dotter tänker uppsöka en abortör. Filmens gynekolog — Arnold Sjöstrand spelar den rollen — vädjar emellertid till de inblandade och som ett argument använder han just den av docent Clason iordningställda kortfilmen, som utarbetats ur ryska och amerikanska vetenskapliga smalfilmer vilka upptagits genom mikrofotografering.

Hur en kvinna blir gravid och så småningom nedkommer med barn är känt, men befruktningsprocessens fortskridande sett ur medicinsk synpunkt är en hemlighet för en större allmänhet. Genom den korta filmen i spelfilmen tänker man, som ett led i den medicinska upplysningen i samband med havandeskap, ge allmänheten en inblick i vad som verkligen sker när spermatozoerna befruktar ägget hos kvinnan.

MYSTERIER

Ett SE-reportage auktoriserat av docent SAM CLASON

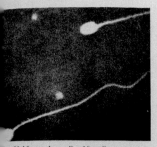
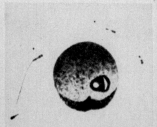
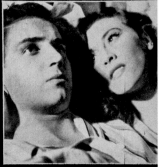

3 Så här ser de manliga könscellerna, spermato-zoerna, ut. Givetvis är de inte så stora i verk-ligheten, men genom mikroskopet kan man tränga ⋅en in på livet och få en klar uppfattning om de-⋅as utseende. Spermatozoerns huvud, som ses till ⋅änster, dirigerar färden, ⋅svansen⋅ håller sig ⋅ingrande i bakgrunden. Den manliga sädescellen ⋅ar en ungefärlig längd av 1 tjugondels millimeter.

4 Här är en tecknad framställning av ägget om-givet av spermatozoer, alltså en motsvarighet till bild nr 2. I den medicinska film, som ingår i Sandrew-Baumans märkliga spelfilm om ungdom och de problem den ställs inför vid ett havande-skap, kan man se hur ⋅listigt⋅ sperman närmar sig ägget — ungefär som kattens lek med råttan.

Här har kanslisekreteraredottern efter ett äkten-skapligt misslyckande med en annan uppsökt sin ungdomskärlek, en ung och fattig medicinare (Carl-Henrik Fant) och resultatet av deras förbindelse blir att hon väntar ett barn. De kan ej gifta sig.

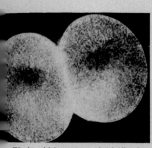
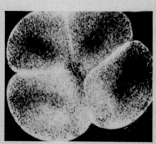
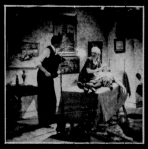

Här har delningsprocessen fortskridit och av det ursprungliga ägget håller en klyvning på ⋅t ske. Om någon sekund har det söndrats i två ⋅zilda delar. Med varje delning fördubblas antalet. ⋅pp till 64 celler är alla likformade, sedan differen-⋅ras de.

8 Fyra celler har uppkommit och sedan fortsät-ter delningen för att till sist bli flera miljar-der. Efter 64 utvecklar sig cellerna till olika väv-nader och olika organ. Redan inom sex veckor har den ensamma cellen blivit en människa i miniatyr.

Med tanke på sitt sociala anseende vill kanslisek-reteraren inte att dottern skall nedkomma med na-got barn och så småningom drivs den unga flickan till en abortör (Georg Skarstedt), som just skall göra ingreppet när polisen spränger hans lya.

⋅Ur denna medicinska film har SE beretts tillfälle att publicera några bilder, ⋅ka återfinnas i mitten på detta uppslag. Bildvalet har utförts av docent ⋅m Clason, vilken dessutom tillmötesgått redaktionens begäran att granska ⋅portaget. Det torde vara första gången ett så unikt bildmaterial från be-⋅uktningsprocessen och celldelningen publicerats.

⋅Huvudfilmen — ⋅Kvinnor i väntrum⋅ är dess arbetsnamn — har regisserats ⋅Gösta Folke och berättar tre episoder ur en kvinnoläkares praktik och de ⋅slag och böner om abort, som han då och då får i mer eller mindre för-⋅ckta ordalag. Det är emellertid långt ifrån någon tråkig propagandafilm, ⋅an en vanlig spelfilm i vilken bl. a. Arnold Sjöstrand, Britta Holmberg, ⋅neta Lagerfeldt, Rudolf Wendblad och Gösta Cederlund medverkar. Sam-⋅igt som den bjuder god underhållning är den ett led i propagandan mot ⋅orter. Också i huvudfilmen har docent Clason medverkat; han står som ⋅dicinsk rådgivare varför man tryggt kan säga att de medicinska detaljerna ⋅riktiga.

⋅å detta uppslag presenterar SE utom de märkliga medicinska bilderna ⋅så några bilder ur huvudfilmen, som beräknas få sin premiär i medio på ⋅ruari. Och då får således även den sensationella kortfilmen sin premiär.

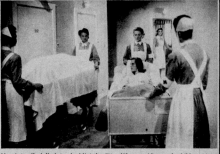

Men inte alla fall slutar lyckligt, berättar läkaren vidare, och skildrar ytter-ligare några fall från sin praktik. Så småningom får han undervisningsrä-det och dottern att överge aborttanken. ⋅Kvinnor i väntrum⋅ heter filmen.

Figure 5.1. The report in the picture magazine *Se*, showing the images of fertilization and cell division that were to be included in *Kvinnor i väntrum* (Women in waiting rooms). Source: "Befruktningens mysterier," *Se*, no. 5 (1946): 6–7.

hygiene films often meant explicit scenes with images taken from medical films showing the effects of venereal disease on the body or childbirth.[23] Narratively, sex hygiene exploitation films often included a gallery of stereotyped characters, whose function was to convey the films' educational message, rather than offer opportunities for identification.[24] While the films can be considered subversive in their challenging of the norms of acceptable cinema and "good taste," their messages were generally very conservative and moralistic.[25]

Mom and Dad was a typical sex hygiene exploitation film in many ways. It tells the story of Joan Blake (played by June Carlson), a teenage girl who gets pregnant by a young man she meets at a dance, Jack Griffin (Bob Lowell), who later dies in a plane crash. The film warns against the pitfalls of poor education about sexual matters, as Joan has received no such education from her parents. Her mother is portrayed as a prudish woman engaged in a local women's club who also helps convince the school to fire a teacher, Mr. Blackburn, for giving lessons on sexual hygiene. When the consequences of Joan's inadequate education have become clear, however, the teacher is reemployed and informs the pupils about sex through two educational films: one about pregnancy and childbirth and one about venereal disease, material that originated from the US Public Health Service. At the end of the film, Joan gives birth to a stillborn child.

Exploitation films were also shown in ways that differed from how mainstream films were presented. Screenings were often segregated by gender and allowed adults only. Moreover, the shows combined the films themselves with lobby displays—which in the case of sex hygiene films could include medical models of the birth process or venereal disease—fake nurses selling books, and extra-filmic events, such as lectures. In the case of *Mom and Dad*, a fictional expert called Elliot Forbes, who was played by different people, interrupted the film with a lecture on sexual hygiene.[26] All this made the audience's experience of an exploitation film very different from that of a mainstream Hollywood film. "The exploitation audience became part of the show, in a limited way, by asking questions and interacting with lecturers, buying books from the 'nurses,' and building on their experience through their engagement with lobby displays," Schaefer writes.[27] In smaller

23 Schaefer, *"Bold! Daring! Shocking! True!,"* 42–95.
24 Schaefer, *"Bold! Daring! Shocking! True!,"* 30–32. See also Kuhn's discussion of audience address in venereal disease propaganda films in *Cinema, Censorship and Sexuality*, 51–56.
25 Schaefer, *"Bold! Daring! Shocking! True!,"* 134–35, 216.
26 Schaefer, *"Bold! Daring! Shocking! True!,"* 119–35.
27 Schaefer, *"Bold! Daring! Shocking! True!,"* 131.

towns, screenings could be conceived as events similar to those of traveling carnivals, circuses, or county fairs.[28] Schaefer describes *Mom and Dad* as "the pinnacle of these exhibition ploys," as it employed all these techniques. In fact, the producer, Kroger Babb, mandated a very specific exhibition program for the film and furthermore used an elaborate promotion strategy as the film traveled from town to town.[29]

The film and its mode of display thus clearly differed from the "wholesome entertainment" of mainstream Hollywood cinema, and its audiences became more active participants in its reception. At the same time, the film's low quality and carnivalesque setting also made it very different from those aimed at more traditional educational contexts, such as school films. Many exploitation films were very profitable, but *Mom and Dad* stands out for its enormous success. Exact audience numbers do not exist, but Schaefer calls it "the most successful sex hygiene film in history," and refers to estimates indicating that it had been seen by twenty million moviegoers by the end of the 1940s and grossed ten times more worldwide by the late 1950s.[30] It also reached large segments of the population, attracting a young middle-class audience that had not previously attended similar films.[31] Like other films of the kind, it also appealed to both men and women. Although later types of "sexploitation" and pornography reached mostly men, classical exploitation films were generally seen by both men and women, and some evidence even suggests that the majority of the audience for sex hygiene films were women.[32] *Mom and Dad* also reached African American audiences, through a "colored unit" that toured the country with Olympic star Jesse Owens as lecturer.[33] The great success of the film attracted the attention of public health authorities. Officials from the US Public Health Service were concerned about the information provided by the film and its use of their material; they responded by expanding their own educational program on venereal diseases.[34]

---

28 Schaefer, *"Bold! Daring! Shocking! True!,"* 132.

29 Schaefer, *"Bold! Daring! Shocking! True!,"* 132–33. See also Suzanne White, "'Mom and Dad' (1944): Venereal Disease 'Exploitation,'" *Bulletin of the History of Medicine* 62, no. 2 (Summer 1988): 252–70, 255.

30 Schaefer, *"Bold! Daring! Shocking! True!,"* 197–98, quotation on 197. For figures about other exploitation films, see 119–21.

31 Schaefer, *"Bold! Daring! Shocking! True!,"* 133; White, "'Mom and Dad,'" 252, 264.

32 Schaefer, *"Bold! Daring! Shocking! True!,"* 124.

33 Schaefer, *"Bold! Daring! Shocking! True!,"* 133; Ghanoui, "Translating Sex Culture," 126–27.

34 White, "'Mom and Dad,'" 267–69.

Mom and Dad and Swedish Film Censorship

Mom and Dad arrived in Sweden in January 1949, imported by the minor film company Svea Film. At the end of the 1940s, the sex education film was well-established in Sweden, and domestically produced feature-length films of this type had also begun to appear in the repertoire. Narratively and stylistically, many of these films were similar to American exploitation films. For instance, stereotyped characters can be noted in the Swedish films, and they sometimes included spectacle in the form of footage of venereal disease and childbirth. However, they were produced by established, sometimes even major, film companies, had higher production values, and often starred well-known Swedish actors. Moreover, they were produced in collaboration with established medical experts.[35]

Meanwhile, films from the United States and other countries continued to be imported to Sweden. Those from the United States were mostly of the exploitation genre. However, Sweden's particular censorship system meant that its cinema culture was less divided into a mainstream and margin than its American counterpart. Even though their place in the cinema was contested, sex education films could be shown in Sweden as part of the regular cinema repertoire. In fact, in the 1940s and 1950s, many sex education films were shown at theaters belonging to Sweden's three major film companies: Svensk Filmindustri, Sandrews, and Europa Film.[36]

Mom and Dad was first submitted to the National Board of Film Censors in January 1949. In their cover letter, the distributor's representatives noted that they intended for a Swedish medical expert to adapt the medical lectures in the film and record them in Swedish.[37] The film was approved for public screenings for an audience over the age of fifteen, provided that a number of cuts were made. First, the censors cut the scenes of Cesarean section in the part about childbirth. Second, a number of scenes showing sores caused by syphilis and children affected by syphilis were cut from the part about venereal disease. The censors had also noted that a full Swedish text list was needed; that more cuts could be made as the final version of the film was scrutinized; that it should be noted in the opening titles that the

35 Björklund, "Most Delicate Subject," 102–11.

36 For a detailed discussion of the relationship between sex education films in Sweden and American exploitation films, see Björklund, "Most Delicate Subject," 80–93.

37 Tore Metzer at AB Svea Film to the National Board of Film Censors, January 11, 1949, series E2, vol. 595, registration number 63/49, archive of Statens biografbyrå (the National Board of Film Censors, hereafter SB), Riksarkivet (National Archives of Sweden, hereafter RA).

film was educational; and that the medical parts should be adapted to the Swedish context.[38]

Perhaps as a response to these many demands, a new version of the film was submitted in March the same year. The distributor noted that the medical doctor Malcolm Tottie would write the Swedish lectures for the film and that he had also edited the part with the Cesarean section. The Swedish title of the film would be *Din kropp är din* (Your body is yours).[39] This time, the censorship decision was a bit more specific. It stated that the film was approved for ages fifteen and up, after a number of cuts were made. The depiction of the Cesarean section showed the incision in the abdomen then omitted everything up to the moment when the opening was sewn back together (basically the entire operation). In the parts about syphilis, the images of male and female genitalia with syphilis, children with syphilis, and male and female nude bodies were cut. It was also stated that the Swedish medical reworking should be sent to the board and that (as previously) it should be made clear in the opening titles that the film contained sex education.[40]

Censors thus demanded that the film be clearly labeled as a sex education film and that the medical parts be adapted to the Swedish context. Moreover, cuts were made in the films-within-the-film. These decisions were not unique to *Mom and Dad*. The censorship card for the Swedish film *Möte med livet* similarly stated that the board presupposed that the opening credits and marketing would clearly indicate that the topic was sex education.[41] Scenes in other films showing Cesarean sections were also cut, for example in the American film *Street Corner* (Albert H. Kelly, 1948), also imported in 1949, and a short film called *The Story of Birth*—which also included a breech delivery. The latter film was first completely banned but later released in a heavily edited version.[42] Films that showed only vaginal births were, however, not cut. The Danish film *Vi vil ha' et barn* (*We Want a Child!*, Lau Lauritzen Jr. and Alice O'Frederiks, 1949), for instance, which received a great deal of attention in the press because of its birth scene, was not cut at all by the censorship board, and neither was *Möte med livet*, mentioned

---

38   Censorship card 74.759, series D1A, vol. 52, SB, RA.

39   Tore Metzer at AB Svea Film to the National Board of Film Censors, March 17 and March 21, 1949, series E2, vol. 599, registration number 724/49, SB, RA.

40   Censorship card 75.065, series D1A, vol. 52, SB, RA.

41   Censorship card 78.438, series D1A, vol. 55, SB, RA.

42   Censorship cards 75.128 (*Street Corner*), 75.719 (*The Story of Birth*), series D1A, vol. 52, and 76.082 (reexamination of *The Story of Birth*), series D1A, vol. 53, SB, RA.

earlier, premiering in 1952.[43] In 1950, Gunnar Klackenberg, the deputy head of the National Board of Film Censors, wrote an article in a journal of psychology and sex education about how the board handled sex education films. Here, he explained the board's reasoning regarding the scenes of childbirth in *The Story of Birth* and *Mom and Dad*:

> A depiction of a naturally occurring delivery has been considered to have a significant value for the general education without at the same time being frightening. We have been more skeptical toward forceps deliveries and Cesarean sections. . . . A depiction of pathological deliveries can of course, like all medical education, serve a good cause, but out of consideration of all women, who are worried enough anyway about the unknown the first time, and all sensitive individuals, for whom medical operations are a shocking experience, these sequences were forbidden.[44]

The decisions taken were thus made out of consideration for women experiencing their first pregnancy and persons who might be shocked by scenes of a surgery. One can argue that this adds new meaning to the norms of mental hygiene governing the censorship board at this time, where films or parts of films considered to be "brutalizing," "exciting," or "confusing the concepts of justice" were to be banned.[45] One reason for the ban could be that the censors surmised that a fear of childbirth could lead women to seek illegal abortions, but Klackenberg's motivation also speaks of a view of censorship concerned with public health issues. Scenes that could frighten a specific group about an experience awaiting them were hence understood as a danger to society.

Reworking the Film for a Swedish Public

Changes to *Mom and Dad* were not made solely in response to demands from the National Board of Film Censors, however. In fact, Malcolm Tottie had been quite engaged in adapting the film to the Swedish context. Tottie, a medical doctor working in Stockholm, specialized in venereology and was

---

43   Censorship cards 75. 808 (*Vi vil ha' et barn*), series D1A, vol. 52, and 78.438 (*Möte med livet*), series D1A, vol. 55, SB, RA. For a discussion of *We Want a Child!* in Sweden, see Björklund, "Most Delicate Subject," 87–89.

44   Gunnar Klackenberg, "Filmcensuren och sexualupplysningen," *Populär tidskrift för psykologi och sexualkunskap* 1, no. 4 (1950): 6.

45   See, for example, Elisabet Björklund, "The Limits of Sexual Depictions in the Late 1960s," in *Swedish Cinema and the Sexual Revolution: Critical Essays*, ed. Elisabet Björklund and Mariah Larsson (Jefferson, NC: McFarland, 2016), 127–28, 131.

a fairly well-known public authority on venereal diseases during these years. Since 1944, he had been the reporting doctor for these issues at the National Board of Medicine, and much engaged in various public health initiatives, not least through his involvement in film production.[46] In the 1940s and 1950s he wrote film scripts, was an adviser for film productions, edited imported films, and acted in films through voice-over or by playing himself.[47] The Swedish lecture that he wrote for the medical parts of *Mom and Dad* was quite different from the original American voice-over. Moreover, new footage was added showing, among other things, scenes from Swedish maternity wards and children's health-care centers.[48] The sequence begins with a statement about women's right to knowledge in the service of mankind:

> Every woman has the right to know how her body works. It is important in order to determine that the complicated human machinery functions properly. There is a rhythm in every woman's life. She matures from girl to woman. By this she becomes biologically fully mature to fulfil her duty for the reproduction of the human race.

This commentary is followed by a section about the menstrual cycle, fertilization, and the development of the fetus illustrated with animated pictures and some microscopic footage of sperm and cell division. The animations depict fertilization of the egg within the fallopian tube, embryonic development within the uterus in cross-section among other organs in the body, and lastly a series of pictures showing the growth of the fetus over a number of weeks through a cross-section of a woman's abdomen, to display the physical changes of pregnancy along with the growth of the fetus.

Tottie proceeds to explain that a woman needs preventive health care during pregnancy and informs the viewer that this can be obtained for free at

---

46   A. Widstrand, ed., *Svenska läkare i ord och bild* (Stockholm: AB Biografiskt Galleri, 1948), 706; Stina Holmberg, ed., *Svenska läkare* (Stockholm: Norstedt, 1959), 776.

47   For example, *Kärlekslivets offer* (Love's victims, Gabriel Alw and Emil A. Lingheim, 1944), *Schleichendes Gift* (Slow poison, Hermann Wallbrück, 1946), *Möte med livet, Rätten att älska* (The right to love, Mimi Pollak, 1956), *Flamman* (*Girls without rooms*, Arne Ragneborn, 1956), and *Eva und der Frauenarzt* (Eva and the gynecologist, Erich Kobler, 1951).

48   My description of the Swedish reworking of the film is based on a German-language version of the Swedish version available in a digitized version at the National Library of Sweden (the analog film is preserved in the archive of the Swedish Film Institute). Thanks to David Pierce for granting permission to digitize the film. The manuscript of Malcolm Tottie's voice-over can be found at the archive of the National Board of Film Censors, series E2, vol. 599, registration number 724/49, SB, RA. My comparison with the American version of the film is based on the Blu-ray distributed by Kino Lorber (2020).

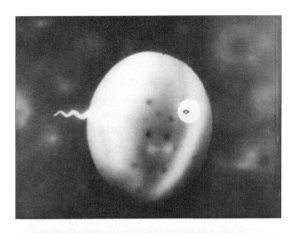

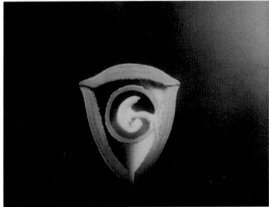

Figures 5.2 to 5.4.
Screenshots from *Mom
and Dad* (Hygienic
Productions/Hallmark,
1944), showing fertilization,
embryonic development,
and fetal growth. Source:
National Library of Sweden.

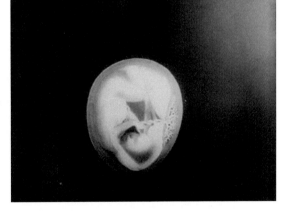

the country's many maternal health-care units. "Don't neglect to make use of society's support agencies!" he says. This exhortation is followed by a section on the advantages of giving birth at a maternity ward in a hospital. Next comes the scene with the vaginal birth, filmed with the camera directed toward the vaginal opening between the spread legs of the anesthetized birthing woman, whose body is completely covered with white cloth.

Following this, a sequence has been added explaining how the newborn baby is taken care of at the hospital—the umbilical cord is cut, and the baby is bathed, clothed, and put to bed. The camera then shows a row of newborn babies in their cribs; Tottie describes them as being both perfect and unique: "Every newborn child has its own type. It can be seen in this . . . parade of small newborn A-children. You cannot say that they look alike. It is possible to see the differences." Clearly part of a eugenic discourse, the term "A-children" was an expression originating in the 1930s, when "A-people"— referring to what was understood as the most healthy and vital group of people in society (in contrast to "B-" and "C-people")—became a concept in various Danish and Swedish advertising campaigns for milk products.[49] This health discourse is developed in the following sections of the film: advice is given that children should be breastfed, while a number of breastfeeding women are displayed. Lastly, scenes from a children's health-care unit are shown; while a doctor examines a small child, Tottie describes the importance of monitoring the children at these units. The section concludes with the words: "Healthy children are the most valuable asset to a nation. Suitable monitoring of and care for the smallest children are one of the ways to take proper care of this fortune."

The part of the film dealing with venereal diseases was also supplemented with Swedish material. Here, a number of images of Swedish informational brochures and some city scenes were added, as well as some depictions of people with venereal diseases. A connection to the health of families can be noted as well. For instance, in the middle part of the section, it is stated that "the venereal diseases can cast a shadow over the home and the family, a shadow that can seriously darken a formerly bright domestic life." The main preventive advice offered by the speaker is a warning against casual encounters and encouragement to seek medical care. Condoms are only hinted at vaguely at the end. The voice-over also explains how a doctor diagnoses the patient and describes the different stages of syphilis to accompanying pictures. These pictures show sores on the body, including some images of the sex organs, but very few compared to the American original. Lastly, it is

---

49   Ylva Habel, *Modern Media, Modern Audiences: Mass Media and Social Engineering in the 1930s Swedish Welfare State* (Stockholm: Aura förlag, 2002), 59–85.

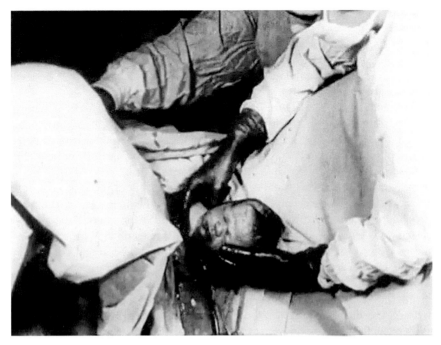

Figure 5.5. Screenshot from *Mom and Dad* (Hygienic Productions/Hallmark, 1944), showing childbirth. Source: National Library of Sweden.

noted that a pregnant woman might transmit the disease to the fetus. The sequence ends with the following statement:

> The venereal diseases are not only prevented by knowledge about their existence and by techniques of prophylaxis. The most important prophylaxis is the individual's way of life. Our living conditions demand that we take responsibility for our lives, our fellow human beings, and the future generation.

The last sentence connects the discussion of venereal diseases with the content about childbirth—and thus reproduction. Thereby, syphilis is constructed as a threat to the health of future generations, in addition to the individual suffering that the disease can lead to. This association also connects the medical parts of the film to the frame narrative of Joan's pregnancy. A possible interpretation of the film's ending is that Joan's child died because of syphilis.[50] But while the Swedish censors cut the images of children with

---

50   See White, "'Mom and Dad,'" 260.

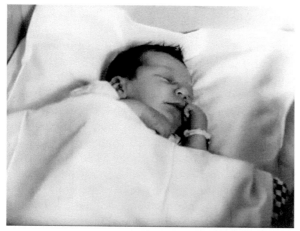

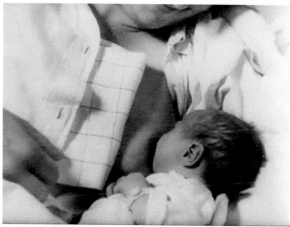

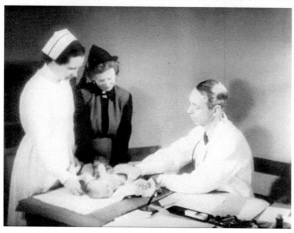

Screenshots from the Swedish version (1949) of *Mom and Dad* (Hygienic Productions/Hallmark, 1944), showing scenes from a Swedish hospital and childcare center. Figure 5.6 (*top*): One of the "A-children." Figure 5.7 (*middle*): A woman breastfeeding her child. Figure 5.8 (*bottom*): A doctor examining a child at a children's health-care unit. Source: National Library of Sweden.

syphilis from the film, stressing children's health in the medical discussion of venereal disease could also support such a view.

The Swedish version thus differs from the American original in its overall stronger focus on the health of children and on informing the viewer about the support that families could receive from society. By eliminating scenes understood to display "pathological" deliveries and the most severe cases of syphilis, censors aimed at diminishing fears of sex and childbirth. Moreover, by adding footage shot in Sweden and a newly written voice-over commentary, the focus of the medical parts of the film shifted from warnings of the consequences of sex to a more positive message about Swedish maternity and childcare and its goal of improved health for children. The new material also communicates eugenic ideas through the use of expressions such as "A-children." The Swedish version of the film thus supported the agenda of educating the audience about their responsibilities as individuals to accept the help offered by society in order to sustain a healthy nation. In this way, the audience of the film was addressed as a public that could be educated into making informed decisions about their sexual and reproductive health.

American Fiction and Swedish Education

When *Mom and Dad* was finally finished and approved for public screenings, the distributor also made decisions that influenced how it came to be discussed. The film was shown at gender-segregated screenings, which received a lot of attention in the press. This practice was common for American sex hygiene films but by 1949 was outdated in Sweden. The National Board of Film Censors still had the power to prescribe gender segregation for certain films but did not do so in the case of *Mom and Dad*. Instead, the decision was taken by the distributor, Svea Film. As I have argued elsewhere, gender segregation in Sweden went from a condition that film owners had to accept in order to get the approval of the censorship authority to a method of self-regulation that film companies sometimes used, perhaps to gain publicity, to meet perceived demands from audiences or because it had become an expected part of the genre.[51] When *Mom and Dad* premiered, this segregation of the audience was, however, not received well. Rather, critics argued that it counteracted the film's purpose of breaking taboos around sexuality.[52] This way of releasing the film thus did not jibe with the efforts to manage its audience into a public, but rather signaled to critics that the

---

51   Björklund, "Most Delicate Subject," 65–78.

52   Berton [Bert Onne], "Aveny," *Afton-Tidningen*, April 5, 1949; A. B. [Allan Beer], "Aveny och Folkan: 'Din kropp är din,'" *Arbetaren*, April 5, 1949.

distributors wanted the film to reach a large audience by hinting that it had sensational content.

Another conspicuous dimension of the discourse around the film when it premiered was the contrast created between its American origin and its Swedish context of reception. The marketing of the film itself highlighted these contrasts. Advertisements announced it as "an American film about the problems of love life," and also mentioned that Malcolm Tottie had edited the Swedish version.[53] A longer advertisement was also printed in many newspapers, in which the film's relevance was connected to the recently published Kinsey report.[54] As Saniya Lee Ghanoui has noted, while such advertisements sensationalized the film through alluring word choices and images, the connection with Kinsey and Tottie's involvement functioned as "backing" for its educational merit.[55] Still, the association with Kinsey did not mean that reviewers connected the film with groundbreaking American sex research. Rather, many highlighted the contrast between what they understood as American backwardness and Swedish progressiveness. *Afton-Tidningen* had sent one female and one male critic to review *Mom and Dad* at different screenings. Both disliked the film. The critic with the byline "Same" wrote:

> What mission a film like "Your body is yours" [*Mom and Dad*] fulfils in our country is hard to see—the USA has in any case publicized itself very badly by exporting it. If prudery, hypocrisy, naivety, and ignorance about the sexual life really occur to that extent in the average American city, then the situation is bad indeed in the "country of progress." In Sweden, where among others the National Agency for Education organizes teaching in sexual hygiene, there are luckily no parallels.[56]

And "Berton" (Bert Onne) wrote: "The film is written for an American audience which ought to be around fifty years behind us in sexual knowledge."[57] Not all reviews were this negative. Some were even positive, finding *Mom and Dad* to be a serious educational film without

---

53 See, for example, advertisements for *Mom and Dad* in *Göteborgs-Posten*, April 2, 1949; *Sydsvenska Dagbladet*, April 4, 1949; and *Afton-Tidningen*, April 4, 1949.

54 See, for example, "Din kropp är din," advertisements for *Mom and Dad* in *Aftonbladet*, April 2, 1949; and *Expressen*, April 2, 1949.

55 Ghanoui, "Translating Sex Culture," 129.

56 Same [*pseud.*], "Folkan," *Afton-Tidningen*, April 5, 1949.

57 Berton [Bert Onne], "Aveny." See also – ng [*pseud.*], "Aveny och Göta: Din kropp är din," *Arbetaretidningen*, April 5, 1949; and Frans B. Liljenroth, "Din kropp är din," *Expressen*, April 5, 1949.

sensational content.[58] However, many reviewers regarded the Swedish parts by Malcolm Tottie as the most praiseworthy. For instance, in *Dagens Nyheter*, the reviewer "J–e" characterized the film as "an American educational film in sexual matters with its greatest value in the parts where our Swedish expert, doctor Malcolm Tottie, objectively and credibly comments on the pictures."[59] Nevertheless, the film seems to have had a wide reception in Sweden. Advertisements and reviews can be found not only in the largest Swedish newspapers based in Stockholm, but also in a large number of local newspapers based in cities and towns across the country.[60]

In 1954, the film was actually imported again, this time by the company Stockholm Film, in a shortened, German-language version. According to the distributor, it was "exactly the same" as the previously imported film, "with Swedish speech in the medical parts by Dr. Malcolm Tottie."[61] This time, the film was exempted from entertainment tax. After the end of World War II, the Swedish tax on cinema revenues had been significantly raised and was a considerable burden for the film industry, but starting in 1952 films could be exempted from this tax if they were judged to be scientific, educational, or enlightening by the National Board of Film Censors.[62] The fact that *Mom and Dad* received this tax exemption means that the film was deemed educational by the board. Despite meeting with some skeptical reviews when it premiered, the film was not generally dismissed as sensational or exploitative in Sweden; rather, a governmental institution regarded it as having serious educational intentions.

---

58   Ten [*pseud.*], "Göta och Aveny: Din kropp är din," *Göteborgs-Posten*, April 5, 1949; Gunn [*pseud.*], "Folkan o. Avenny: Din kropp är din," *Stockholms-Tidningen*, April 5, 1949.

59   J–e [*pseud.*], "Aveny och Folkan: 'Din kropp är din,'" *Dagens Nyheter*, April 5, 1949. See also Heed [*pseud.*], "Din kropp är din på Folkan – Aveny," *Aftonbladet*, April 5, 1949, and U. S–m [*pseud.*], "Aveny, Folkan: Din kropp är din," *Svenska Dagbladet*, April 5, 1949.

60   This is based on searches made in the Swedish digitized newspaper database at the National Library of Sweden, "Svenska dagstidningar," https://tidningar.kb.se/. This database covers a limited number of Swedish digitized newspapers, which means that the film was probably shown in other places as well.

61   Censorship card 85.185, series D1A, vol. 60, SB, RA; Sture Sjöstedt at AB Stockholm Film to the National Board of Film Censors, October 26, 1954, series E2, vol. 705, registration number 2384/54, SB, RA. Quotation from the letter by Sjöstedt.

62   See Björklund, "Most Delicate Subject," 78–80.

Conclusion

Discussing historical visualizations of pregnancy in public requires detailed attention to the various contexts and media in which these visualizations were displayed to fully grasp the consequences of their being public. The case of *Mom and Dad* in Sweden is illustrative in this regard because it highlights how the transnational circulation of medical imagery of pregnancy and childbirth transformed the meanings produced by these images. While the film was shown in public in both the United States and Sweden, in the sense that it appeared in commercial cinemas, the different institutional, regulatory, and cultural frameworks surrounding these screenings resulted in different versions of the film connected to different ways of understanding and addressing the audience.

It is of course difficult to reconstruct how cinemagoers in the late 1940s reacted to a film like *Mom and Dad*. However, it is reasonable to believe that the film that audiences encountered in the United States was understood quite differently from the edited version that premiered in Sweden in 1949. Despite differences between the various local contexts where the film was shown within the United States, it was arguably more marginalized in relation to the mainstream film culture there than it was in Sweden. This contrast can be explained in many ways, not least through the definition of cinema as a place for entertainment rather than education, established in the United States through the Production Code. This difference is illuminated by the ways in which various actors representing governmental or public health interests responded to the film. While American health officials were concerned about the film and responded by increasing their own educational efforts, the strategy in Sweden was to transform the film into acceptable education aligned with society's goals of producing healthy citizens. The censorship board consequently demanded that the educational framework of the film be made clear, and cut scenes understood to create undesirable psychological effects in the viewer. Furthermore, through the engagement of a real medical expert with an established reputation, the medical content was reframed as offering enlightenment about society's efforts to support families and improve the health of mothers and children. Thus, the Swedish audience seems to have been addressed as a public to a greater extent than its counterpart in the United States, as the new version of the film tied its message closer to the rights and responsibilities of citizens. At the same time, the censorship efforts speak of a paternalistic view of this public as being vulnerable and in need of care and protection.

When the film moved from one national context to another, its content changed in very concrete ways, which both reflected and affected ideas about its audience. At the same time, the gender-segregated screenings—a practice that for many decades had been connected with sensationalism—met with skepticism from many critics. In the reception, a clear line was also drawn between what was perceived as American ignorance—represented by the fictional story in the film—and Swedish modernity, which was represented by the additions by the Swedish medical doctor Malcolm Tottie. This in itself can be said to have constructed the Swedish audience as an educated public, far ahead of people in the United States. The irony of this is that while the strategy of creating a Swedish version of the film made images of pregnant and birthing bodies more available in mainstream cinemas in Sweden, many people who saw the film in more marginal spaces in the United States viewed scenes of birth and disease that were censored for Swedish audiences. One could thus debate whether the audience in Sweden was really viewed as an independently thinking public, or rather as a group of people in need of discipline and guidance from authorities.

Finally, following the circulation of images of pregnancy and childbirth through a film like *Mom and Dad* and paying attention to how the visual material was reused and edited throughout also raises other questions, not least ethical ones. From our contemporary perspective, for example, it is difficult not to wonder to what extent the women who gave birth on camera had given consent to being filmed. Even if they agreed to participate, it was probably difficult for them to anticipate that the footage would circulate far beyond the medical institutions where it was made, showing up in exploitation and sex education films viewed by millions in the United States and faraway countries. Not unlike how Lennart Nilsson's fetal images were appropriated by various political interests decades later, these medical childbirth films were reused and edited in new contexts that gave them new meanings—meanings that the birthing women were probably unaware of.

Chapter Six

The Drama of the Fetoplacental Unit

Reimagining the Public Fetus of Lennart Nilsson

Solveig Jülich

Over the years, many different kinds of images have been discussed in relation to the "public fetus."[1] But one that returns in these conversations is the stunning color picture of a "Living 18-week-old fetus" by Swedish photographer Lennart Nilsson featured on the cover of the American magazine *Life* in April 1965. Enveloped in the white amniotic sac, the fetus was depicted as an astronaut floating gravity-less in a starry sky. The magazine promised to reveal, for the first time, the "Drama of Life before Birth," and Nilsson's photo-essay included close-ups of fertilization as well as embryos and fetuses of various ages.[2] According to Barbara Duden, this publication was a turning

1   The author wishes to thank Anne Fjellström at Lennart Nilsson Photography for her generous help and support in providing material for this study. The work is part of the research program "Medicine at the Borders of Life," funded by the Swedish Research Council (registration number 2014-1749).

2   Lennart Nilsson and Albert Rosenfeld, "Drama of Life before Birth," *Life*, April 30, 1965. available at https://books.google.co.uk/books?id=UVMEA AAAMBAJ&printsec=frontcover&source=gbs_ge_summary_r&cad=0#v=on epage&q&f=false (last accessed May 8, 2023). The photograph on the *Life* cover was also reproduced on the cover of different language editions of the pregnancy advice book *A Child Is Born*, including the 1967 Spanish edition, see figure 7.3 in Santesmases's chapter in this volume. For the first Swedish edition, see Lennart Nilsson, Axel Ingelman-Sundberg, and Claes Wirsén, *Ett barn blir till: En bildskildring av de nio månaderna före födelsen: En praktisk rådgivare för den blivande mamman* (Stockholm: Bonnier, 1965).

point in the proliferation of fetal pictures in popular culture.[3] Other feminist researchers have also demonstrated how the composition of these images facilitated arguments for fetal personhood put forward by American and British antiabortion activists in the 1970s and 1980s. They state that the depiction in *Life* of embryos and fetuses in free-floating solitude helped to justify the view of the fetus as an individual, autonomous from its mother, with its own rights. Indeed, we learn that the pregnant woman has been completely erased from Nilsson's visual universe.[4]

Yet, there is still much that remains to be explored about Nilsson's public fetus. In particular, we are left wondering how he was able to produce the spectacular photographs for "Drama of Life before Birth." The unwillingness of the photographer to share his story as well as the deliberate strategies of Nilsson's publishers and editors to conceal information about the background of the images have created productive theories as well as misunderstandings and ignorance.[5] For instance, the photograph that appeared on the cover of *Life* has mistakenly been described as a picture of a fetus inside the womb, whereas all the others in the photo-essay are claimed to portray dead embryos and fetuses outside the body.[6] The management of the publicity surrounding the photographer can also help explain why he has often

3   Barbara Duden, *Disembodying Women: Perspectives on Pregnancy and the Unborn*, trans. Lee Hoinacki (Cambridge, MA: Harvard University Press, 1993), 14.

4   Sarah Franklin, "Fetal Fascinations: New Dimensions to the Medical-Scientific Construction of Fetal Personhood," in *Off-Centre: Feminism and Cultural Studies*, ed. Sarah Franklin, Celia Lury, and Jackie Stacey (London: HarperCollins Academic, 1991), 190–205; Sandra Matthews and Laura Wexler, *Pregnant Pictures* (New York: Routledge, 2000), 195–98; Carol A. Stabile, "Shooting the Mother: Fetal Photography and the Politics of Disappearance," *Camera Obscura* 10, no. 28 (1992): 179–205. For a discussion of the "maternal erasure" theory, see Rebecca Whiteley, *Birth Figures: Early Modern Prints and the Pregnant Body* (Chicago: University of Chicago Press, 2023), 66–69, 291, and chapter 12 in this volume.

5   Solveig Jülich, "Lennart Nilsson's *A Child Is Born*: The Many Lives of a Pregnancy Advice Book," *Culture Unbound* 7, no. 4 (2015): 627–48.

6   See, for instance, Lauren Berlant, *The Queen of America Goes to Washington City: Essays on Sex and Citizenship* (Durham, NC: Duke University Press, 1997), 105; Donna Haraway, *Modest_Witness@Second_Millennium. FemaleMan©_Meets_OncoMouse: Feminism and Technoscience* (New York: Routledge, 1997), 178; Meredith W. Michaels, "Fetal Galaxies: Some Questions about What We See," in *Fetal Subjects, Feminist Positions*, ed. Lynn M. Morgan and Meredith W. Michaels (Philadelphia: University of Pennsylvania Press, 1999), 113–32.

been thought of as inventor of his own techniques and equipment.[7] In fact, creating this reputation has been part of the founding myth propagated by Nilsson himself and his publishing house.[8]

In previous research, I have shown that Nilsson's early photographs of human development were produced in collaboration with prominent doctors who campaigned against Swedish abortion legislation in the 1950s and 1960s. Publishers and editors in the popular press supported him financially, commissioning fetal pictures that were published as shocking testimony to the effects of abortion. The embryos and fetuses depicted in the images were increasingly aestheticized and their human traits emphasized.[9] Coinciding with the publication of "Drama of Life before Birth" in *Life* and the pregnancy advice book *Ett barn blir till* (*A Child Is Born*) Nilsson's later photoessays started to express a more positive view of women's right to abortion.[10] From the mid-1960s, many of his photographs were used as material for sex education in schools as well as promotion for Sweden's progressive society.[11]

To complicate this story further, the present chapter examines, for the first time, the creation of Nilsson's pictures of human reproduction in the context of 1950s and 1960s Swedish fetal research. Although many doctors and researchers opposed abortion, they were mostly in favor of using aborted fetuses for medical experiments. This attitude was also in line with a state interest in tapping into reproductive research to develop new contraceptives and abortion methods—in order to improve national reproductive health services as well as to address global overpopulation.[12] The endocri-

---

7   See, for example, Sarah Franklin's discussion in Suzanne Anker and Sarah Franklin, "Specimens as Spectacles: Reframing Fetal Remains," *Social Text* 29, no. 1 (2011): 107–8.

8   This approach is developed in my book manuscript, *Photographing Life and Death: Lennart Nilsson, Medicine and the Media in Sweden, ca. 1940–2020.*

9   Solveig Jülich, "Picturing Abortion Opposition: Lennart Nilsson's Early Photographs of Embryos and Fetuses," *Social History of Medicine* 31, no. 2 (2018): 278–307.

10   Nilsson, Ingelman-Sundberg, and Wirsén, *Ett barn blir till.* The first American edition of *A Child Is Born* was published in 1966 by Delacorte Press and the first British edition in 1967 by Allen Lane/The Penguin Press. See Solveig Jülich, "The Making of a Best-Selling Book on Reproduction: Lennart Nilsson's *A Child Is Born*," *Bulletin of the History of Medicine* 89, no. 3 (2015): 491–525.

11   Solveig Jülich, "Fetal Photography in the Age of Cool Media," in *History of Participatory Media: Politics and Publics, 1750–2000,* ed. Anders Ekström et al. (London: Routledge, 2011).

12   Morag Ramsey, *The Swedish Abortion Pill: Co-producing Medical Abortion and Values, ca. 1965–1992* (Uppsala: Acta Universitatis Upsaliensis, 2021), chapter 2.

nologist Egon Diczfalusy, in retrospect, spoke of "the rise of the fetoplacental empire" to describe the international leadership in fetal research that
Sweden achieved during the 1960s but later lost. In his view, the novelty of
this research lay in the understanding of the hormonal symbiosis between
the woman, the fetus, and the placenta during pregnancy: "the fetoplacental
unit."[13] Nilsson, encouraged by his publishing house, took advantage of and
helped to market this powerful alliance between medical, media, and governmental actors.[14]

Drawing on fresh empirical material, including interviews, this chapter
aims to demonstrate how Nilsson collaborated with medical, scientific, photographic, and technical experts to produce the famous pictures of embryos
and fetuses that later circulated in the press and across visual culture.[15]
Importantly, most of the images were dependent on induced or spontaneous abortions, and he photographed the embryos and fetuses outside (ex
utero) or inside the womb (in utero). Building on the history of visual and
material culture of reproduction, I show that a focus on material resources,
techniques, and practices is crucial for understanding the profound impact of
Nilsson's embryonic and fetal pictures over time.[16] I highlight how Nilsson
and his team developed three different styles for visualizing human reproduction: the embryo and fetus in isolation, the fetus in bits, and the fetoplacental unit or, in popular terms, the fetal astronaut.[17] The term "style"

13　Egon Diczfalusy, "My Life with the Fetal-Placental Unit," *American Journal of
Obstetrics and Gynecology* 193, no. 6 (2005): 2025–29.

14　I develop this theme in *Photographing Life and Death.*

15　This chapter draws on the author's semistructured interviews with three doc-
tors and researchers (Egon Diczfalusy, March 16, 2009; Ingemar Joelsson,
October 10, 2008; and Björn Westin, January 26, 2009), a nurse (Maj-
Britt Reinhold, February 16, 2009), and a photographer (Carl O. Löfman,
December 19, 2008) who helped or in other ways supported Nilsson with the
photographing of embryos and fetuses.

16　Important work includes Tatjana Buklijas and Nick Hopwood, *Making
Visible Embryos* (online exhibition), 2008–10, http://www.hps.cam.ac.uk/
visibleembryos/ (last accessed May 27, 2023); Nick Hopwood, *Haeckel's
Embryos: Images, Evolution, and Fraud* (Chicago: University of Chicago Press,
2015); Lynn M. Morgan, *Icons of Life: A Cultural History of Human Embryos*
(Berkeley: University of California Press, 2009); María Jesús Santesmases,
"Circulating Biomedical Images: Bodies and Chromosomes in the Post-
eugenic Era," *History of Science* 55, no. 4 (2017): 395–430; and studies cited
elsewhere in this volume.

17　In her pioneering work from 1984, Ann Oakley drew a parallel between representations of the fetus as "cosmonaut" and the concept of "the fetoplacental
unit" in medical textbooks, but she did not mention Nilsson's pictures in this
context. See Ann Oakley, *The Captured Womb: A History of the Medical Care*

is employed to denote the long-lasting visual effects of techniques as well as of aesthetic and commercial considerations in the making of these particular pictures. The notion of style also points to groups of viewers who either favor or reject a certain visual trend.[18] In conclusion, this chapter suggests that the variation in visual technique, style, and sleight of hand is important to take into account when considering the political power and audience appeal of Nilsson's public fetus. It reveals that the famous images of embryos and fetuses he produced were anything but truthful or objective.

The focus on the making of Nilsson's fetal imagery also calls attention to ethical issues. The medical experiments on pregnant women and their embryos and fetuses that are described in this chapter took place during a period when principles for informed consent had not yet been established in Sweden. As elsewhere, research ethical committees were initiated at university hospitals in the mid-1960s, but in practice there were few restrictions on this research. The introduction of the Transplantation Act in 1995 regulated for the first time the use of aborted fetuses for scientific research, and from that point it has required the consent of the woman. Before 2006 there were no specific guidelines or legislation that regulated the use of fetoscopy or other prenatal diagnosis. Instead, it was ruled by general medical praxis.[19] This situation opened a window of opportunity for Nilsson to photograph embryos and fetuses in a way that was almost impossible elsewhere.

The Rise of the Fetoplacental Empire

After World War II, fetal research became a prominent feature of medicine in Sweden. This research built on a longer history (as will be elaborated below) and was connected to an international community of medical and biomedical researchers. Most studies in other countries had to rely on animal models since access to human embryos and fetuses was restricted or prohibited for various reasons. In Sweden, where abortion had been decriminalized in

---

of *Pregnant Women* (Oxford: Blackwell, 1984), 174–78. For a more recent discussion on the "fetal astronaut," see Margaret Carlyle and Brian Callender, "The Fetus in Utero: From Mystery to Social Media," *KNOW: A Journal on the Formation of Knowledge* 3, no. 1 (2019): 56.

18 For a helpful discussion, see Kim Beil, *Good Pictures: A History of Popular Photography* (Stanford, CA: Stanford University Press, 2020), 4–8.

19 Helena Tinnerholm Ljungberg, "The Moral Imperative of Fetal Research: Framing the Scientific Use of Aborted Fetuses in the 1960s and 1970s," and Anna Tunlid, "The Moral Landscape of Prenatal Diagnosis," both in *Medicine at the Borders of Life: Fetal Knowledge Production and the Emergence of Public Controversy in Sweden*, ed. Solveig Jülich (Leiden: Brill, 2024).

1938 and was permitted on medical, eugenic, and humanitarian grounds, and from 1946 on socio-medical indications, there were plenty of aborted fetuses.[20] The newly established Swedish Medical Research Council urged researchers to use this material for scientific studies:

> We do not know how long the current abortion law will last. It would be a remarkable waste of unique scientific material if this was not used for extensive studies of chemical and physiological problems for which similar conditions there probably exist nowhere in the world.[21]

This advantage was emphasized over and over again in official policy documents describing the conditions for medical research in postwar Sweden. Yet this interest in conducting studies that involved aborted fetuses did not automatically mean that researchers and doctors took a positive view of Swedish abortion law. Quite the opposite; many of them were explicitly against abortion unless the woman's life was at stake. But since the damage had already been done, they reasoned, it was better to use material from abortions for research that could benefit science and humanity. In many areas, including pediatrics, gynecology, and endocrinology, fetal research emerged as an important subfield and was sponsored by the American National Institutes of Health and the Ford Foundation, among others.[22]

It was not only access to an infrastructure of aborted fetuses that made Swedish medical research unique in an international context. Crucially, the fetuses acquired from abortions were often from midterm pregnancies and well preserved. In part this had to do with the fact that getting a legal abortion in 1950s and 1960s Sweden was by no means simple. The application process usually took considerable time since it involved visiting and obtaining approval from two doctors and a social worker (or the decision rested with the social-psychiatric committee at the National Board of Medicine). Many women who underwent abortion were between the thirteenth and eighteenth week of pregnancy. For these abortions the most common methods used were vaginal and abdominal hysterotomy (sometimes referred to as vaginal Cesarean section and abdominal Cesarean section). This was also the case for abortions performed on eugenic indications in combination with sterilization. By the late 1960s, vacuum aspiration and saline injections gained in demand, which meant that the aborted embryo or fetus was extracted in pieces through the cervix. These destructive techniques made

---

20   Solveig Jülich, "Historicizing Fetal Knowledge Production, Reproductive Politics, and Conflicted Values," in Jülich, *Medicine at the Borders.*

21   Arvid Wallgren and Gunnar Ågren, "Förslag ang. bildandet av en subkommitté för human foetalfysiologi och kemi den 11/10 1950." F2: 10. Medical Research Council archive, National Archives, Sweden.

22   Jülich, "Historicizing Fetal Knowledge."

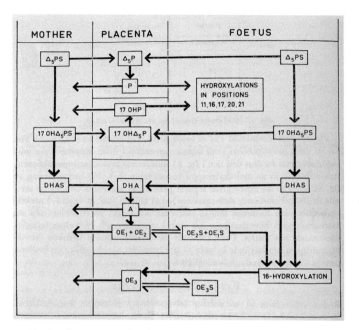

Figure 6.1. An illustration of "the fetoplacental unit": the complex hormonal interrelationships between the placenta, the fetus, and the woman during pregnancy. From Egon Diczfalusy, "Människofostrets roll vid graviditetens endokrina reglering," in *20 års medicinsk forskning: Statens medicinska forskningsråd 1945–1965*, ed. Yngve Zotterman (Stockholm: Norstedt, 1965), 372.

the abortion material useless for the kind of investigations and methodologies that interested many reproductive researchers at the time.[23]

Karolinska Institute, the medical university in Stockholm and home of the Nobel assembly, became a central hub for fetal research and a major beneficiary of international grants. At its two obstetrics and gynecology clinics, located at Sabbatsberg Hospital and Karolinska Hospital, researchers worked out various methods for studying living or dying fetuses. Led by Egon Diczfalusy, a so-called perfusion technique was developed that made it possible to keep human fetuses "alive" for a short time after the abortion operation. Above all, the researchers were interested in acquiring basic knowledge about the interaction between the fetus, placenta, and "mother,"

---

23   Jülich, "Historicizing Fetal Knowledge." The abortion techniques are described in Ramsey, *Swedish Abortion Pill*, 49–50. For early abortions another surgical technique was used: dilation and curettage (D&C).

a system that was conceptualized as "the fetoplacental unit." Expectations of practical benefits were high. For instance, perfusion studies on aborted fetuses were performed to test new contraceptives and abortion methods, and it was anticipated that a new thalidomide scandal could be prevented by investigating how and with what effects drugs were transferred from the pregnant woman to the fetus.[24]

Postwar fetal research in Sweden or, in the words of Diczfalusy, "the rise of the fetoplacental empire" became intermingled with Nilsson's visual enterprise. Unexpectedly, the freelance press photographer, whose formal education had ended with elementary school, became involved with doctors and researchers at Karolinska Institute, and for a while he was a member of Diczfalusy's team.[25] But it was embryology that first caught Nilsson's attention and led to these collaborations.

The Embryo and Fetus in Isolation

Nilsson first developed a style that portrayed the embryo and fetus laid bare and separated from the pregnant body. This was not something new. The wet specimens prepared by the Dutch anatomist Frederik Ruysch in the late seventeenth century could show more or less of the maternal body, depending on which audience the preparator wished to address. Midwives under training in the eighteenth century were interested in seeing the fetus within the womb, whereas embryologists of the late nineteenth century often preferred to view the fetus in isolation, to facilitate comparative analysis between humans and across species. But in all cases the fetuses were dead, and the reproductive organs came from dissected women.[26] Nilsson also relied on ex utero material, and he took his inspiration from embryological studies where the developing human was in focus.

As elsewhere in Europe and the United States, larger embryological collections had been built at many university hospitals in Sweden during the

---

24   Jülich, "Historicizing Fetal Knowledge." Thalidomide was a drug prescribed to pregnant women under the name of "neurosedyn" in Sweden that caused severe deformities in the children born to these women.

25   Diczfalusy, "My Life with the Fetal-Placental Unit"; Diczfalusy, interview with the author.

26   Ray, this volume; Nick Hopwood, "Producing Development: The Anatomy of Human Embryos and the Norms of Wilhelm His," *Bulletin of the History of Medicine* 74, no. 1 (2000): 29–79.

decades around 1900.[27] Human material was not easily obtainable. By establishing collegial networks of physicians and midwives, the medical researchers were able to collect products from women's miscarriages, ectopic pregnancies, and other losses. The decriminalization of abortion in 1938 made it easier to get access and increased the number of fetal bodies collected for research and education. However, after World War II embryological collections gradually lost their scientific importance as new experimental methods for culturing living cells became more attractive and available to research laboratories.[28]

Nilsson first encountered embryological specimens when, working as a freelance press photographer, he was commissioned to take a portrait of the controversial professor and chief physician Per Wetterdal at the women's clinic of Sabbatsberg Hospital in Stockholm in 1952. Wetterdal had refused to carry out approved abortions at the clinic, and he had recently delivered a speech from the pulpit of Matteus Church against the existing law on abortion. During his visit, Nilsson was shown objects from the hospital's embryological collection. According to contemporary sources, it was not uncommon that doctors kept human specimens in jars in their consulting rooms to persuade abortion-seeking women who came to see them to reconsider their choices. Many in the medical profession were opposed to abortion at the time. This visit to the women's clinic resulted in both a photograph of Wetterdal, portrayed in a priestlike manner, and a series of pictures of dead aborted fetuses featured in Sweden's foremost picture magazine, *Se* (See), under the headline "Why Must the Fetus Be Killed?" This 1952 antiabortion article became a gateway for Nilsson to the medical community, which usually kept "sensationalistic" press photographers at arm's length.[29]

Nilsson worked for several years to document human development at Sabbatsberg Hospital. In the beginning he borrowed specimens and brought them to his photographic laboratory, which was located close to the hospital. Later he was offered one of the rooms in the research section of the clinic, where he could keep his cameras, flashguns, microscopes, and other technical

27   On the United States, see Morgan, *Icons of Life*; on Germany, see Hopwood, *Haeckel's Embryos*; on Sweden, see Solveig Jülich, "Embryology and the Clinic: Early to Mid-Twentieth Century Stories of Pregnancy, Abortion, and Fetal Collecting," and Eva Åhrén, "Visualizing the Early Stages of Life: Embryology and Fetal Anatomy at Karolinska Institute, 1820s–1920s," both in Jülich, *Medicine at the Borders*.

28   Jülich, "Embryology and the Clinic"; Solveig Jülich and Isa Dussauge, "Fetuses as Instruments of Health: Polio Vaccine and the Nation in the Postwar Period," in Jülich, *Medicine at the Borders*.

29   Karl E. Hillgren and Lennart Nilsson, "Varför måste fostret dödas?," *Se*, no. 28 (1952): 13–17. For a discussion, see Jülich, "Picturing Abortion Opposition."

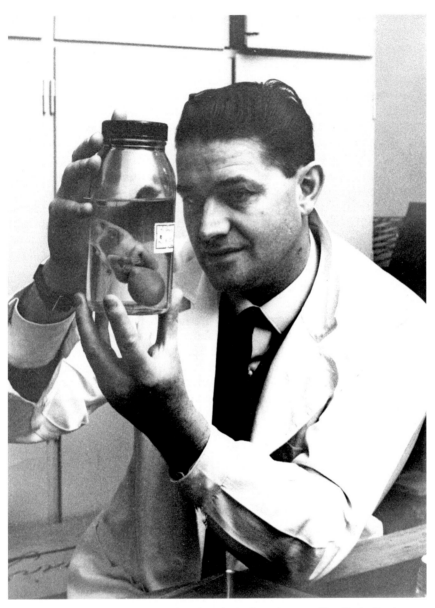

Figure 6.2. Lennart Nilsson with embryological specimen at Karolinska Institute in 1965. From "Lennart Nilsson, Kanske inte världsbäst men . . . Fosterlandets främste!," *Arbetet*, February 10, 1968. Photo: Tore Ekholm. Courtesy of Bilder i Syd, Sweden.

equipment. As the project grew, he managed to make similar arrangements with heads of clinics and chief physicians at other hospitals in Stockholm. He was courted by magazine editors who asked for more spectacular pictures as well as his publisher, who suggested that he make a pregnancy advice book with the photographic material. There was thus an expanding market for Nilsson's work.[30]

Photographs of embryological specimens had begun to be published in international picture magazines. In 1950, *Life* featured a series of "remarkable" pictures of the development of a human being from an unfertilized egg cell to an almost fully developed fetus. Most of these specimens, which also included fetal skeletons at various stages of growth, came from the Carnegie Institution of Washington's famous Department of Embryology in Baltimore. There were similarities between these anatomical pictures in *Life* and Nilsson's first fetal photographs in *Se*. He had placed the black-and-white pictures of enlarged specimens in sequence, which was an established convention in embryological textbooks. The embryos and fetuses had been completely freed from membranes and the placenta, except for a forty-day embryo in *Life* that was shown in cross-section inside its amniotic sac. In both cases, the specimens had been photographed against a black background that enhanced contrast and clarity but also gave many of them a clinical, even macabre look. However, there was no mention of abortion in the *Life* story.[31]

The picture of the forty-day embryo in *Life* must have triggered Nilsson's interest, because in a few years' time his "portrait" of a human embryo after six weeks of development, enlarged eighty-five times, appeared in the same magazine. According to *Life*, in comparison to the previous pictures the magazine had published, this one was outstanding for its clarity in showing how a "tiny human" took shape.[32] Crucially, Nilsson was a highly skilled and technically driven photographer, whereas other images had probably been produced on a more routine basis by assistants at medical and scientific institutions.

As explained by Nilsson in his 1955 book *Reportage* (Reports), it was quite challenging to take this picture of the eighteen-millimeter-long embryo. With the help of a fellow reporter at *Se*, he placed the specimen in a laboratory watch glass with a little fluid, but the least vibration from trams

30 Jülich, "Making of a Best-Selling Book."

31 "The Human Embryo," *Life*, July 3, 1950, 79–81; Hillgren and Nilsson, "Varför måste fostret dödas?"

32 Lennart Nilsson, "Embryo's Face," *Life*, March 30, 1953, 115. It was also published in Swedish; see Karl E. Hillgren and Lennart Nilsson, "Verklighetens svindlande saga," *Se*, no. 1 (1953): 10–11.

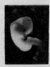
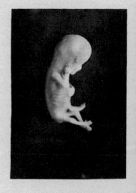

FOSTRETS UTVECKLING

Tidsangivelsen avser graviditetsmånader, som omfattar fyr...

Andra månaden

Tredje månaden

Ovanstående foster är sex veckor gammalt, drygt 15 mm långt och väger ca 1 gram. I detta stadium har utvecklingen redan gått så långt att övre delen av svalget börjat bildas. Skelettet anlägges i form av brosk. Sköldkörteln utbildas och blodet pulserar i blodkärlen. Genom de ännu tunna yttre delarna av huvudet skimrar hjärnhinnorna.

Fostrets liv och utveckling startar i och med att en sädeskropp intränger i ägget. När detta befruktats inträder en snabb delning av äggcellen i två celler, som sedan vardera delar sig i två o. s. v. Efter några få dagar har det befruktade ägget övergått i en samling celler som alla befinner sig i delning. Cellmassan differentierar sig i tre principiellt skilda celltyper, arrangerade i tre lager: ektoderm (av grek. *e'ktos* = utanför, och *de'rma* = hud), mesoderm *(me'sos* = i mitten befintlig) och entoderm *(ento's* = inom). Inom cellskivorna uppkommer veckningar, instjälpningar, avsnörningar och utbuktningar, som utgör de första anlagen för kroppens olika organ.

Från ektodermet utvecklas bl. a. överhuden och nervsystemet. Från början skivformigt böjer sig ektodermet runt så att ytterkanterna förenas och omsluter de övriga groddbladen. Härigenom uppkommer kroppens spolform.

Från mesodermet utvecklas hjärta, blodkärl och stödjevävnader (bindväv, brosk). Från entodermet utvecklas mag-tarmkanalen med bukspottkörteln, levern, körtlarna i magsäckens och tarmarnas väggar.

Det befruktade ägget ger också upphov till de hjälporgan med vilka fostret fäster sig i livmodern och hämtar sin näring från modern. Moderkakan är fästad vid livmoderns vägg. Mellan moderkakan och fostret löper blodkärl i navelsträngen, som förbinder fostret med moderkakan. Under tidigaste fosterstadiet är navelsträngen tämligen tjock i förhållande till fosterkroppen. Navelsträngen fäster sig i bukväggen och härifrån föres blodet till och från fostrets hjärta. I moderkakan syrsättes fostrets blod (som inte kommunicerar med moderns) och erhåller näringsämnen för fostret. Via blodkärl i navelsträngen föres blodet till fostrets hjärta och pumpas därifrån ut i dess organism. Sedan går det genom hjärtat och navelsträngskärlen åter till moderkakan för att lämna ifrån sig ämnesomsättningsprodukterna som upptagits i fosterkroppen och för att syrsättas på nytt.

Det ofullständigt utvecklade, i fosterhinnor vatten simmande embryot har blivit en cm lång varelse med tydligt mänskliga dr Vikten är c:a 20 gram. Redan en yttre un sökning kan nu avgöra om fostret är en po eller en flicka. (Mikroskopiskt kan könskörtla skiljas från varann då embryot är 2 cm långt.

Detta är en flicka. I hennes kropp har marna utvecklats och tarmrörelser börjar u träda. Lungorna har fått sitt slutliga utsee och andningsrörelser kan förekomma. Hjärt klaffar och valvler fungerar. Man kan få fr olika reflexrörelser och iakttta spontana röre av extremiteterna. Hjärnvindlingarna utveck Ur det tidigare anlagda brosket startar benb ningen och benmärgen börjar ingripa i b bildningen. Vissa endokrina körtlar (av gr *e'ndon* = invärtes, och *kri'nein* = avsöndra) kommit igång, bl. a. bukspottkörtelns insu producerande faktor. Levern är kraftigt utveck (den utgör 1/10 av fostrets hela vikt). Gallb och gallgångar är utdifferentierade.

Under tredje månaden växer fostret hast Längden från hjässan till svansbasen ökar f 3 till 7 cm och vid slutet av månaden är kropp ungefär 9 cm lång. Proportionerna ändras kroppsdelarna nalkas sin definitiva form. I an månaden har fostret hand- och fotplattor tredje månaden föres blodet till fostrets hjärta o fötterna i mera fullständigt skick och nag börjar uppträda. Huvudet är fortfarande re tivt stort, bäckenparti och benanlag relativt sn Ögonen, förut sidoriktade, riktas småningom a mera framåt och ögonlocksvecken sammanväx

Av 1.000 legala aborter i Sverige utfördes	Av 1.000 legala aborter i Sverige utfördes
23	**217**
vid graviditet med foster i detta stadium.	vid graviditet med foster i detta stadium.

Figure 6.3.
Photographs intended to demonstrate "The development of the fetus up to the point of viable life." Spread from Karl E. Hillgren (text) and Lennart Nilsson (photo), "Varför måste fostret dödas?," *Se*, no. 28 (1952): 16–17. Courtesy of Lennart Nilsson Photography.

TILL GRÄNSEN FÖR LIVSDUGLIGHET

jämna veckor. Fotografierna visar fostren i naturlig storlek

Fjärde månaden

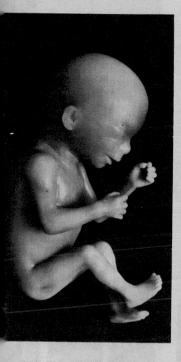

Femte månaden

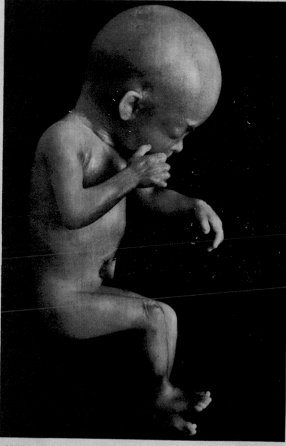

Fostret företer alltmer mänskliga drag och man har i fjärde månaden ett starkt intryck av att fostret är en människa i miniatyr. Ansiktet är nu så utvecklat att detta uttryck motiveras. Näsborrarna öppnas. I pannan börjar korta, färglösa hårfjun att sticka fram. Ytterörat tar form, svett-körtlarna och underhudsfettet utvecklas, huden blir fastare och rosafärgad. Blodkärlen syns genom huden och deras banor motsvarar redan nu de som finns hos den utvecklade människan. Rörelseförmågan är ytterligare ökad och flera reflexer kan frambringas. Foster på detta stadium bär individuella drag. Till och med hos tvillingar kan i detta stadium individuella egenheter skönjas.

De inre organen har fortsatt att växa i takt med de yttre och deras funktion fullkomnas alltmer. Som exempel kan nämnas att matsmältningsenzymn börjar uppträda i tarmen. Enzymer är de aktiva faktorerna i sekretet från matsmältningskörtlarna. Vid slutet av fjärde månaden är fostret c:a 16 cm långt och väger c:a 120 gram. Kvinnan börjar nu känna fosterrörelser.

Längden har ökat till 25 cm och vikten till c:a ½ kg. Fostrets rörelser har blivit så starka att de tydligt uppfattas av modern. Benen har vuxit i förhållande till kroppen i övrigt. De s. k. lanugohåren som är så karaktäristiska för nyfödda barn utvecklas över hela kroppen. Nervbanorna i ryggmärgen fullständigas. Levern producerar galla och bukspottkörteln producerar äggvitenedbrytande enzym.

Den fortsatta utvecklingen över femte månaden företer inte så språngvisa drag som tidigare. De flesta organ är nu också utvecklade. I sjätte månaden förkalkas tandkronorna. Fostret är vid månadens slut 30 cm långt. I sjunde månaden förlängas huvudhåren, underhudsfettet utvecklas ytterligare och ögonlockens tidigare sammanväxning upphör så att ögat kan blottas. Fostret är nu 35 cm långt och står på gränsen till livsduglighet utanför moderns organism. — Det fullgångna nyfödda barnet är c:a 50 cm långt.

> Av 1.000 legala aborter i Sverige utfördes
> **403**
> vid graviditet med foster i detta stadium.

> Av 1.000 legala aborter i Sverige utfördes
> **297**
> vid graviditet med foster i detta stadium.

> Motsvarande siffror för sjätte och sjunde månaden:
> **57** resp. **3**

SLUT

in the street outside made the object move, which resulted in blurred photographs. After many unsuccessful attempts they found out that they could steady the specimen on a piece of plasticine. The watch glass was then put on a flask that was strongly lit from below by a projector. The camera was designed for micro- and macro-photography, and the pictures were taken with a yellow filter and special plates that had been made sensitive to all colors except red and orange, so-called orthochromatic plates. It required an exposure of nearly a minute, but finally Nilsson succeeded in getting all the details: "the cerebral hemispheres, the rudiments of a mouth, a nose and ears, as well as arms and legs." This result took a week to accomplish.[33]

Apart from this report, there exist few testimonies from Nilsson on how he produced the embryonic and fetal images or where the human materials came from. But he was dependent on access to the hospitals' specimen collections for reaching his goal to visualize all the stages of development from fertilization to birth. According to several persons who worked at Sabbatsberg Hospital in the 1960s it was actually for Nilsson's sake that the collection, consisting of some hundreds of jars, was still maintained. Newly delivered dead embryos and fetuses from surgical operations were prepared and conserved by nurses or doctors at the ward and then saved for the photographer. No one else paid much attention to the collection at this time.[34]

However, the specimens within hospital collections had clear disadvantages. First, many of the fetuses had been collected for the education of midwives and had severe deformities and defects of various kinds. Nilsson wanted normal, healthy objects. Another problem was that the material was undeniably not alive. Certain characteristics like, for example, discolorations could not be concealed by lighting or retouching.[35] For this reason, in parallel to photographing embryological specimens, Nilsson collaborated with researchers and photographic specialists to develop techniques for taking pictures of living fetuses inside as well as outside of the pregnant body.

The Fetus in Bits

In the 1950s, Nilsson started to develop a second style that revealed the fetus, not as a figure comparable to portrait photography, but in smaller bits and parts within the uterus. This kind of imaging was made possible by the development of endoscopic instruments and wide-angle lenses. Physicians in many countries had long used endoscopes, various types of tubes carrying

33   Lennart Nilsson, *Reportage* (Stockholm: Bonnier, 1955), 53–54, 122.
34   Joelsson and Reinhold, interviews with the author.
35   Joelsson explained this during the interview.

light, to examine gynecological and obstetrical problems. But it was not until the postwar period that techniques of looking inside women's reproductive bodies started to become more routinely used, such as culdoscopy and laparoscopy.[36] In yet another technique, hysteroscopy, an endoscope was introduced through the vaginal and cervical canal for visualization of the uterus. As miniature cameras as well as color film technology improved, endoscopic pictures of the womb and the surrounding area were produced for diagnostic and scientific uses. It took longer for what is today called fetoscopy, an invasive and risky method for viewing the fetus inside the uterus, to be introduced into medicine. The technique had its peak in the 1970s, after which ultrasound was often preferred to diagnose fetal abnormalities.[37]

Björn Westin at Sabbatsberg Hospital performed one of the first fetoscopic examinations in the world. In 1954 he reported having carried out a "hysteroscopy in early pregnancy" with a McCarthy's panendoscope, an instrument originally designed for looking inside the bladder. This endoscope, as the name indicates, had a wide-angle lens that gave a better view of the inside of the organ or, in this case, the living fetus. However, it was used not for diagnosis but rather in the investigation of fetal physiology as well as in the new field of fetal medicine. When Westin inserted the panendoscope through the cervix of women who were going to have legal abortions, he could observe how the fetuses moved inside the womb and how one of them

---

36   On the history of endoscopy, see Laurits Lauridsen, *Laterna Magica in Corpore Humano: From the History of Endoscopy* (Aarhus: Steno Museum, 1998); and Michael J. O'Dowd and Elliot E. Philipp, "Laparoscopy," in *The History of Obstetrics and Gynaecology* (New York: Parthenon, 2000), 417–26. For a cultural history, see José van Dijck, *The Transparent Body: A Cultural Analysis of Medical Imaging* (Seattle: University of Washington Press, 2005), 64–82. Culdoscopy was performed with an instrument that was inserted via the vagina through the peritoneum up into the abdominal cavity in order to investigate suspicions of sterility or extra-uterine pregnancy. In laparoscopy the instrument was inserted through the abdominal wall into the abdominal cavity, which made it possible to discover pathological changes, take tissue samples, and carry out certain types of surgical operations. In Sweden, laparoscopy was introduced in the early 1950s at the women's clinic in Lund, while it was used only in a limited fashion at the Sabbatsberg women's clinic. See Mats Ahlgren, "Laparaskopin 100 år: Förr vid gynekologisk diagnostik nu också vid kirurgi," *Läkartidningen* 94, no. 3 (1997): 162–64.

37   Olivia Mandile, "Endoscopic Fetoscopy," *Embryo Project Encyclopedia* (July 18, 2017), http://embryo.asu.edu/handle/10776/12563. Oakley, *Captured Womb*, 171–72.

swallowed several times. When he compressed the umbilical cord, the movements and the swallowing ceased after two minutes.[38]

When Nilsson heard about Westin's fetoscopic observations, he became
very interested. Was it technically feasible to connect a camera to the endoscope and take pictures of the fetus inside a woman's uterus? Nilsson confided
to Westin that he had a large sum of money from his publisher that could be
used to finance the project. In addition, his assistant Werner Donné, an engi-
neer specializing in optics and flash technology, could help to improve and
rebuild McCarthy's panendoscope for their specific needs. Westin, for his
part, saw collaboration with the photographer as an opportunity to compare
his earlier results from perfusion experiments on aborted fetuses outside the
uterus with conditions in utero documented in pictures (see below).[39]

First of all, Westin designed an endoscope that was then built by Donné.
They decided to use the wide-angle optics from the panendoscope and then
affixed an electronic flash designed by Donné. After that they did a series of
test runs, which showed that a number of factors affected the photographic
result: everything from the distance between the film and the object and
the sensitivity of the film to the kind of light source that was used. To solve
these photographic problems, they consulted Helmer Bäckström, professor
of photography at the Royal Institute of Technology in Stockholm, and two
of his colleagues from the same department. These three were paid for their
services, and the arrangement included the loan of some supplementary
photographic equipment from Bäckström. Altogether six medical, photographic, and technical experts were thus involved in the work of developing
what Westin called "hystero-photography."[40]

When they had finished these preparations, the investigation began. The
women chosen for the study were to have their abortions in the fourteenth
to the eighteenth week of pregnancy. Their identities are unknown, but they
probably came from a variety of socioeconomic backgrounds, since health-
care facilities such as gynecological clinics were subsidized for all citizens. A
local anesthetic was given but no general anesthesia, most likely because this
would have affected the fetus. The endoscope was inserted into the cervix—
on one occasion also through the abdomen—and by means of a knife inside
the tube the membrane of the fetus was punctured. When this had been
done, the knife was replaced by the optical system and the flash. According

38   Björn Westin, "Hysteroscopy in Early Pregnancy," *Lancet*, October 23, 1954,
     872.
39   Westin, interview with the author.
40   Björn Westin, "Technique and Estimation of Oxygenation of the Human Fetus
     in Utero by Means of Hystero-Photography," *Acta Paediatrica* 46 (March
     1957): 117–24; Westin, interview with the author.

to Westin the vision was "extremely good," and it was possible to examine the fetus, the placenta, and the umbilical cord in detail. No lack of oxygen could be observed; the skin of the fetus was pink, and several glandular openings were discernible. After that, Nilsson took the pictures. When the fetus had been removed, Westin extracted a piece of the umbilical cord, which was placed in a saline solution, perfused, and photographed at roughly the same distance as the pictures taken inside the body.[41]

After comparison it turned out that there were marked differences between the photographs taken inside the body and those taken outside. The photographs of fetuses in the womb had a blue tinge that was perceived as "artificial" in relation to the endoscopic observation. This was an effect due to the fact that Donné's flash contained krypton gas, which emitted blue light. The amniotic fluid served as a red filter, however, and reduced the blue tones. But to get the same hue in the pictures taken in the saline solution outside the womb, it was necessary to use photographic filters. On the basis of the photographic material, Westin could deduce that the oxygenation of the umbilical vein was stronger in the fetus than after the birth. The photographs thus confirmed his earlier studies and, he thought, indicated new ways of acquiring knowledge of the physiology of the fetus. Nilsson, for his part, gained valuable knowledge of photographic techniques that would benefit him in his subsequent work.[42]

The resulting pictures were not, however, as sensational as the photographer had hoped. What Nilsson most wanted to capture was the face of the human fetus, and on one occasion when he had the unique opportunity to photograph a fetus that was sucking its thumb, Donné's flash did not work.[43] Instead he had a series of very small, circular pictures of body parts that were almost impossible to identify without the accompanying text, including details of the ear, the skin, the placenta, and the umbilical cord. This is why they were only published in a scientific journal, together with Westin's report.[44]

---

41   Westin, "Technique and Estimation of Oxygenation."

42   Westin, "Technique and Estimation of Oxygenation."

43   See the interview with Nilsson that was made by the American television program NOVA (WGBH/PBS) and published on their homepage: "Behind the Lens: An Interview with Lennart Nilsson," http://www.pbs.org/wgbh/nova/odyssey/nilsson.html (last accessed March 25, 2022).

44   Westin, interview with the author. The earliest fetoscopic photographs were probably taken by the Japanese photographer Chie Mohri and the gynecologist Takaaki Mohri in 1954. On these experiments, see Rafael F. Valle, "Development of Hysteroscopy: From a Dream to a Reality, and Its Linkage to the Present and Future," *Journal of Minimally Invasive Gynecology* 14, no. 4 (2007): 413.

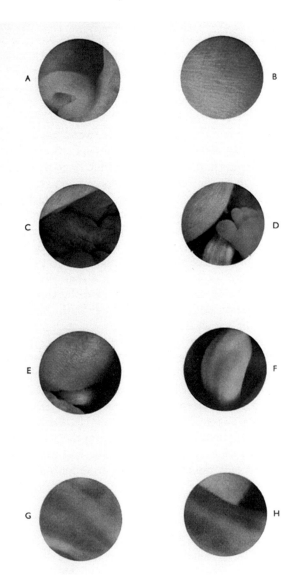

Figure 6.4. Nilsson's endoscopic pictures of living fetuses inside the body (A–G). Views showing: (A) the ear and one upper limb, (B) the fetal skin, (C) central part of the placenta, (D) the toes, (E) the placenta at the left margin, (F) the umbilical cord, (G) umbilical vein. The last picture (H) shows a piece of the umbilical cord outside the body after perfusion. From Westin, "Technique and Estimation of Oxygenation,"117–24. Photo: Lennart Nilsson. Courtesy of Lennart Nilsson Photography, and John Wiley and Sons.

By the beginning of the 1960s, Nilsson owned or could borrow several endoscopes of different types and from different manufacturers. Yet it was only later that the German instrument maker Karl Storz's endoscopes with fiber optics and a Hopkins lens system became available and transformed the market.[45] The endoscopes that Nilsson used alternated between the older technique with the light source inserted in the organ and a newer technique with "cold light" outside the body, although this was not yet fiber optics. Some of them had been rebuilt by his assistant Donné, who continued to develop wide-angle optics as well as flash technology. Thanks to the shorter focal length of Donné's lenses, in comparison to McCarthy's panendoscope, it was possible to get a wider angle of view and thereby, using an electronic flash, to capture a larger part of the embryo or fetus. Nilsson used his Leica camera to take color pictures, and attempts were also made to film the movements of the fetus inside with movie cameras.[46] However, technical difficulties seem to have obstructed the photographer's dream of capturing fetal life before death, for only one image reached a wide audience in the 1960s: the introductory picture to the photo-essay "Drama of Life before Birth."

Most probably, Donné's improved endoscope was used for "the first portrait ever made of a living embryo inside its mother's womb," published in *Life* in 1965. The accompanying text made it clear that this picture had been taken using an endoscope equipped with a wide-angle lens and a flash. By reading the text carefully it was also possible to conclude that the other photographs showed embryos and fetuses outside the body since these had been "surgically removed for a variety of medical reasons."[47] Some of these, as already discussed, were likely specimens from hospital collections that had been photographed in one of Nilsson's photographic laboratories, at home or close to the ward. But others were produced in the operating room immediately after abortion operations and other surgery on pregnant women. This resulted in ex utero pictures as well, but the embryos and fetuses looked more vivid and natural than the ones of specimens. Tracing the history of this visual style will take us back to Westin's early experiments at Sabbatsberg Hospital.

But first it is worth mentioning that fetoscopy was in some respects a dead end for Nilsson. Although technological standards improved in the decades following the 1960s, doctor's growing ethical awareness made it much harder for the photographer to get permission to take pictures during fetoscopic

---

45   Joelle Bentley, "Photographing the Miracle of Life," *Technology Review* 95 (November/December 1992): 58–65.

46   This is discussed in more detail in Jülich, *Photographing Life and Death*.

47   Nilsson and Rosenfeld, "Drama of Life before Birth," 54–55.

examinations.[48] Sometimes he could also use his specially designed, wide-angled endoscopes from Jungner Instrument AB in Stockholm to simulate a view of the fetus in utero. The second edition of *A Child Is Born*, published in the mid-1970s, pointed out that a series of photographs taken with the unique Jungner lens had made it possible to visualize for the first time how the fetus lay enclosed in the womb. The captions, along with the circular form of the wide-angle pictures, worked together in drawing the viewer into the image and creating an impression of transparency: that the photographs showed a living fetus inside the body of a woman.[49] This was not the case, however. The fetus had been removed from a deceased woman and then placed in a round bowl in the forensic laboratory at Karolinska Institute, where Nilsson took his pictures.[50]

The Fetoplacental Unit

In parallel with the endoscopic experiments, Nilsson came to develop a style that pictured the living fetus connected to, or at least with traces of, the pregnant body, such as the umbilical cord and the placenta. The idea of using ex utero, living human fetuses that came from the operating room for research and preparing exceptional specimens was not a complete innovation. Early twentieth-century American embryologists had injected fixate fluids into living embryos and fetuses in order to study blood vessels and the lymph system with greater care. Also in the United States, between 1932 and 1958, the neuroanatomist Davenport Hooker performed neurological tests on fetuses obtained from miscarriages and induced abortions. He used a movie camera to record the reflexes of the fetuses and assembled the footage into a silent educational film called *Early Fetal Human Activity* (1952). Some of these images were later reproduced in science writer Geraldine Lux Flanagan's best-selling book *The First Nine Months of Life* (1962). There

48   It is instructive to compare the 1965 picture in *Life* with a fetoscopic image of the face of a fetus in Lennart Nilsson et al., *A Child Is Born: New Photographs of Life before Birth and Up-to-Date Advice for Expectant Parents*, 2nd American ed. (New York: Delacorte, 1977), 125. The latter is significantly blurrier than the former.
49   Lennart Nilsson et al., *A Child Is Born*, 116–17, 120–21. Also see Lennart Nilsson, "Through a Unique Lens," *Sweden Now* 10, no. 5 (1976): 79. For a discussion, see Solveig Jülich, "Lennart Nilsson's Fish-Eyes: A Photographic and Cultural History of Views from Below," *Konsthistorisk tidskrift/Journal of Art History* 84, no. 2 (2015): 75–92.
50   Löfman, interview with the author.

were other experiments on ex utero living fetuses in the United States and Britain, but they were rare.[51]

From the end of the 1940s researchers at Karolinska Institute conducted studies that involved living aborted fetuses, including a small team of gynecologists at Sabbatsberg Hospital led by Westin. Like Hooker, they preferred hysterotomy as an abortion method, and the embryos and fetuses delivered to their laboratories were quickly immersed in warm saline solution. But Hooker had experimented in vain with various techniques to slow down asphyxia and death, which occurred between seven and twenty minutes. Westin and his team were able to develop a perfusion apparatus that made it possible to keep the fetuses alive for up to twelve hours after oxygenized blood had been injected by means of a catheter in the umbilical vein. It was described as an "artificial placenta" and consisted of a chamber of glass (specially made by the medico-technical company Kifa in Stockholm) and an "oxygenerator"—a machine that produced oxygen. The fetus was placed in the chamber, which was filled with an "artificial amniotic fluid" at a temperature of 77° F. Westin envisaged that this research would be of value in the treatment of premature babies and also reduce the risk of cerebral palsy and other forms of grave postdelivery brain damage in fully developed babies that were asphyctic and "apparently dead."[52]

However, the primary value of Westin's perfusion apparatus was its use in experimental studies of the "fetoplacental unit." Drawing on this technique, Diczfalusy and his team at Karolinska Hospital systematically explored the fetal, placental, and maternal interrelations in the formation of steroids during pregnancy. In connection with legal abortion operations, the intact fetus was removed from the uterus and placed in a bath of artificial amniotic fluid. The placenta, still attached to the fetus via the umbilical cord, went into a separate vessel containing blood. By tagging tiny molecules with radioactive labels and then setting them adrift in the fetal and placental circulation, Diczfalusy was able to discover where and

51 Morgan, *Icons of Life*, 198–99; Emily K. Wilson, "Ex Utero: Live Human Fetal Research and the Films of Davenport Hooker," *Bulletin of the History of Medicine* 88, no. 1 (2014): 132–60; Johanna Schoen, *Abortion after* Roe (Chapel Hill: University of North Carolina Press, 2015), chapter 2.

52 Björn Westin, Rune Nyberg, and Göran Enhörning, "A Technique for Perfusion of the Previable Human Fetus," *Acta Paediatrica* 47 (July 1958): 339–49; Bo Vahlquist and Björn Westin, "Utvecklingsforskning: 1. Fosterforskning—den foeto-placentära enheten," in *20 års medicinsk forskning: Statens medicinska forskningsråd 1945–1965*, ed. Yngve Zotterman (Stockholm: Norstedt, 1965), 376.

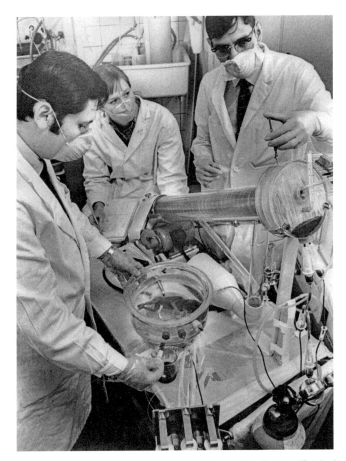

Figure 6.5. Diczfalusy's team at Karolinska Institute with the "artificial placenta," the perfusion apparatus, around 1970. Photo: Lennart Nilsson. Courtesy of Lennart Nilsson Photography.

how the crucial hormones that help maintain pregnancy were constructed, what they did, and what happened to them.[53]

---

53   Egon Diczfalusy, "Människofostrets roll vid graviditetens endokrina reglering," in Zotterman, *20 års medicinsk forskning*, 367, 373; Oscar Harkavy and John Maier, "Research in Reproductive Biology and Contraceptive Technology: Present Status and Needs for the Future," *Family Planning Perspectives* 2, no. 3 (June 1970): 5–13. On the life and career of Diczfalusy, see Giuseppe Benagiano and Mario Merialdi, "Egon R. Diczfalusy, the Discovery of the

Westin's perfusion apparatus was also decisive for Nilsson's development of a new style of visualizing embryos and fetuses. The in utero pictures taken with the endoscope during their collaborative experiments in the mid-1950s had been promising, but the most important result came from comparing them with photographs of the umbilical vein in a saline solution. The picture of the umbilical vein was not particularly remarkable in itself, visually speaking, but the method of photographing embryos and fetuses in fluid pointed in a new direction. Westin's "fetus chamber" could be exchanged for a water tank or an aquarium-like vessel. Through the tests run by the photography experts participating in the experiments, Nilsson knew what specific arrangements and technical equipment, such as photographic filters, were needed to make the objects placed under water look (what was perceived as) natural and alive.[54]

After Westin had left Sabbatsberg Hospital for a research visit abroad, Nilsson established contact with Ingemar Joelsson, who was assistant physician at the women's clinic between 1961 and 1965. He had a room adjoining Nilsson's, and it was he who supplied the photographer with "fresh fetuses," as they were called at that time. In an interview with Joelsson that I conducted some years ago, he described how the photographing was done. As soon as a patient came to the hospital for a miscarriage or an extra-uterine pregnancy, one of the staff called Nilsson, who came and looked for suitable objects: embryos and fetuses of all sizes, from the early stages of development to as late pregnancies as possible—the whole range of fetal development. If small embryos were concerned, he would take them with him and photograph them through the microscope in his room at the ward. But apart from the fact that everything happened very quickly, there was often also a lot of hemorrhaging in spontaneous abortions, which made it more difficult to take pictures. Therefore, Nilsson preferred to take his pictures in connection with legal abortions, when it was easier to control the whole process.[55]

When an induced abortion was to be carried out, Nilsson was notified beforehand and was present in the operating room with his camera and all

---

Fetoplacental Unit and Much More," *Contraception* 84, no. 6 (2011): 544–48.

54 Westin, "Technique and Estimation of Oxygenation"; Westin, interview with the author.

55 According to Joelsson, if there was enough time, the women were asked for permission to photograph their embryos and fetuses. He did not recall that anybody declined; they were thankful for the "help with the abortion." No ethical guidelines existed at the time, and it was the professors who decided what was allowed and what was not. When interviewed by the author, the nurse, Reinhold, could not remember that the women were asked for permission. She said there were no routines for asking.

the equipment. After a fetus had been taken out, it was put on a green cloth, and the opaque chorion was removed. In the beginning this was something that Joelsson or a nurse helped Nilsson with, but later he learned to do it himself. The veil-like amnion he often left in place—sometimes also the umbilical cord and the placenta. The embryo or fetus was immersed in the solution-filled tank, which was brought into the operating room. Light sources were placed so that they lit the tank from behind and from the sides, which gave a soft light with fewer reflections. In addition to black-and-white film, Nilsson used color film, which was in high demand by international picture magazines. If not too much time had passed, a certain amount of blood circulation remained in the bodies and was registered in the photographs.[56]

This rearrangement of the operating room at the women's clinic into a photographic studio was a prerequisite for the creation of the pictures that came to be included in "Drama of Life before Birth." The "space" that the embryos and fetuses were said to float in was not the inside of a body but a tank filled with water, and the details in the picture that resembled faraway stars and planets were bubbles in the water and particles from the placenta. Along with the color, the lighting and the water contributed to the pictures' soft, warm look. The fact that many embryos and fetuses still lay in their amnions and were seemingly anchored to the uterus by the umbilical cord strengthened the impression that they had been photographed inside the body.[57]

We see here why the human placenta is so prominent in "Drama of Life before Birth." The picture at the right of the "Spaceman" shows a placenta immersed in the water tank before one side of it was peeled off to make the embryo inside accessible.[58] In a separate section, under the heading "The Marvels of the Placenta," *Life*'s Albert Rosenfeld described it as "an extraordinary organ" whose "remarkable abilities" only recently had come to be appreciated by scientists. Without naming any individuals, Rosenfeld's reporting that the placenta, the fetus, and the mother formed a functional unit and that each participated in the production of hormones during pregnancy resembled the basic results of Westin's and Diczfalusy's perfusion studies.[59]

---

56   Joelsson and Reinhold, interviews with the author.

57   For a detailed analysis, see Jülich, *Photographing Life and Death.*

58   Nilsson and Rosenfeld, "Drama of Life before Birth," 65, available at https://books.google.co.uk/books?id=UVMEAAAAMBAJ&printsec=frontcover&source=gbs_ge_summary_r&cad=0#v=onepage&q&f=false (last accessed May 7, 2023).

59   Albert Rosenfeld, "The Marvels of the Placenta," *Life*, April 30, 1965, 73.

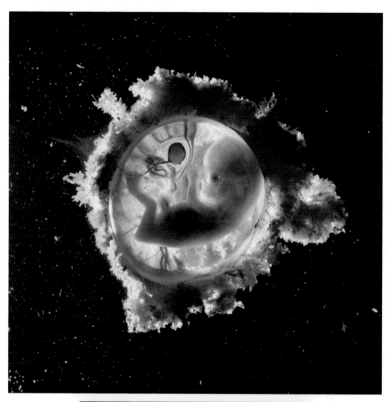

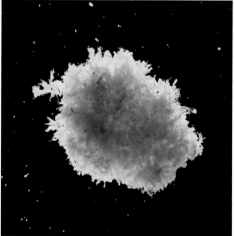

Figures 6.6 and 6.7. The picture on the top first appeared in *Life* in 1965 and was later dubbed the "Spaceman." Below is the placenta, which played a central role in the story. Photographs by Lennart Nilsson. Courtesy of Lennart Nilsson Photography/SPL.

According to Diczfalusy, the "fetoplacental empire" came to an end in the early 1970s, when prostaglandins were introduced in Sweden for the termination of pregnancy, which made hysterotomy "unethical."[60] However, the fall of the "empire" may equally have been an effect of increased public and parliamentary debates about fetal research both in Sweden and in the United States, where Sweden was often presented as a bad example. In addition, the conditions for performing perfusion studies on living fetuses changed when abortion on demand was introduced in 1975 and midterm abortions became less frequent.[61] At any event, Nilsson no longer had unlimited access to living, aborted fetuses for his photographs.

Reimagining Nilsson's Public Fetus

This chapter has addressed the misconceptions and lack of transparency surrounding Nilsson's photographs of human reproduction. The confusion of the in utero and ex utero images has inadvertently contributed to the mystifying—or indeed, the mythifying—of the photographer and his work. Moreover, to nuance the feminist criticism of the erasure of the maternal body from Nilsson's pictures, the woman on the cover of the 1965 issue of *Life* never disappeared, because she was never there. Or rather, the pregnant body was not erased from the pictures; she and the fetus had been separated at an earlier stage. The majority of Nilsson's images show ex utero embryos and fetuses from legal abortions.

Contrary to popular belief, Nilsson was not a scientist, and his images were only rarely published as elements of research articles in scientific journals. However, he collaborated with reproductive researchers who, at least initially, had expectations of the scientific use and value of the photographs they produced in partnership. After a certain time, they were frequently offered pictures for illustrative, educational, and marketing purposes or as gifts in the form of signed artworks.[62] Neither was Nilsson an inventor of scientific instruments or photographic lenses. He made enough money from selling the images in order to afford specially built endoscopes and exclusive wide-angle lenses. In addition, he hired technical and photographic experts who helped him improve existing instruments as well as supporting him with the handling of the equipment.

---

60   Diczfalusy, "My Life with the Fetal-Placental Unit," 2028. Prostaglandins later became a component of medical abortion. See Ramsey, *Swedish Abortion Pill.*

61   Jülich, "Historicizing Fetal Knowledge."

62   I elaborate on this in *Photographing Life and Death.*

Insights into the processes of photographic production also help to counteract the notion of a universal fetus. Key is the understanding of how Nilsson, always with his commercial interests in mind, creatively developed a stylistic repertoire for representing human life. First, he drew on a style from scientific, embryological imaging that depicted the developing embryo or fetus in isolation. But embryological specimens were dead and in fact looked dead. Thus, second, he used endoscopic instruments and wide-angle lenses to experiment with a style that offered (or simulated) circular views of bits of the living fetus in utero. However, the promise of photographing living embryos and fetuses inside the body was never fulfilled, for technical as well as ethical reasons. Third, he developed an innovative style that presented the ex utero living (or dying) fetus with the umbilical cord and the placenta. This last category can be seen in light of Diczfalusy's concept of the role of the fetus, the placenta, and the mother during pregnancy: the fetoplacental unit. Accordingly, what is featured on the *Life* cover is not so much the "Drama of Life before Birth" but rather the "Drama of the Fetoplacental Unit." This variation in visual style and trick effects demonstrates clearly that the universal, natural, and objective fetus is another myth that has been built around Nilsson's photographic work.

Paying attention to diversity of styles also helps to make sense of the social, cultural, and commercial flexibility of Nilsson's fetal pictures, including their contradictory uses in antiabortion campaigns and sex education in schools. Audiences have appreciated or dismissed images of fetuses in black-and-white or color, in bits or showing whole bodies, isolated or connected to the pregnant body, for a range of different reasons, thereby affecting the life courses of these representational styles. History shows that visual trends come and go but sometimes vanish. Some of the visual conventions and material that first inspired Nilsson—such as photographing embryological specimens—may seem outdated but have recently been revived through the advancement of digital technology.[63] Fetoscopic images have become ubiquitous in visual culture but are still showing only smaller parts of the fetus in the womb.[64] Pictures of the fetoplacental unit, on the other hand, were only possible to produce for a short period, at least in the style that drew from medical experiments on living fetuses. Nonetheless, representations of the fetus as an astronaut have become immensely popular. In various ways, this

---

63   As discussed by Lynn M. Morgan, the digitization of the Carnegie Human Embryo Collection has created a new "life" for these historical specimens. See Morgan, *Icons of Life*, 208–11.

64   Deborah Blizzard, *Looking Within: A Sociocultural Examination of Fetoscopy* (Cambridge, MA: MIT Press, 2007), chapter 3.

ambiguous imagery has shaped the visual culture of pregnancy and abortion from the 1960s onward.[65]

It seems ironic that Swedish medical research on aborted human fetuses aiming for new contraceptives and abortion methods came to be used—through the mediation of Nilsson's pictures—in support of antiabortion activism. But then again Diczfalusy never spoke of fetal "personhood." His claim was that the fetus, the placenta, and the mother interact as a functional unit, dependent on each other. Even if the pregnant body could not be included in the picture, the placenta is there, symbolizing the link to the living woman. The public fetus of Lennart Nilsson emerged from this feto-placental empire.

---

65 Carlyle and Callender, "The Fetus in Utero," 57. Also see the web exhibit "The Fetus in Utero," curated by Carlyle and Callender, University of Chicago, https://the-fetus-in-utero.rcc.uchicago.edu/ (last accessed August 23, 2022).

Chapter Seven

The Public Fetus in Franco's Spain

Women, Doctors, and Feminists in the Circulation of Pregnancy Images

María Jesús Santesmases

In Spain, the late 1960s saw the rise of the fetus as a living subject. Fetal images contributed to the creation of a visual culture of pregnancy associated with that of the fetus.[1] In the middle of Francisco Franco's dictatorship (1939–75), with censorship in force, women's rights erased, and the *pill* to be banned as a contraceptive, images of the inner pregnant body were received by government censors as medical content, and by publishers as an opportunity. Photographs of naked people were not allowed in magazines, newspapers, or books, but images of the naked unborn, as this chapter shows, circulated easily and widely in Spain. Their unimpeded distribution was due to the fact that such representations were included in books conceived, marketed, and regarded as scientific, medical information.

As messengers for this culture of representing pregnancy through fetal images, a group of pregnancy guides were published in Spain from 1963 onward, whose images coproduced what Barbara Duden has called the

1   Thanks to Lori Gerson for translation of an earlier and shorter version and to Joanna Baines for her English copyediting. Research for this chapter was funded by the Spanish Ministry of Science and Innovation (PID2019-106971GB-I00).

"public fetus."[2] Two of these books were translated into Spanish—Geraldine Lux Flanagan's *Los primeros nueve meses de la vida* (*The First Nine Months of Life*), from English, appeared in 1963, and Lennart Nilsson's pregnancy advice book *Un niño va a nacer* (*Ett barn blir till*), in 1967. *La madre que espera* (*The Expectant Mother*), edited by Spanish Catholic activist María Salas Larrazábal, was also published in 1967. And in the same year, feminist cartoonist Núria Pompeia issued her graphic guide to pregnancy, *9 Maternasis*, simultaneously in Spain and France. In it she acknowledged feelings of discomfort and astonishment as the belly grows, in contrast to the happy and tranquil pregnant women depicted in the books by Flanagan, Salas Larrazábal, and Nilsson. Pompeia's feminist awareness would counteract any romantic view of those scientifically and medically based pregnancy guides.

Focusing on these books, this chapter explores how fetal images circulated in Spain, from abroad and within. The processes of translation, publication, and distribution enable reflection on the circulation of visual cultures of pregnancy and the human fetus in Spain. As containers for images, these books were mobile depositories for the culture of the fetus, depositories of a visual culture of pregnancy.[3] This printed material is regarded here as having established a gendered visual epistemology of pregnancy—a naturalization of womanhood through motherhood. The popularization of the fetus entailed the disappearance of mothers and their bodies in three of these books, while one focuses exclusively on a woman's pregnant body. These two cultures, one focused on fetuses, and the other on the woman's body, demonstrate the open nature of these cultures of pregnancy. A plurality of cultures shared a particular period of time, the last third of the twentieth century, and circulated between political regimes—between Western democracies and Franco's dictatorship. These images bring the history of biology and biomedicine to successive political and cultural times and geographies, gendered precisely by practices regarding pregnancy and its visual cultures.[4] Following these new images of the photographed fetus from the United States and Sweden into

---

2   Barbara Duden, *Disembodying Women: Perspectives on Pregnancy and the Unborn*, trans. Lee Hoinacki (Cambridge, MA: Harvard University Press, 1993).

3   Inspired, and in discussion with, Robert Darnton, "'What Is the History of Books?' Revisited," *Modern Intellectual History* 4, no. 3 (2007): 495–508; Robert Darnton, "What Is the History of Books?," *Daedalus* 111, no. 3 (1982): 65–83.

4   This is insightfully displayed in chapter 12, this volume.

Spain through their reproduction in translated books, this chapter shows that they coexisted with feminist cultures that brought women's bodies fully into focus, as Pompeia's book does, placing the complete body of a pregnant woman and her feelings at the core of a pregnancy narrative.

By focusing on those narratives and reflecting on audiences—wide or restricted, women and society at large, censored in Spain under Franco's dictatorship yet reflecting a diversity of women's cultures—these twentieth-century fetal scenes can be followed through the circulation of images in journals and books. With this aim, the chapter first presents a reconstruction of the images included in Flanagan's and Nilsson's books and their Spanish translations; the political circumstances of such translations, intended to control the publication of books in a dictatorial regime; and the classification of these books and Salas Larrazábal's pregnancy guide as scientific works with implicitly nonpolitical contents.[5] The chapter also discusses Pompeia's work in the same decade as a contribution to a visual style of pregnancy. Pompeia's eloquent lines expressed a disconnect between her own experiences and these idealized discourses. Final reflections relate to the diversity of cultures of the public fetus era—pregnancy as a public and scientific event—the social life of whose imagery shows the coexistence of a feminist view and that of the medicalized unborn. Thus, a historical reconstruction of the circulation of fetal images in Spain is presented in a wider landscape, placing the public fetus in the context of the emergence of second-wave feminism in Pompeia's drawings and collages.

Pregnancy and Consumption in Franco's Dictatorship

The images in the books by Flanagan, Salas Larrazábal, and Nilsson are representations that evoke biology, a display of human embryology that moves from sperm to the fetus. The fetuses are shown in solitude, isolated, even though only a human presence could have made the portrait and witnessed the last few minutes of these premature births in motion.

Representations of pregnancy in Spain emerged not only from the clinic but also from the Catholic Church, and from the combination of these authorities with the dictatorship's repressive ideology. Novel medical

---

5   In addition to the historiography cited in the introduction to this volume, this chapter is inspired by Teresa Ortiz-Gómez and Agata Ignaciuk, "The Fight for Family Planning in Spain during Late Francoism and the Transition to Democracy, 1965–1979," *Journal of Women's History* 30, no. 2 (2018): 38–62; Agata Ignaciuk and Teresa Ortiz-Gómez, *Anticoncepción, mujeres y género: La "píldora" en España y Polonia (1960–1980)* (Madrid: Catarata, 2016).

technologies that could affect women and fertility were seen as technical developments, as long as they did not interfere with pronatalist policy.[6] The disciplining effect of obstetrics and gynecology, as Ann Oakley has termed it, played its part.[7] According to Teresa Ortiz and Agata Ignaciuk, the aim of the Franco regime's National Catholic ideology "was, on the one hand, to enhance natality in a country mutilated by the civil war and, on the other hand, to promote a gender regime in which women's bodies were symbolic and material sites for the reproduction" of the new Spanish nation.[8] As historian Aurora Morcillo has phrased it, women "would be saved by motherhood," as beings that reproduced without passion.[9] Franco's dictatorship offered women the opportunity to achieve salvation by becoming prolific mothers, in what Morcillo has termed a "nationalization of motherhood."[10] Women had an active role in this environment of absent freedom, at least from the dictatorship's second decade in the 1950s onward, as they managed their spaces in the new consumer society. At the suggestion of the regime's Sección Femenina (Women's section), which in its newsletter created a feature titled "Women Want to Work," single and married women left the home to become educated and contribute to household finances. Potential roles classified as female included—in addition to domestic work in their own or someone else's home—nursing, assisting in offices, laboratories, shops and schools, and journalism. These freedoms to consume and work outside the home, however, could never be allowed to oppose or obscure women's role as reproductive bodies.

In the 1960s Spanish social life, though developing economically, still took place under the practices imposed by the dictatorship over the previous decades. The population was able to keep abreast of lifestyles in Western consumer society, with cars, telephones, and household appliances of all kinds occupying public and private spaces and creating styles of clothing,

---

6   This was the case with the pill: Esteban Rodríguez-Ocaña, Agata Ignaciuk, and Teresa Ortiz-Gómez, "Ovulostáticos y anticonceptivos: El conocimiento médico sobre 'la pildora' en España durante el franquismo y la transición democrática (1940–1979)," *Dynamis* 32 (2012): 467–94.

7   Ann Oakley, *The Captured Womb: A History of the Medical Care of Pregnant Women* (Oxford: Basil Blackwell, 1984).

8   Ortiz-Gómez and Ignaciuk, "Fight for Family Planning," 38.

9   Aurora G. Morcillo, *The Seduction of Modern Spain: The Female Body and the Francoist Body Politics* (Lewisburg, PA: Bucknell University Press, 2010), 29. On "reproduction without passion," see Clare Hanson, *A Cultural History of Pregnancy: Pregnancy, Medicine and Culture, 1750–2000* (Basingstoke, UK: Palgrave Macmillan, 2004), 60.

10   Morcillo, *Seduction*, 155.

communication, and mobility.[11] Spanish society exhibited a double life. On the one hand, it was subjected to censorship practices by the Franco regime and inspired by images in official No-Do (acronym of Noticiario y Documentales) newsreel—compulsorily exhibited in cinemas before each screening. On the other hand, films, television, and tourism transmitted modernity from abroad.[12] This double-faced message was distributed throughout Spain by the publishers and distributors of the books analyzed in this chapter as pregnancy books, as if pregnancy itself were fully embedded in this consumer society while women were kept in a permanent condition of unemancipated minorhood.

Ex Utero Fetuses in Motion

Geraldine Lux Flanagan was a progressive woman, one of the founders of the International Childbirth Education Association in the United States, and an activist for informed pregnancies and births. Her book on the first nine months of life, published in 1962, was very popular in the United States.[13] Clear, informative, and targeted at young mothers and fathers who wished to know about "the growth of their baby" (as Flanagan wrote to feminist medical anthropologist Lynn Morgan), the book provided detailed information on developments occurring in a woman's uterus during pregnancy. The number of photographs included was unprecedented in this genre of publications, as was their quality. Flanagan preferred photographs of "living" fetuses, thereby avoiding pictures of those immersed in alcohol in so many anatomical museums. She contacted the neuroanatomist Davenport Hooker, who, with his colleague Tryphena Humphrey, studied "the prenatal function of the central nervous system in living aborted fetuses." The photographs Hooker provided came from experiments he had conducted with prematurely born fetuses, from miscarriages or "operations to conserve the lives of pregnant women."[14]

---

11   Morcillo, *Seduction*, 352.

12   Rosa M. Medina-Doménech and Alfredo Menéndez-Navarro, "Cinematic Representations of Medical Technologies in the Spanish Official Newsreel, 1943–1970," *Public Understanding of Science* 14, no. 4 (2005): 393–408.

13   Geraldine Lux Flanagan, *The First Nine Months of Life* (New York: Simon & Schuster, 1962). On Flanagan's biography and work for this book, see Lynn M. Morgan, *Icons of Life: A Cultural History of Human Embryos* (Berkeley: University of California Press, 2009), 197–204.

14   Morgan, *Icons of Life*, 197, and the quotation by Davenport Hooker on 199; Emily K. Wilson, "Ex Utero: Live Human Fetal Research and the Films of Davenport Hooker," *Bulletin of the History of Medicine* 88, no. 1 (2014):

Although books on the unborn had been published using photographs of embryos preserved in organic solvents, Flanagan's book was created with the intention of displaying live fetuses, at the height of the baby boom being experienced in Spain as in many other Western societies during this era of economic growth. The tiny bodies shown in the photographs were alive when filmed, just a few minutes before dying outside the womb.

The Spanish version of Flanagan's book was translated by María Luisa Borrás, an author of works on art history and a professor at the Autonomous University of Barcelona, who also translated novels and history books from English.[15] With a stated print run of five thousand copies and a second edition in 1967, the cover of the pocket-sized, paperback Spanish version has the title printed over the photograph of a sad-looking young woman in an advanced stage of pregnancy: brooding and in profile, she grasps the seat back with one hand (figure 1).[16] This photograph—the name of the photographer does not appear among the copyright holders—appears to suggest it is possible to alleviate any concerns a pregnant woman may have. The pregnant woman seems to have feelings about her condition.[17] She certainly looks unhappy, as if worried about the unknowns of being pregnant; the ignorance that produces such unhappiness appears to be taken for granted, and the biological details on the book's pages, it is implied, could alleviate her discontent. She is perhaps sad to be pregnant; such sadness is a challenging representation for the dictatorship's policy of promoting motherhood. This troubled woman could overcome her unhappiness with a scientific narrative of her unborn, the main agent of her pregnancy, or so the cover photograph suggests. Scientific photographs included in the book provide

132–60; Rosalind Pollack Petchesky, "Fetal Images: The Power of Visual Culture in the Politics of Reproduction," *Feminist Studies* 13 (1987): 263–92; Johanna Schoen, *Abortion after* Roe (Chapel Hill: University of North Carolina Press, 2015), chapter 2.

15 Geraldine Lux Flanagan, *Los nueve primeros meses de la vida*, trans. María Luisa Borrás (Barcelona: Seix y Barral, 1963). María Luisa Borrás is listed among authors and translators in the catalogue of the Biblioteca Nacional de España (Madrid).

16 See the application form submitted by the publishers of Flanagan's book in Spanish in Madrid, October 29, 1962; Archivo General de la Administración (General Archive of the Spanish Administration), Alcalá de Henares, Madrid. Fondo del Ministerio de Cultura, Delegación Nacional de Prensa, Propaganda y Radio (hereafter AGA), AGA 21/14219. On the Spanish censorship archives, see Daniel Gozalbo Gimeno, "Historia archivística de los expendientes de censura editorial," *Creneida: Anuario de literaturas hispánicas* 5 (2017): 8–34.

17 Petchesky, "Fetal Images," 277.

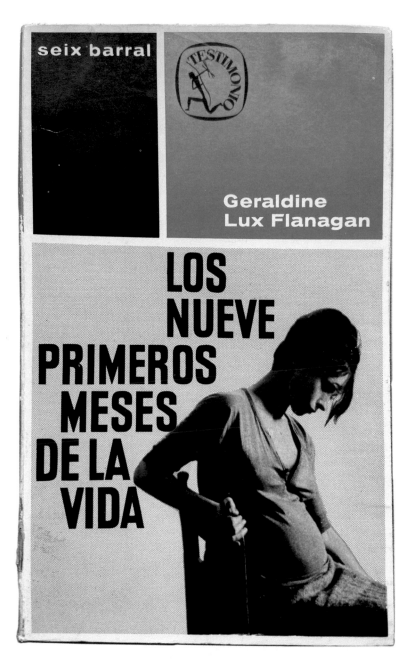

seix barral

Geraldine
Lux Flanagan

LOS
NUEVE
PRIMEROS
MESES
DE LA
VIDA

Figure 7.1. The cover of Flanagan's *Los nueve primeros meses de la vida*, trans. María Luisa Borrás (Barcelona: Seix y Barral, 1963).

certainty about embryological development and happiness to come, shown
by the four photographs of the mother's wide smile in the last chapter.

The Influence of Geraldine Lux Flanagan's Book

The contribution of Flanagan's book to the visual and narrative discourse on
pregnancy is reflected in the fact that some of the photographs within were
reproduced in a book published in 1967, edited by the Spanish Catholic
activist María Salas Larrazábal, with a second edition in 1971, under the title
La madre que espera (*The Expectant Mother*).[18]

A writer, essayist, and cofounder of the Seminario de Estudios sociológicos de la mujer (Seminar on women's sociological studies), created in
1960 in Madrid and led by feminist activist María Lafitte (also known as the
Countess of Campo Alange), Salas Larrazábal participated in the seminar's
studies on the changing situation of women in Spain. She is best known for
her book *Nosotras, las solteras* (*We Single Women*), published in 1959, which
asserts the visibility, respect, and recognition of women in this civil state.[19]
This Catholic and self-attributed feminism shows the variety of social and
cultural practices that existed under the dictatorship and were produced by
women in Spain at the time. Groups of middle- and upper-class women created networks to study and promote the presence of women beyond their
role as mothers and childhood educators. Many were already working outside the home, as did numerous other women from low-income families.[20]

Women and their bodies are fully in focus in *La madre que espera*, which
includes images of the developing embryo and fetus and is also a pregnancy
guide. A large, square, coffee-table book, thirty centimeters across and 169

18   Mary Salas [María Salas Larrazábal] ed., *La madre que espera* (Madrid:
      Alameda, 1967).
19   María Salas Larrazábal, *Nosotras las solteras* (Barcelona: Juan Flores Editor,
      1959); Begoña Barrera López, "El Seminario de Estudios Sociológicos
      de la Mujer (1960–1986): Investigación y reivindicación feminista del
      Tardofranquismo a la Transición," *Bulletin hispanique* 118 (2016): 611–28;
      Rosa M. Medina Doménech, *Ciencia y sabiduría del amor: Una historia cul-
      tural del franquismo (1940–1960)* (Madrid: Iberoamericana Vervuert, 2013);
      Rosa M. Medina-Doménech, "'Who Were the Experts?' The Science of Love
      vs. Women's Knowledge of Love during the Spanish Dictatorship," *Science as
      Culture* 23, no. 2 (2014): 177–200; Concha Borreguero et al., *La mujer espa-
      ñola: De la tradición a la modernidad (1960–1980)* (Madrid: Tecnos, 1986).
      On María Lafitte, see Begoña Barrera López, *María Laffitte: Una biografía
      intelectual* (Sevilla: Universidad de Sevilla, 2015).
20   Barrera López, "Seminario de Estudios Sociológicos," 614–15.

pages long, with hard red covers and white flyleaves, it was written by a team under the direction of Salas Larrazábal, with religious and medical guidance. Mentioned in the credits are a priest (José María Javierre), an illustrator (Asun Balzola), a designer (Francisco Izquierdo), a medical overseer (Francisco Bonilla, professor of gynecology at the University of Valencia), and the person recognized as the main medical source (José Botella Llusiá, professor of gynecology at the University of Madrid, and an academic authority on gynecology and medicine during the Franco regime).

The text deals with women's emotions and provides information about their bodies, genitals, and birth, as well as hygiene, nutrition, and psychology. In the second chapter, "The First Feeling of the Child," after drawings of female genitalia, a section on "Intrauterine Life" was included. It reproduced, without credit, five photographs from Flanagan's book.[21] The biopolitics of the body from Flanagan's book are incorporated into the tome by Salas Larrazábal.[22] The images are identical; only the captions vary slightly. The fetal biography is summarized from its first moments—"Human life begins when the male germ (sperm cell) penetrates into the egg"—to the ninth month, when the "housing" has become so small that the child can only turn on its side. These pages move from the body of a woman to embryology and fetal growth as a scientific-medical complement to the experience of pregnancy. "Human progenitor cells begin their union," and "after six days the fertilized egg, by successive divisions, has given rise to 150 cells"; in the third week, the "embryo is one millimeter long and hardly noticeable to the naked eye"; in the fifth month, "the mum clearly notes its movements," declare the captions to these reproduced photographs. Not one image of a fetus in motion from Flanagan's book was included, however.

The book by Salas Larrazábal, comprehensive, informative, accurate, and including clinical information, indicates the source of authority concerning gestation in its third chapter: "The best thing, go to the doctor."[23] The photographs, advice, and recommendations suggest the work is aimed at educated women, informed and curious, a similar audience to Flanagan's, although here a social and humanistic approach is taken. "Women are totally

---

21 Salas, *La madre que espera*, 20–21, includes six photographs identical to those in Flanagan, *Los nueve primeros meses de la vida*, 22, 34, 41. Salas Larrazábal's book attributes the image of a supposed nine-month fetus (21)—"the home has become so small that the baby can only turn to its side"—to an identical image in Flanagan (76), whose caption describes it as a fetus "at the beginning of the 5th month."

22 On the Franco dictatorship's biopolitics, see Salvador Cayuela Sánchez, *Por la grandeza de la patria: La biopolítica en la España de Franco* (Madrid: Fondo de Cultura Económica de España, 2014).

23 Salas, *La madre que espera*, 29.

fulfilled" by motherhood, the text declares; "Women without Children" are also addressed, under a separate heading.

The fact that some of the photographs from Flanagan's book are shown here may have arisen from the source of medical guidance. Flanagan's book is likely to have circulated among medical professionals as well as public audiences—a dozen copies are preserved in Spanish university libraries.[24] And the images it contains helped establish the visual culture of contemporary pregnancy, represented in the photographs of embryos and fetuses, in addition to women's bodies, bellies, and partners; the married couple is also displayed in Salas Larrazábal's book. The book situates fetal photographs within the political culture of the Franco regime, praising motherhood and emphasizing the need to overcome women's supposed ignorance regarding scientific facts and knowledge.

Nilsson's Photographs

In the United States in April 1965 *Life* magazine published an article, "Drama of Life before Birth," in which pregnancy was shown in a set of color images of embryos and fetuses throughout their development and up to birth.[25] Created by Swedish photographer Lennart Nilsson, the images were displayed as if a camera had been given access to a pregnant uterus, and in an order representing an embryo's development to the size and shape required for a healthy birth. Although all but one of these photographs were of dead fetuses, which Nilsson had photographed after miscarriages and surgical procedures, the images were presented as a depiction of ongoing life before birth, as the headline claimed.[26] The story and images were published in weekly newspapers in other countries: in France, *Paris Match* ran the article in April 1966, and in Spain, *Gaceta Illustrada* included it in one of its May issues in 1965 and in 1966. Nilsson also published a book of his photographs in 1965, accompanied by a text by Swedish doctors Claes Wirsén and

---

24   According to the catalogue of the Spanish network of University Libraries, REBIUN, https://rebiun.baratz.es/rebiun/search?q=Geraldine+Lux+Flanagan (last accessed April 25, 2023).

25   As is discussed in detail in chapter 12 in this volume, the main reference and inspiration concerning the visual cultures of the public fetus is Duden, *Disembodying Women*.

26   Solveig Jülich, "The Making of a Best-Selling Book on Reproduction: Lennart Nilsson's *A Child Is Born*," *Bulletin of the History of Medicine* 89, no. 3 (2015): 491–526; Solveig Jülich, "Picturing Abortion Opposition in Sweden: Lennart Nilsson's Early Photographs of Embryos and Fetuses," *Social History of Medicine* 31, no. 2 (2018): 278–307.

Axel Ingelman-Sundberg from the Karolinska Institute in Stockholm.[27] By that time, the Nobel Prizes, and the Karolinska Institute's authority within the committees responsible for selecting from the nominations, had garnered popularity and acclaim for both the awards and the institute.

The book was published in Spanish as *Un niño va a nacer*, translated by Juan Masoliver, in 1967 by Aymá (Barcelona) and slightly later the same year by Círculo de Lectores (Barcelona).[28] The jacket included the same photograph as the Swedish edition: a mother and a baby (figure 2). A picture of a fetus appears on the back cover. Women's bodies were absent. The fetal portraits, space age in appearance, have a dark background and inspired the shot of the fetus in Stanley Kubrick's *2001: A Space Odyssey*, which premiered in Spain in October 1968.[29] The immaculate little bodies portrayed by Nilsson in no way evoked the pain and suffering of delivery, either spontaneous or induced, or the blood lost by a mother during labor. These were new images in their coloring, precision, and cleanliness. Clean as steel tools, the images of embryos and fetuses glow like futuristic space technologies promising motherhood.

Censorship and Medicine

All publications—periodicals of any kind, books, and films—were controlled by censorship laws in Spain during the Franco dictatorship.[30] Until 1966,

---

27   Lennart Nilsson, Axel Ingelman-Sundberg, and Claes Wirsén, *Ett barn blir till: En bildskildring av de nio månaderna före födelsen: En praktisk rådgivare för den blivande mamman*, 1st Swedish ed (Stockholm: Bonnier, 1965).

28   Although I could not find definitive evidence, the translator could be the renowned Catalan intellectual Juan Ramón Masoliver, recognized for his translations of poetry and fiction. On his receiving the national award for translation in 1989, see Áurea Fernández Rodríguez, "El Premio Nacional a la Obra de un Traductor y el perfil de los premiados," *Transfer* 12 (2017): 29–55. AGA 21/18636, Expediente 10364; and AGA 21/18597, Expediente 9822.

29   On this analysis, situating the solitary fetus in the middle of a nowhere very similar to the night sky, see, in addition to Petchesky, "Fetal Images," Lynn M. Morgan and Meredith W. Michaels, eds. *Fetal Subjects, Feminist Positions* (Philadelphia: University of Pennsylvania Press, 1999); Scott F. Gilbert and Rebecca Howes-Mischel, "'Show Me Your Original Face Before You Were Born': The Convergence of Public Fetuses and Sacred DNA," *History and Philosophy of the Life Sciences* 26, no. 3–4 (2004): 377–94, 477–79. See also Hopwood's chapter and Jülich and Björklund's conclusion in this volume.

30   On the censorship archives during Franco's dictatorship, see J. Andrés de Blas, "El libro y la censura durante el franquismo: Un estado de la cuestión y otras

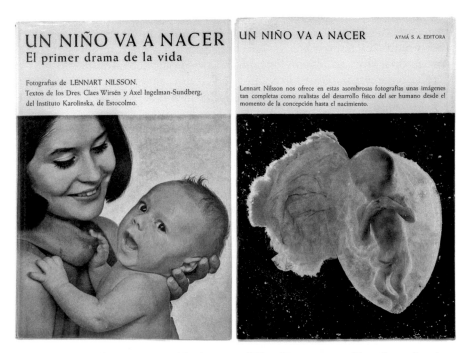

Figures 7.2 and 7.3. Front and back cover of *Un niño va a nacer* (Barcelona: Aymá, 1967). Courtesy of Lennart Nilsson Photography and Bonnier Rights.

material intended for publication had to be reviewed by a "reader" (the term coined for censors) from the Oficina de Orientación Bibliográfica (Office of bibliographic orientation) of the Ministerio de Prensa y Propaganda (Ministry of Press and Propaganda). From 1966 onward, all books underwent censorship control, either after printing, by being rejected by the censor and withdrawn from the market, or through self-censorship practiced by publishers and authors to avoid such a risk. "Readers" completed a form in which a manuscript's ideological values were evaluated to verify whether they respected "the dogma and moral requirements of the Catholic Church and its ministers," the political regime and its institutions, and the people who collaborated or had collaborated with the authorities. Even if the work as a whole was accepted, paragraphs could be removed if the censors recommended it.

consideraciones," *Espacio tiempo y forma: Serie V, Historia contemporánea* 12 (1999): 281–301; see also Gozalbo Gimeno, "Historia archivística."

In October 1962, the Spanish translation of Flanagan's book was presented in manuscript to the Ministerio de Prensa y Propaganda; it was approved in September 1963.[31] Classified under "scientific-technical works," this singular pregnancy guide was authorized for circulation.[32] With this brief statement, the review was completed without further explanation. The book was published by Barcelona's Seix Barral in 1963, the same year as the first British edition.[33]

Four years later, on December 4, 1967, the publishing house Aymá presented the book *Un niño va a nacer*, whose authors were listed as "Lennart Nilsson and others," to the same Oficina de Orientación Bibliográfica. Permission for publication was awarded two days later. Such swift evaluations were possible under the new law, which considerably shortened control and monitoring processes. A second edition with identical title and contents was presented on December 20 of the same year by the publisher Círculo de Lectores and, as the previous edition from Aymá had already been reviewed, accepted.

The book *Un niño va a nacer* was defined as "accepted" for circulation following its classification as "Obstetrics."[34] Describing its contents, the reader noted, "A vision in still images, in black and color, of the genetic process (*proceso genésico*), accompanied by the technical explanation, from fertilization to the days following childbirth, through the story of a couple and their reactions to the woman's pregnancy." In the following paragraph he added: "Publishable." This approval of texts taken as illustrated guides to pregnancy, with images classified as scientific and medical—obstetrics in this case—suggests that medicine and science were not regarded as challenging the political regime and motherhood; rather, they fully promoted pregnancy as a policy for women. Spain was not unique in its pronatalism, an attitude that was strong in many European countries from at least the 1930s.[35]

---

31   AGA 21/14219, Expediente 5816-62.

32   AGA 21/14219, qualified as "Obra científico-técnica" (scientific-technical book) in the report signed by the chief of the Sección de Circulación y Ficheros (Unit of Circulation and Files) of the Oficina de Orientación Bibliográfica.

33   Geraldine Lux Flanagan, *The First Nine Months of Life* (London: Heinemann, 1963). The book was reprinted in Britain at least five times up to 1978.

34   AGA 21/18636, Expediente 10364; and AGA 21/18597, Expediente 9822.

35   Gisela Bock and Pat Thane, introduction to *Maternity and Gender Policies: Women and the Rise of the European Welfare State*, ed. Gisela Bock and Pat Thane (London: Routledge, 1991), 12–13.

Circulation of Fetal Photographs

The two books written by Flanagan and Salas Larrazábal included fetal imagery in texts presented as guides for pregnancy. They prepared the cultural landscape for Nilsson's book. Distributed widely, first in Sweden and immediately thereafter in the United States and other Western countries, Nilsson's photographs gained immense international prominence.

In Spain, *Un niño va a nacer* was marketed by Círculo de Lectores, a publishing house created in 1962.[36] The number of copies of *Un niño va a nacer* declared to the Ministry of Press and Propaganda in December 1966 was ten thousand.[37] In 1969, Círculo de Lectores had more than half a million subscribers to its quarterly catalogue, composed of promotional texts about selected books that caught the eye like news items. Through this catalogue, which covered some 350 titles per year and was distributed by a network of agents throughout the country, Círculo stayed in contact with its subscribers. In 1970, Círculo de Lectores reached one million subscriptions. As a mail-order catalogue, the periodical dedicated its pages to successive new publications. Sales agents became instrumental in catalogue dissemination, and through personal contact with customers, they offered advice and provided chosen titles. In this way, those who lived in areas without bookstores or libraries could buy a certain number of books per year on a subscription basis. This payment ensured purchases, with customers selecting the titles that most grabbed their attention. Thus the composition, design, and color of some of the most eye-catching information was a major influence on customers attempting to get the most out of their subscription.

Un niño va a nacer was publicized on a full page in Círculo's catalogue in January 1968. From 1968 to the end of 1970, at least one fetal photograph was included in each catalogue, an intense three-year circulation of Nilsson's photographs among a high number of subscribers. Short texts promoting the book remained in the catalogue until 1978. Issues could be shared by entire households, so the actual circulation far exceeded the number of subscribers,

---

36 Círculo de Lectores was launched in 1962 as a publishing house co-owned by two other publishers: the German Bertelsmann and Spanish Vergara. Raquel Jimeno Revilla, "El proyecto artístico-cultural de Círculo de Lectores: La creación de un nuevo público lector" (PhD diss., Universidad Autónoma de Madrid, Facultad de Filosofía y Letras, 2015). Part of this dissertation has been published in Raquel Jimeno Revilla, *Círculo de Lectores: Historia y trascendencia de un proyecto cultural* (Buenos Aires: Ampersand, 2020). I am grateful to Raquel Jimeno for having shared her PhD dissertation materials with me.

37 AGA Box 21/18636, form submitted by Círculo de Lectores, Barcelona.

including people of all ages, from children to grandparents. Raquel Jimeno, author of a detailed and compelling historical reconstruction of Círculo de Lectores, remembers the "excitement when the catalogue arrived" at her home, always delivered by the publisher's agent.[38]

Under the (translated) title "The drama of the life that is born through the most wonderful series of photographs," a full-page promotion of Nilsson's book appeared with three photographs of fetal hand formation and an embryo inside its membrane. Given the spectacular nature of these images, which had never previously been seen in this new publishing market, the space occupied by Nilsson's fetal photographs must have had an effect on sales figures, not to mention the fact that a million subscribers saw them in 1970. Even if they did not select the book, they received the fetal photographs. Thus, the catalogue itself became an agent in the circulation of these images, participating in the cultures of the public fetus and making it more public than any other means of distribution.

From homes to public libraries, their dissemination suggests that Nilsson's fetal photographs became part of popular culture, at least for people with access to culture and books, in rural as well as urban settings. Successive editions sold this way can be found today in the catalogues of more than one hundred public libraries, in thirty-six universities, and seventy municipal libraries throughout Spain. Since many municipal and regional public libraries dispose of old collections and, in recent years, seldom-requested books to make room for new titles, it is reasonable to suggest that these copies have survived from a larger number that circulated in earlier decades.

The book's content, and everything that was absent from it, suited the rules imposed by the dictatorship, complementing its pronatalist policy during the years with the highest birth rates in Spain's history.[39] All of this illustrates the intensity with which a gendered order of things prioritizes, classifies, and represses.

These were the last few years of the dictatorship's Catholic Spain: many women still wore a veil in church, school classrooms were segregated by gender, and contraceptives were only permitted to regulate menstruation. In this environment, Nilsson's pristine fetal images could have been received

---

38   Jimeno Revilla, "El proyecto artístico-cultural," 1.

39   On its relation to early fetal cytogenetics, see María Jesús Santesmases, "Circulating Biomedical Images: Bodies and Chromosomes in the Post-eugenic Era," *History of Science* 55, no. 4 (2017): 395–430; María Jesús Santesmases, "Women in Early Human Cytogenetics: An Essay on a Gendered History of Chromosome Imaging," *Perspectives on Science* 28, no. 2 (2020): 170–200.

as evoking the purity of pregnancy and motherhood, an unusual display of clean bodies yet to be born. Evidence from the images took on immense explanatory power based on the authority that expert scientific knowledge enjoyed throughout the twentieth century, especially after World War II. In this way, a visual culture of pregnancy was naturalized. Construction of a fetal ontology put biomedical images of uterine gestation into circulation within a culture of gender representation, inserting women's bodies into contemporary reproductive policies.

Feminist Representations of Pregnancy and the Unborn

In 1967, the journalist and cartoonist Núria Pompeia (a pseudonym for Núria Vilaplana Buixons) published a portrait of pregnancy in her book *9 Maternasis*.[40] Unpaginated, *9 Maternasis* is made up of full-page drawings and collages. The images are drawn in simple black lines, the only color being the page background. Black contours show the features of a woman going through successive stages of her pregnancy until childbirth. The woman is alone on every page, always with her mouth covered by her hand or by an object in her hands, without text or any other characters: each page reflects a step, or stage, beginning with a tranquil scene in which she reads alongside a stack of books, a cup, and a coffeepot. Solitude is the main impression, accompanied, as the book progresses, by amazement at the growing belly and discomfort during a medical consultation on a stretcher. An expert in avoiding happy endings, Pompeia presents pregnancy as an invasive and disconcerting process: the protagonist appears stunned and silent. In 1968, the book inspired a four-minute animated film with the same title and story line.[41]

Pompeia is also considered a pioneer feminist in feminist graphic art.[42] From the late 1960s onward, she collaborated in the earliest feminist

40 Núria Pompeia, *9 Maternasis* (Barcelona: Kairós; Paris: Pierre Tisné, 1967).

41 Jan Baca and Toni Garriga, *Maternasis* (1968), animation by Marga Llauradó and Ana María Serrahima, YouTube, https://www.youtube.com/watch?v=bicbvv-CgOQ&t=8s (accessed October 18, 2021).

42 On Pompeia, see Claudia Jareño and Anne-Claire Sanz-Gavillon, "Dibujar el feminismo: la obra temprana de Núria Pompeia," *Filanderas: Revista interdisciplinar de estudios feministas* 3 (2018): 59–76; María Teresa Arias Bautista, "El humor feminista de Nuria Pompeia," *Más igualdad, redes para la igualdad: Congreso Internacional de la Asociación Universitaria de Estudios de las Mujeres* (Seville: Arcibel, 2012), 21–32.

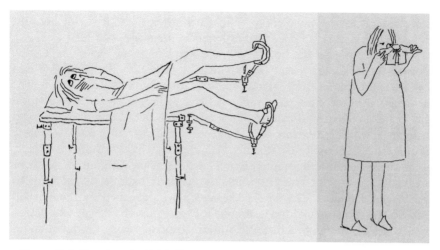

Figure 7.4. Drawings by Núria Pompeia, *9 Maternasis* (Barcelona: Kayrós; Paris: Pierre Tisné, 1967). Reproduced with permission kindly granted by Núria Pompeia's heirs.

periodicals and initiatives such as associations and cultural programs, while her cartoons were published by progressive magazines. The pages dedicated to labor and birth are represented in black with no drawings, thus suggesting not only a dark space—a metaphor for the lack of public images and knowledge about childbirth—but also a dark, difficult, perhaps painful time in her own life. Throughout the book, it is the fully expressive eyes that reveal this woman's feelings. Collages are introduced to reflect either wishes or fears: cut-outs of a superman, a saint, Einstein's formula $E = mc^2$, are pasted on the woman's womb. On the final page, the head of a crying newborn is pasted by the woman's bedside; her eyes look surprised by this presence.

The hand that covers the protagonist's face in every page expresses the silence of the book itself, which, with its visual style, counteracts any romantic visions of pregnancy disseminated elsewhere, including the guides by Flanagan, Salas Larrazábal, and Nilsson. Pompeia's eloquent line drawings express the discrepancies with these idealized discourses. Such romantic images are also embodied in the biomedicine of pregnancy: as Emily Martin has insightfully demonstrated, the encounter between egg and sperm has been conceptualized as a love story.[43] By contrast, Pompeia's book does not

43   Emily Martin, "The Egg and the Sperm: How Science Has Constructed a Romance Based on Stereotypical Male-Female Roles," *Signs: Journal of Women*

represent any love or coupledom; no partner appears, and it is only her solitary self, reflected in her eyes, that experiences pregnancy and birth.

When working on the book, Pompeia was reading *Le Deuxième Sexe* by Simone de Beauvoir, while *The Feminine Mystique* by Betty Friedan and *La dona a Catalunya* by Maria Aurèlia Capmany were in circulation.[44] Pompeia's own reconstruction suggests her drawings were generated within this feminist climate and culture of the late 1960s, when feminism emerged in Spain, at least in some intellectual and social circles, during this late decade of the long, repressive dictatorship.[45] Pompeia's visual narrative counteracted the message promoted and circulated by Franco regime policies for pregnancy, birth, and very large families (a yearly national award went to the biggest families). This book, like later ones published by the Catalan cartoonist (who attended the well-known Escola Massana for art and design in Barcelona), brings together the author's experiences as a woman and a mother.[46] Pompeia's drawings challenge the gendered social order by representing the suffering it produced for women. Her humoristic cartoon drawings were "a defense in the face of an aggressive world, of the bad and the unpleasant . . . a weapon, not an attack weapon but a defense against how stupid, terrible, and grotesque the world could be."[47] Together with

in Culture and Society 16, no. 3 (1991): 485–501.

44   Jarreño and Sanz-Gavillon, "Dibujar el feminism," 60. It is highly likely that she read Simone de Beauvoir's book in French, or the first Spanish translation published in Buenos Aires, Argentina (Leviatán), in 1952, and in Mexico, in 1965 (Siglo XXI), or she maybe knew about the Catalan translation to be published in 1968 (Edicions 62). See Isabel Morant, "Lecturas de 'El segundo sexo' de Simone de Beauvoir," *Descentrada* 2 (2018): e053; and Gloria Nielfa Cristóbal, "La difusión en España de El segundo sexo, de Simone de Beauvoir," *Arenal. Revista de historia de las mujeres* 9 (2002): 151–62.

45   For early testimonies and studies of feminism in Spain at the time, see Geraldine Scanlon, *La polémica feminista en la España contemporánea* (Madrid: Akal, 1976); Monica Threlfall, "The Women's Movement in Spain," *New Left Review* 151 (May/June 1985): 44–74.

46   Jareño and Sanz-Gavillon, "Dibujar el feminismo," 64.

47   Juan José Navarro Arisa, "La seriedad de dos humoristas gráficos. Nuria Pompeia y Quino han publicado dos nuevos libros," *El País*, April 25, 1983, https://elpais.com/diario/1983/04/25/cultura/420069615_850215.html (last accessed May 27, 2023). Quoted in Arias Bautista, "El humor feminista," 21.

her husband, she founded the publishing house Kayrós, which produced *9 Maternasis* and Pompeia's later feminist cartoons.[48]

Published simultaneously in France by Pierre Tisné, *9 Maternasis* was reviewed by the French weekly *L'Express*. Barcelona daily *La Vanguardia* associated it with the author's husband, Salvador Pániker, and with a combination of humor and tenderness stripped the book of its criticist tone.[49] Pompeia later published full-page vignettes from the Metamorphosis series in the weekly *Triunfo*, criticizing the state of society and the economy at the end of the Franco regime. She also published other books in which she developed her critical vision of fantasies relating to marriage and women's lives: *Y fueron felices comiendo perdices* (1971), *Por los siglos de los siglos* (originally in Catalan, 1971), *Mujercitas* (1972), and with Manolo V el Empecinado (a pseudonym for the well-known writer and journalist Manuel Vázquez Montalbán), *La educación de Palmira* (1975). Pompeia drew for many other critical and humorous periodicals, contributing to the Spanish feminist movement of the late 1960s, which operated outside—or rather, against—the official culture. During the last years of the dictatorship, many publications included texts in which criticism of the absence of freedom could be read between the lines, which, at times, was tolerated.

Pompeia's trajectory is representative of feminism during the late Franco regime. By including her book among its examples, this chapter shows the diversity of discourses and practices by women for women in the last decade of the dictatorship. Science and feminism appeared as mutually challenging, even if avoiding any direct confrontation—two strategies that coexisted in social and women's cultures in Spain at the time.

Circulation of the Public Fetus and Its Cultures: Scientific Images, Romantic Love, Feminism

Preceding ultrasound fetal images displayed on the screen and page, the public fetus analyzed by Barbara Duden joined a culture of pregnancy focused on an image of promise, a child-to-be. While women's bodies have come in and out of focus within the social cultures of pregnancy, the unborn has had a starring role in the emotional, physical, and medical knowledge of

---

48 Claudia Jareño and Anne-Claire Sanz Gavillon, "Núria Pompeia: Metamorfosis de una obra (1967–1985)," *Otras miradas, voces y formas de la creación feminista desde los años 60 en el Estado español*, ed. Claudia Jareño Gila and Anne-Claire Sanz Gavillon (Manresa: Bellaterra, 2021), 65–90, 70.

49 Jareño and Sanz-Gavillon, "Dibujar el feminismo," 65.

pregnancy from the 1960s onward, in Spain as, at least, in Western Europe and North America. It was the practice and circulation of fetal photography that stabilized the unborn as a medical and cultural subject. The images that became cultures of the public fetus circulated in books, and thus the travels of these cultures were also those of books. This chapter has presented four such books, authored by three women and a man, one of them a cartoon of pregnancy without fetal images. The four books were contemporaneous, published in Spain between 1963 and 1967. The work by the American science writer Geraldine Lux Flanagan includes stills from films of newly aborted fetuses, alive and moving ex utero. The collection edited by the Spanish Catholic activist María Salas Larrazábal includes a few of the same photographs, reflecting their impact: it appears that a book on pregnancy could no longer avoid including this kind of image. The work of the photographer Lennart Nilsson and doctors from the Karolinska Institute, Axel Ingelman-Sundberg and Claes Wirsén, circulated in Spain not only as a book but in the newsletter catalogue distributed by its publishers. The cartoon by Núria Pompeia exhibits, by contrast, a personal feminist history of emotions and anxieties, a woman feeling alone throughout her pregnancy.

The texts in the books by Flanagan, Salas Larrazábal, and Nilsson are thorough and detailed, and include the most current knowledge on reproductive biology at that time. Their key contribution was photography. Evaluated by the censors as medical content, the images adapted to the values of decency, marriage, and love as rites and prerequisites for gendered behaviors, both public and private. As precise and extremely clean descriptors of the process of motherhood, visual evidence transformed pregnant women into biology and, as biology invaded the feeling of the body awaiting a child, culture and biology exchanged meanings. The result of this exchange was the representation of pregnancy as a scientific fetal biography.[50] Biology became evidence, replacing the mother as a source of identity and representation of gestation. Added to the biologization of this process were scientific explanations, instructions on food, drinks, medicines, and the feelings of pregnant women themselves, adapting to what Salas Larrazábal called the "living space" of the fetus. The fetus, as it begins to grow, undergoes uterine constraints and prepares to leave, endowed with autonomous will in respect to the physiology of the maternal body.

The circulation of the images in these books is shown by their existence in library catalogues even today: Nilsson's is the most widely distributed in public libraries, while those by Salas Larrazábal and Flanagan can now be

---

50   Pregnancy as a fetal biography is suggested by many feminist authors, including Petchesky, "Fetal Images"; Schoen, *Abortion after* Roe; Wilson, "Ex Utero."

found only in Spain at the Biblioteca Nacional de España (Spanish national library) in Madrid. Pompeia's book is available in some public libraries, and the state of the copy I borrowed suggests it has been read often: it is not well preserved. Out of print for many years, it was republished in 2021 by Kayrós.

This chapter has shown how fast and easily images circulated in books, from the United States and Sweden into Spain, once approved by the dictatorship's censors, who regarded Flanagan's as "scientific" and Nilsson's to be on "obstetrics." Of the two books produced in Spain, the one edited by Salas Larrazábal was the product of consensus between a set of contributors—among them, a gynecologist, a priest, and a medical reviewer—coordinated by a Catholic activist for some women's rights. Pompeia's book on pregnancy is solely about a woman, the changes in her pregnant body, and her states of mind, including surprise, anxieties, and fears about the future of what she carries within her womb. These images have been preserved by the books that contain them, in libraries and their catalogues: in this respect, Nilsson's has attracted the most public attention and recognition regarding its agency in manufacturing the public fetus.

No matter the political regime, whether the democracies in the United States and Sweden, or the dictatorship of Spain, these fetal images and the books that contained them circulated widely across time and geography. This culture of woman-meaning-mother has made pregnancy an event that unveils women through a social epistemology fully focused on the child-to-be. As part of the same culture, fetal photographs fit effortlessly in a conception of women's bodies as the transitory spaces of any lineage. Even if they were "of Woman born," to retrieve the influential feminist text by Adrienne Rich, all fetal images analyzed here originally appeared as solo portraits, as if these tiny bodies at some point floated in the universe as autonomously clean, pure bodies to be received or observed as a dramatic twentieth-century biological scene.[51] Such selective visual cultures have been described by feminist studies as belonging to a long-standing patriarchy and its visual social epistemology.[52]

---

51 Adrienne Rich, *Of Woman Born: Motherhood as Experience and Institution* (New York: Norton, 1976); Lynn M. Morgan, "A Social Biography of Carnegie Embryo no. 836," *Anatomical Record Part B: The New Anatomist* 276 (2004): 3–7.

52 From Rich, *Of Woman Born*, and Elisabeth Badinter, *L'amour en plus: Histoire de l'amour maternel, XVIIe–Xxe siècle* (Paris: Flammarion, 1980), to more recent works, such as Gloria A. Franco Rubio, ed., *Maternidades desde una perspectiva histórica* (Barcelona: AEIHM-Icaria, 2019), a whole historiography of maternity and maternal love has been joined by Marga Vicedo, *The Nature*

As this starring role for the fetus emerged, it coexisted with a burgeoning feminist approach to pregnancy that placed women at the core. This feminist culture openly regarded pregnancy as a time of astonished anxiety and birth as a painful event to be represented in black, followed by the company of a newborn. Books are taken here as agents in the circulation of fetal cultures of pregnancy as well as feminist cultures of women's bodies. As the contents of the group of books analyzed here show, the public fetus also belongs to a wider culture of pregnancy and women, one that includes women's perceptions of their own bodies as knowledge and as practices of representation.

---

and Nurture of Love: From Imprinting to Attachment in Cold War America (Chicago: University of Chicago Press, 2014), among many others.

Chapter Eight

Visual Strategies of Antiabortion Activism and Their Feminist Critique

The Public Fetus in the United States

Nick Hopwood

There is reason to doubt the common assumption that the Swedish photographer Lennart Nilsson's pictures in *Life* magazine took the fetus public in 1965.[1] On the one hand, audiences of millions had long seen images of human embryos and fetuses, and political argument already invoked the unborn.[2] On the other, the term "public fetus" appeared in print only in 1987, when the political scientist Rosalind Petchesky coined it in the journal *Feminist Studies.* Invoking the art critic John Berger's distinction between "public photographs" and those "which belong to private experience," Petchesky expressed concern that the exploitation of Nilsson's photos and of ultrasonography in the antiabortion activism of the New Right could "obstruct or harass an abortion decision" as sonograms became routine.

---

1   I thank the editors for the opportunity and their support, and Silvia De Renzi, Solveig Jülich, Jesse Olszynko-Gryn, and two anonymous press readers for comments on drafts.

2   Tatjana Buklijas and Nick Hopwood, *Making Visible Embryos* (online exhibition), 2008–10, http://www.hps.cam.ac.uk/visibleembryos/ (last accessed May 27, 2023); Natasha Zaretsky, *Radiation Nation: Three Mile Island and the Political Transformation of the 1970s* (New York: Columbia University Press, 2018), 36–43.

She warned activists and scholars of "the power of visual culture in the politics of reproduction."[3]

Petchesky wrote after what she called "a decade of fetal images," though she found "the earliest appearance of these photos in popular literature" in 1962. Her essay catalyzed cross-disciplinary scholarship on a category previously limited to obstetrics and to commentary on art.[4] Historians have worked since then to extend the timeline in an appropriate way. Certain features of the public fetus can be found in the eighteenth century, notably the illusion of growth independent of a pregnant body. But the phenomenon in the strict sense can best be understood as beginning in a set of extraordinarily politicized episodes within a long revolution in visualizing human origins before birth.[5]

A large European "family" of unborn entities is usually presented as having been reduced to serial representations of progressively more advanced embryos and fetuses—and embryological visions did become dominant in ways no premodern one ever was. Yet even moderns have worked to bring "egg," "embryo," "fetus," "abortus," "miscarriage," "products of conception," "fruit," "malformation," and "baby" together, or to keep them apart. The antiabortionist icon stands out among these subjects and objects for the power with which it projects onto earlier stages an autonomous, rights-bearing already-baby. Two who made it potent, John and Barbara Willke of the US National Right to Life Committee, advised allies "never, never use the word 'fetus,'" which "pro-abortionists" had cast as a "non-human glob." The Willkes acknowledged "fetus" as "the proper medical term," but wrote that "if you are convinced that this is a human life, . . . speak of the 'unborn,'

3   Rosalind Pollack Petchesky, "Fetal Images: The Power of Visual Culture in the Politics of Reproduction," *Feminist Studies* 13, no. 2 (1987): 263–92, on 280–81, 285. The article expanded a chapter that appeared under the same title in Michelle Stanworth, ed., *Reproductive Technologies: Gender, Motherhood and Medicine* (Cambridge: Polity Press, 1987), 57–80.

4   Petchesky, "Fetal Images," 268; Lynn M. Morgan and Meredith W. Michaels, eds., *Fetal Subjects, Feminist Positions* (Philadelphia: University of Pennsylvania Press, 1999).

5   Barbara Duden, "Anatomie der guten Hoffnung. Darstellungen des Ungeborenen bis 1799," Habilitationsschrift, Universität Hannover, 1993; Duden, "Zwischen 'wahrem Wissen' und Prophetie. Konzeptionen des Ungeborenen," in *Geschichte des Ungeborenen. Zur Erfahrungs- und Wissenschaftsgeschichte der Schwangerschaft, 17.–20. Jahrhundert*, ed. Duden, Jürgen Schlumbohm, and Patrice Veit (Göttingen: Vandenhoeck & Ruprecht, 2002), 11–48; Buklijas and Hopwood, *Making Visible Embryos*; for a survey focused on the law: Sara Dubow, *Ourselves Unborn: A History of the Fetus in Modern America* (New York: Oxford University Press, 2011).

'pre-born,' or 'developing child' or 'baby.'"[6] To write, rather, of the public fetus is to encompass the weaponizing of medical images against abortion-law reform and feminist critiques of that strategy.

This chapter critically synthesizes the literature on fetal images, including analyses scattered through general histories of abortion, in light of my own research on visualizing human development. I thus place the public fetus—the visuals and their rejection—in a long-term history of imaging prenatal life that pays the powers of series special attention. Ordering pictures of embryos and fetuses that died at various times created the illusion (not necessarily a deception) that viewers were seeing a single organism developing from one stage to the next. The public fetus subverts developmental series with its essential feature, an insistence that earlier stages represent a baby endowed with rights. I analyze how this was done through tactics including backward viewing of the series and focusing on a single fetal stage; generating the effect of life and contrasting this with death; selecting anticipations of the final form; and, not least, magnification and removing connections to the pregnant body. All have precedents, but brought together in antiabortionism produced a new entity that a political movement made influential.[7] I focus on the fetus because the role of in vitro fertilization in publicizing early embryos is another huge story; on the United States because the phenomenon has mattered most in America's abortion wars and their shaping of global reproductive health care; and on the period since World War II because that is when images of living fetuses went public.

The debut of neither the public fetus nor sexual liberation can be dated quite so precisely as in the English poet Philip Larkin's claim that "Sexual intercourse began / In nineteen sixty-three / (which was rather late for me)," but if much was already there around 1950, a great deal would change in the following tumultuous decades.[8] Visual innovation in representing

---

6   Dr. and Mrs. J. C. Willke, *How to Teach the Pro-Life Story* (Cincinnati, OH: Hayes, 1975), 25.

7   I take approach and material from my book manuscript, *The Embryo Series: Seeing Human Development Before Birth*; for previous work along similar lines: Nick Hopwood, "Producing Development: The Anatomy of Human Embryos and the Norms of Wilhelm His," *Bulletin of the History of Medicine* 74 (2000): 29–79; Hopwood, *Embryos in Wax: Models from the Ziegler Studio* (Cambridge: Whipple Museum of the History of Science, 2002); Buklijas and Hopwood, *Making Visible Embryos*; Hopwood, "A Marble Embryo: Meanings of a Portrait from 1900," *History Workshop Journal* 73 (Spring 2012): 5–36; Hopwood, *Haeckel's Embryos: Images, Evolution, and Fraud* (Chicago: University of Chicago Press, 2015).

8   Larkin is quoted in Simon Szreter, "Victorian Britain, 1831–1963: Towards a Social History of Sexuality," *Journal of Victorian Culture* 1, no. 1 (1996): 136–49, on 139.

the unborn came out of the intersections of the medical management of human procreation and the communications industry.[9] Novelty had once been driven by anatomy collaborating with obstetrics and gynecology, the industrialization of printing, the reinvention of wax modeling, and the rise of exhibitions. Now it was produced where the medicalization of reproduction—increasing antenatal surveillance, abortion-law reform and controversy, more sex education—relied on a visual turn involving color photography, television, video, and sonography. The crucial postwar shift was from drawings and models of dead specimens to photos, films, and scans of fetuses that were alive, or were claimed to be, and then that might develop into babies. Mobilized in welfare reform, workplaces, and clinics, and above all in the backlash against liberalization of the antiabortion laws, as well as in a reevaluation of miscarriage, the images became intensely personal as well as extraordinarily public. In part as a result of these transformations, readers may find some of the practices I discuss to be disturbing.

The antiabortionist fetus became entrenched in conservative milieux as it shaped policy, experience, and identity from before *Roe v. Wade* (1973), the US Supreme Court decision that generalized abortion rights, to *Dobbs v. Jackson Women's Health Organization* (2022), which repealed this protection. Yet that fetus never swept all before it. Mainstream representations have provided alternatives, while abortion providers have challenged their opponents' gaze even in clients' preabortion viewing of sonograms and postabortion viewing of fetal remains. A long-term view makes it possible to grasp the power of the public fetus and to recognize its limits.

"The First Generation . . . to Have a Clear Picture"

Images of developing embryos and fetuses came to stand for the course of a pregnancy when nineteenth-century anatomists and artists used material collected from miscarrying and aborting women, from postmortems, and later also from gynecological operations, to construct developmental series that ever wider audiences saw in books, museums, and magazines. In the process, clumps in blood, interpreted by the women who passed them as either waste material or children to come, were reframed as embryos and fetuses. Turned into vivid pictures and arranged in series of incrementally

<hr>

9   On reproduction: Nick Hopwood, Rebecca Flemming, and Lauren Kassell, eds., *Reproduction: Antiquity to the Present Day* (Cambridge: Cambridge University Press, 2018); on communication: Nick Hopwood, Peter Murray Jones, Lauren Kassell, and Jim Secord, "Introduction: Communicating Reproduction," *Bulletin of the History of Medicine* 89, no. 3 (2015): 379–405.

more advanced preparations, they were taken out of narratives of health, illness, and pregnancy loss and used to convey the effect of development. The most heated image wars were sparked by tendentious comparisons of vertebrate embryos, their early similarity evidencing the claim that humans evolved from other animals. Early twentieth-century campaigns for maternal health, infant welfare, and birth control made embryos and fetuses still more visible.[10] Progress was the dominant theme, though symbolist artists used the fetus as a (misogynist) symbol of procreative and creative failure. As pregnancy became a respectable conversation topic, books, charts, models, and wet specimens took embryos and fetuses to the first mass audience. World's fairs staged large-scale, public, family viewing in the 1930s in the United States. After 1945 images of human development entered schools on a significant scale, especially through coy sex-education films.[11]

By this time the center of research in human embryology, the Carnegie Department at Johns Hopkins University in Baltimore, was promoting Chester Reather's "amazing photographs" in picture-led, ad-heavy magazines. In "How Life Begins," in McGraw-Hill's short-lived *Science Illustrated*, recently described monkey material stood in for the earliest stages, still unseen in humans. At seven days after fertilization "perhaps the earliest human embryo ever photographed" came from an ongoing program that would be deemed unethical today: collecting specimens from the first two weeks of development from patients who had charted their periods and had sex at known times before clinically indicated hysterectomies. The series continued to the tenth week and another focused on "development of the embryo foot" (figure 8.1). Photos of mother and baby and obstetrician and baby bookended the story, but those of embryos and fetuses were here, as often though by no means always, isolated from pregnant bodies, let alone the larger processes of reproduction.

The most important magazine was *Life*, the optimistic, progressive, corporate portraitist of the United States and its place in the world to urban

---

10   Hopwood, "Producing Development"; Hopwood, *Embryos in Wax*; Buklijas and Hopwood, *Making Visible Embryos*; Hopwood, *Haeckel's Embryos*.

11   Buklijas and Hopwood, "Visual Culture" and "Rationalizing Reproduction," *Making Visible Embryos*, http://www.sites.hps.cam.ac.uk/visibleembryos/s4_3.html and http://www.sites.hps.cam.ac.uk/visibleembryos/s4_4.html; Rose Holz, "The 1939 Dickinson-Belskie Birth Series Sculptures: The Rise of Modern Visions of Pregnancy, the Roots of Modern Pro-Life Imagery, and Dr. Dickinson's Religious Case for Abortion," *Journal of Social History* 51, no. 4 (2018): 980–1022; Lara Freidenfelds, *The Myth of the Perfect Pregnancy: A History of Miscarriage in America* (New York: Oxford University Press, 2020), chapter 4; "Sex Education," *Life*, May 24, 1948, 55–62.

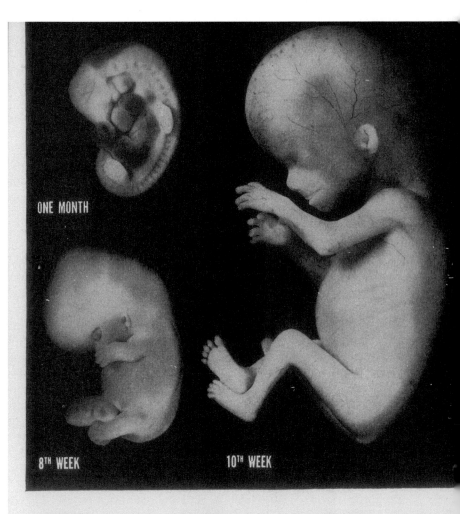

ONE MONTH

8TH WEEK

10TH WEEK

ONE MONTH

Here is Reather's close-up of the 28-day embryo shown on the preceding page. The buds protruding from the side of the body will soon become arms and legs. The bulbous organ around which the head and neck appear to be wrapped is the heart, which at this stage protrudes from the body. In the neck can be seen four bronchial grooves, reminiscent of the gill slits of a fish; these and other similarities between the human embryo and embryos of other animals are among the most striking evidence that we have in support of the theory of evolution.

8TH WEEK

Now unmistakably human, the embryo is almost an inch in height. The head still comprises nearly half the total bulk. The toes and fingers are still webbed. But facial rudiments, arms and legs, hands and feet are all clearly formed. Note that limb buds have rotated a full 90 degrees from their retracted position at one month. (For more about hands and feet, see opposite page.) Within, the nervous system is developing rapidly; lung bulbs have begun to grow, and liver is just getting started at its task of manufacturing red blood cells.

10TH WEEK

The embryo has taken on most of the external appearance of a human baby, and is now called a fetus. The legs can kick. The blood vessels in the head are clearly visible through the still transparent "skin" of the fetus. Months must elapse before the fetus is ready to be born; but these months are occupied primarily in growth in size and in the further development of internal organs. But as even the naked eye can see in this remarkable photograph, a single cell has changed almost into a baby in ten short weeks.

18

Figure 8.1. Spread of photos by Chester Reather of the Carnegie Department of Embryology from "How Life Begins." We see development from one month to the tenth week, by which time "a single cell has changed almost into a baby,"

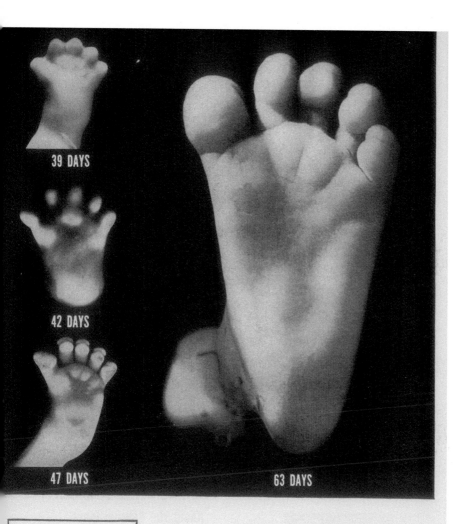

39 DAYS

42 DAYS

47 DAYS

63 DAYS

DEVELOPMENT OF THE EMBRYO FOOT

These photographs show that the embryo does more than merely grow, for with its enlargement new organs appear and begin to take form.

All four limbs start as simple buds of tissue which protrude from the side of the trunk; an arm is indistinguishable from a leg except by position. As the buds grow, the shape of the limb emerges, and by the sixth week the digits are seen as small bumps at the end of the limb.

But hand and foot are still very similar. In the next weeks, as the limbs grow, the hands develop long, strong fingers, while the toes of the foot remain the rather undeveloped digits that they are in man. Instead, the foot develops a long arch of bones between heel and toes, and by the ninth week has its characteristic shape.

Later, the finer details emerge, and in the tenth week toenails develop from thickened areas of skin on the toes. The foot is by now well formed; later fetal stages involve only the hardening of the bones. Architecturally, it is already designed to support great weight, foreshadowing its future task of carrying a full-grown human being.

and of the foot from 39 to 63 days. The previous spread covered the not-yet-fertilized egg to 28 days. Halftones from *Science Illustrated* 1, no. 4 (July 1946): 18–19.

and suburban, middle-class, largely White America. In 1950 a photo-essay began with Reather's prize-winning photo of a forty-day Carnegie embryo and more results of that daring collecting program. The pictures were still opaque, anatomical, and black-and-white; the next pages in this series even included fetal skeletons from the University of California. But soon *Life* featured photos by the gynecologist Landrum Shettles that claimed to show human fertilization and "the actual process of life at the earliest stage ever observed."[12]

In 1962 this photojournalism was consolidated by "Dramatic Photographs of Babies before Birth" in *Life*'s rival *Look*, and the book this advertised, former *Life* reporter Geraldine Lux Flanagan's *The First Nine Months of Life*. The pages were modern, with large black-and-white photos bled to the edge and set off with blank space. The claim to novelty was bold: "We are the first generation . . . to have a clear picture of the course of our development from a single cell to an individual, active, and responsive to our environment long before birth. We are . . . the first to know the full history of our earliest hours and days."[13]

Lack of direct evidence for the first two weeks had not stopped countless depictions of human development over the previous century and a half; chicks and domestic mammals often stood in. As much as new sights, change was about heightened demand for photos, which embryologists had begun producing in the late nineteenth century. Flanagan's book included four main kinds: Shettles's pictures of development from fertilization to a cluster of cells, which although becoming controversial among specialists, had cornered the market; the standard Carnegie embryos; stills from the films that the anatomist Davenport Hooker took of the reflex responses of dying fetuses, then widely viewed without demur; and some framing photos of a happy White mother and baby from a book on natural childbirth.[14] Around

---

12 "The Human Embryo," *Life*, July 3, 1950, 79–81; "The Start of Life," *Life*, September 21, 1953, 81–82 (quotation). On the Carnegie Department: Lynn M. Morgan, *Icons of Life: A Cultural History of Human Embryos* (Berkeley: University of California Press, 2009); on Shettles: Robin Marantz Henig, *Pandora's Baby: How the First Test Tube Babies Sparked the Reproductive Revolution* (Boston: Houghton Mifflin, 2004).

13 Geraldine Lux Flanagan, "Dramatic Photographs of Babies before Birth," *Look*, June 5, 1962, 19–23; Flanagan, *The First Nine Months of Life* (New York: Simon and Schuster, 1962), 9.

14 On Hooker's films: Emily K. Wilson, "Ex Utero: Live Human Fetal Research and the Films of Davenport Hooker," *Bulletin of the History of Medicine* 88, no. 1 (2014): 132–60.

the same time post-Sputnik reforms brought human embryos into high-school textbooks with more-detailed accounts of procreation.[15]

Though about to be cast into the shade by Nilsson's icons, photos of human embryos and fetuses were thus already on show as never before.[16] Innovations in communication and in reproduction then made his sensational representations of "life before birth."

"Drama of Life before Birth"

To stage a spectacle, Nilsson exploited the access provided to patients, from the early 1950s, by Sweden's liberal abortion law and collaboration with engineers, editors, and especially a team of antiabortionist gynecologists who were researching the fetus and placenta. Solveig Jülich has reconstructed this context and a shift to using the photos in sex education, but the reproductions in most countries are still largely unexplored.[17] The exception is their US debut, in the photo-essay "Drama of Life before Birth" in the April 30, 1965, issue of *Life* magazine and the advice book *A Child Is Born*, on which we have had much comment but little research.[18] With a longer view that allows a sharper focus on the question of novelty, I look again.

Life's claim that the photos were "unprecedented" rested primarily on the use of endoscopy, that is, "a super-wide-angle lens and a miniature flash attached to a surgical probe." This produced only one photo, which

15 Buklijas and Hopwood, "Public Embryology," *Making Visible Embryos*, http://www.sites.hps.cam.ac.uk/visibleembryos/s6_4.html.

16 On the obscuring effect of iconic images: Hopwood, *Haeckel's Embryos*.

17 Solveig Jülich, "Fetal Photography in the Age of Cool Media," in *History of Participatory Media: Politics and Publics, 1750–2000*, ed. Anders Ekström et al. (London: Routledge, 2011), 125–41; Jülich, "The Making of a Best-Selling Book on Reproduction: Lennart Nilsson's *A Child Is Born*," *Bulletin of the History of Medicine* 89, no. 3 (2015): 491–525; Jülich, "Picturing Abortion Opposition in Sweden: Lennart Nilsson's Early Photographs of Embryos and Fetuses," *Social History of Medicine* 31, no. 2 (2018): 278–307; Jülich, this volume. On, for example, Japan: Kinoshita Chika, "Taiji ga mitsuryo surumade: Gensuibaku kinshi undo to seiseiji" [The embryo hunts in public: Anti-nuclear movements and biopolitics], in *Taiko bunkashi* [A history of oppositional cultural politics], ed. Tsuboi Hideto and Unoda Naoya (Osaka: Osaka University Press, 2021), chapter 4; on Spain: Santesmases, this volume.

18 For example, Suzanne Anker and Sarah Franklin, "Specimens as Spectacles: Reframing Fetal Remains," *Social Text* 29, no. 1 (2011): 103–25, on 107–9; and other studies cited in this chapter.

generated anticipation in a newspaper ad.[19] The more general innovations were the aestheticization of embryos and fetuses in huge, lifelike photos by an established magazine photographer (not a specialist medical one), and the platform these received as a cover story for the forty million readers of America's "family album."[20]

Science Illustrated had depicted and described how "a microscopic gray blob . . . changes into a fetus, with limbs and organs and a face."[21] Twenty years later Nilsson bid for beauty as well as liveliness, setting off warm bodies against cool or dark backgrounds using color filters and negatives retouched also to remove reflections.[22] Cars, cigarettes, and drinks still took most of *Life*'s color, the ads reassuringly domestic amidst the wars, protests, strikes, and disasters. Following a young woman showing her legs around Chrysler's Dodge Coronet, Nilsson's drama unfolded across eight uninterrupted center spreads, an oasis of calm to match "the tranquillity of his mother's womb." Then the fetus was "shoved out . . . into the hostile world," and readers saw "seamless flooring" and the Ford XL. The essay cast embryo and fetus as noncommercial, even as it advertised them.[23]

The shots of surgically isolated fetuses in chambers of saline solution were lit from the back and sides to bring out their translucent delicacy. As the embryo grew and the magnification went down, headings tracked time in numbers of weeks and evoked key transformations: "Weightless Ride in a Salty Sac," "All of the Body Systems Formed and at Work," "A Thumb to Suck, a Veil to Wear." The astronaut reference was deflated—"The starlike spots . . . are merely bubbles in a fluid the photographer has used to support the amnion"—without reducing the effect. Developmental anatomy had long focused on body parts (figure 8.1), and in 1953 *Life* reproduced Nilsson's black-and-white portrait of "embryo's face."[24] Now close-ups of resonant structures looked forward more tantalizingly to the

19   "The Drama of Life Before Birth," *New York Times*, April 26, 1965, 64. *Life* admitted after publication that in Japan Chie and Takaaki Mohri had already filmed the fetus in utero: "Letters to the Editors," *Life*, May 21, 1965, 27.

20   Lennart Nilsson and Albert Rosenfeld, "Drama of Life before Birth," *Life*, April 30, 1965, 54–72A, available at https://books.google.co.uk/books?id=U VMEAAAAMBAJ&printsec=frontcover&source=gbs_ge_summary_r&cad=0 #v=onepage&q&f=false (last accessed May 7, 2023); on *Life*: Erika Doss, ed., *Looking at* Life *Magazine* (Washington, DC: Smithsonian Institution Press, 2001).

21   "How Life Begins," *Science Illustrated* 1, no. 4 (July 1946): 15–20, on 15.

22   Jülich, "Making of," 509; Jülich, this volume.

23   Nilsson and Rosenfeld, "Drama," 70–71.

24   Nilsson and Rosenfeld, "Drama," 61, 65, 68; "Embryo's Face," *Life*, March 30, 1953, 115.

baby-to-be—dangling feet, hands ready to clasp, a sucked thumb, an open eye—though not in this family magazine the genitals that embryologists had pictured separately, too.[25] It was a commonplace to find "drama" in "life before birth," but the new stress on active life chimed with reports of medical explorations into "prenativity."[26]

Feminist critics of the male gaze would indict Nilsson's photos for identifying with the embryo and fetus as the individualized, spaceman hero of a story that erased the pregnant body. Yet some pictures show the placenta, and the text, which used "baby" less than Flanagan and others, did not explicitly gender embryo or fetus until "his" replaced "it" in a separate essay about the placenta at the end. The embryos and fetuses were described as if inside the womb's safe haven, where there were dangers, but thanks to the placenta no overwhelming threat; German measles is mentioned as an exception. The language signals that the ideological pressure was still low, but these lively, colorful portraits made embryos and fetuses vivid as well as conspicuous subjects of their own development.[27] To judge from the published reactions, previously unexplored, many viewed the photos as if they had never seen a human embryo or fetus before.

"Locked in the . . . Womb with the Secret of Life"

Orchestrating a response three weeks later, *Life* constructed the publication as a milestone in its own brave history of breaking taboos with public support: "The majority of those who wrote in admired the pictures," expressing "awe" at the "miracle" of life. "The remainder thought them 'disgusting' or 'repulsive.'" Of fifteen initially published letters, seven men, three of them MDs, prized the "sheer beauty and daintiness" of "some of the most remarkable photographs in the history of photography." The women in favor wrote as mothers or mothers-to-be; one reported "the most stimulating and provocative questioning I have ever encountered in my three youngest children, aged 10, 11 and 14—a not-soon-to-be-forgotten sharing of delicate beauty and truth." A third of correspondents, all women, objected to the topic as

---

25 On synecdoche: Celeste Michelle Condit, *Decoding Abortion Rhetoric: Communicating Social Change* (Urbana: University of Illinois Press, 1990), 88–89; for genitals, for example, Hopwood, *Embryos in Wax*, 38.

26 "Control of Life," *Life*, September 10, 1965, 59–79.

27 Carol A. Stabile, "Shooting the Mother: Fetal Photography and the Politics of Disappearance," *Camera Obscura* 10, no. 1 (1992): 179–205; Duden, *Disembodying Women: Perspectives on Pregnancy and the Unborn*, trans. Lee Hoinacki (Cambridge, MA: Harvard University Press, 1993), 10–20; for Nilsson as representing the fetoplacental unit: Jülich, this volume.

inappropriate in a magazine that children saw: "What next? The mating process on the cover?" Only Mrs. Walter Gerules referenced abortion—"the most beautiful pictures of murder"—though another picked this up the next month.[28] There was no feminist analysis and would not be for a while.

The photos became iconic by copying; remediation elevated them for new audiences and made their miracles routine. A few gained individual fame, but more succeeded as a group or by inaugurating a style, while the endoscopic image, once crucial to the claim to novelty, dropped out of sight. When Nilsson won a competition, newspapers printed his "dramatic photograph of a human fetus" at sixteen weeks. *Life* would use another internal photo in yet more ads, while the cover one, with still more of the placenta, built anticipation for publication of the advice book *A Child Is Born* in January 1967.[29]

Pregnancy guides had included embryos; popular embryologies had tracked the progress of development. Now a pregnancy book put the fetus in charge while aligning its development with milestones in a tale of a couple having a child—a story that substituted for those of the women who would not carry the pictured embryos and fetuses to term. Textbooky diagrams and black-and-white shots bulked out the color photos. Faithful to the Swedish publisher Bonnier's playbook for the original, published fifteen months before, Delacorte Press invited readers "to witness a miracle . . . as old as time and as new as this moment . . . through the magic of modern science."[30]

In Sweden, a leading gynecologist had tempered the positive response by dissent from what he recognized as formerly antiabortion propaganda, but this was not yet an issue in America.[31] Many appreciated "the deeply moving story of a young couple," White and working class, which framed the book and made the racial coding explicit, complete with conventional advice on

---

28   "Editors' Note, 1938: Birth of a Baby; 1965: Drama of Life," and "Letters to the Editors," *Life*, May 21, 1965, 3, 27; "Letters to the Editors," *Life*, June 11, 1965, 25. In response to the 1950 "Human Embryo" essay, *Life* printed one letter for, one against: "Letters to the Editors," *Life*, July 24, 1950, 8; compare the negative comments on Nilsson's black-and-white, antiabortionist photos in Sweden in 1952: Jülich, "Picturing Abortion Opposition," 294.

29   For example, "Pictures," *Cincinnati Enquirer*, May 8, 1966, "Pictorial Enquirer," 28; "Everybody's Been Here. We Brought Back Pictures," *New York Times*, March 4, 1968, 20; "You Are Invited to Witness a Miracle . . . ," *New York Times*, January 22, 1967, "Book Review," 33. Fetoscopy was also a "dead end" for Nilsson himself: Jülich, this volume.

30   "You Are Invited" (quotation); Lennart Nilsson, Axel Ingelman-Sundberg, and Claes Wirsén, *A Child Is Born* (New York: Delacorte, 1966); on Bonnier: Jülich, "Making of."

31   For the dissent: Jülich, "Making of," 519–21.

regimen and doctors' visits—but "some of the most amazing photographs ever taken" stole the show. As the *Yazoo Herald* noted from Mississippi, "It's a fairly familiar story to those of us who have had a little biology"—which most were receiving by this time—"but never before has it been told in the company of such remarkable photographs. It's hard to say just what happens, but when the pictures and text of *A Child Is Born* are looked at together, we suddenly lose that old classroom feeling. It's not like a textbook or a lecture. We . . . see and feel . . . the million miracles of birth . . . in human terms."[32]

Two prime-time documentaries screened in March 1968. Based on Nilsson's images, Swedish TV's *Så börjar livet* (*The Beginning of Life*, 1965) aired on the public National Educational Television with a panel discussion. ABC's *How Life Begins* included five minutes of Shettles's shots of alleged fertilization and Nilsson's photos, which loomed large in the advertising, but *The Beginning of Life* was more immersive: "Viewers who tuned [in] Monday could have only been left with an overwhelming feeling of having been locked in the same womb with the secret of life."[33]

The following month Stanley Kubrick's science-fiction blockbuster, *2001: A Space Odyssey*, culminated in a "star child" representing the next phase of human evolution. Nilsson's fetal photos partly inspired the shot of a model baby in an amnion-like bubble with hand to lips.[34] Participatory practices amplified commercial strategies when viewing in magazines and newspapers and on TV was extended by a *Life* educational reprint, slides, and filmstrips that allowed more flexible usage in classrooms and with other groups.[35] Textbooks and exhibits reproduced Nilsson's photos; teachers put up bulletin boards; photographers imitated him.[36]

---

32 James L. Dertien, "Where the Action Is . . . Your Library," *Daily Republic* (Mitchell, SD), January 28, 1967, 3; "Book Review," *Yazoo Herald*, February 2, 1967, 19.

33 Harold Schindler, "2 Views on Miracle of Reproduction, Both Good," *Salt Lake Tribune*, March 21, 1968, 4B; on *The Beginning of Life*: Solveig Jülich, "Televising Inner Space: Lennart Nilsson's Early Medical Documentaries on the Interior of the Human Body," in *Representational Machines: Photography and the Production of Space*, ed. Anna Dahlgren, Dag Petersson, and Nina Lager Vestberg (Aarhus: Aarhus Universitetsforlag, 2013), 149–69.

34 Eric Grundhauser, "The Cosmic Fetus of '2001: A Space Odyssey' Hasn't Aged a Day," *Atlas Obscura*, May 23, 2018, https://www.atlasobscura.com/articles/kubrick-2001-star-child-prop.

35 Jülich, "Fetal Photography," stresses this intersection.

36 Rebecca Ross Dechow, "Ideas for Bulletin Boards," *American Biology Teacher* 42, no. 5 (1980): 308–9; for imitations: Roberts Rugh and Landrum B. Shettles, *From Conception to Birth: The Drama of Life's Beginnings* (New York:

Prior sex education had perhaps lacked impact although increasingly universal; now the aestheticized, undidactic style in a range of colorful new media, and the opportunities for appropriation created sensations. Embryos and fetuses had never been more visible or looked more beautiful. The activist backlash against what during the 1960s was claimed as a woman's right to abortion would restore antiabortionism as a frame.

"When We Use Slides, We Win"

Though evolutionists and sex reformers had taken the lead in promoting embryological visions of life, photos had been deployed against abortion, such as when physicians tried to dissuade unhappily pregnant women.[37] The rising prominence of human development had yet to make fetuses legal or political subjects. The disarmament organization SANE might appear as "defenders of the unborn," but it focused on children, as did the most shocking images from the Vietnam War.[38] Then antiabortionists changed strategies.

In the late 1960s, as US states passed increasingly liberal abortion laws, Christian opponents sought wider support by arguing less for the sanctity of fetal life and more for fetal rights, less with religious than with medical authorities.[39] They extended the visual rhetoric that medics had used on individual women and groups. In 1967 a former president of the Catholic Physicians Guild showed bottled fetuses to Colorado senators in an attempt to have them repeal the first reformed abortion law.[40] By 1968 antiabortionists were recruiting Nilsson's photos to personify the fetus in state-level

---

Harper & Row, 1971); Claude Edelmann, *Les premiers jours de la vie* ([Paris]; Taillandier, 1971), a book based on the film of the same name.

37 Edwin Bradford Cragin, *Obstetrics: A Practical Text-Book for Students and Practitioners* (Philadelphia: Lea & Febiger, 1916), 513; Leslie J. Reagan, *When Abortion Was a Crime: Women, Medicine, and Law in the United States, 1867–1973* (Berkeley: University of California Press, 1997), 84–85.

38 Dawn E. Johnsen, "The Creation of Fetal Rights: Conflicts with Women's Constitutional Rights to Liberty, Privacy, and Equal Protection," *Yale Law Journal* 95, no. 3 (1986): 599–625; Finis Dunaway, *Seeing Green: The Use and Abuse of American Environmental Images* (Chicago: University of Chicago Press, 2015), chapter 1; Zaretsky, *Radiation Nation*, chapter 1; quotation from the hostile article, "How Sane are the SANE?" *Time*, April 21, 1958, 13–14.

39 Condit, *Decoding Abortion Rhetoric*, chapter 4.

40 Jennifer L. Holland, *Tiny You: A Western History of the Anti-Abortion Movement* (Oakland: University of California Press, 2020), 58–61.

battles against reform. In 1970 *Life* pictured a lawyer holding *A Child Is Born* open at a four-month-old fetus and declaring, "This is my client."[41] In October 1971 lawyers with Americans United for Life submitted fetal photos, signed by over two hundred physicians, to the US Supreme Court in *Roe v. Wade* and the companion case *Doe v. Bolton*.[42]

Antiabortionists also started displaying a second kind of image. Catholic authors had once censured discussion of the details of abortion as in bad taste, and Nilsson's photos owed their success to aestheticization. Now activists collected shots of dismembered fetuses discarded after abortion and set them up to evoke disgust. The priest, Benedictine monk, sociologist, and liberal Democrat Paul Marx, who showed students a film of a vacuum abortion in April 1970, inspired those "symbolic entrepreneurs" of antiabortionism, the Catholic physician and nurse couple John ("Jack") and Barbara Willke of Cincinnati. From 1971 they worked for the major antiabortion organization, the National Right to Life Committee, which John Willke served as president in the 1980s. They developed the devastating visual strategy outlined in the bible of the "pro-life" movement, their *Handbook on Abortion*, and further explained in the manual *How to Teach the Pro-Life Story*. They proved it in campaigning to defeat abortion-repeal referenda in Michigan and North Dakota in November 1972 (figure 8.2).[43]

"With rare exceptions," the Willkes advised, "never lecture or debate in front of a live audience without slides" because "when we use slides, we win."[44] Slides and packs of photos were most popular, as well as bottles and films, and the Willkes also recommended TV documentaries, exhibits with flyers, blown-up photos in TV interviews, postcards, billboards, bumper stickers, decals, tapes, jewelry, lapel buttons, Christmas cards, stationery, and T-shirts. Silent magnification enhanced the significance of the fetus,

41   *The Terrible Choice: The Abortion Dilemma* (New York: Bantam, 1968); Beth Day and Margaret Liley, *The Secret World of the Baby* (New York: Random House, 1968); "ZPG," *Life*, April 17, 1970, 32–37.

42   Daniel K. Williams, *Defenders of the Unborn: The Pro-Life Movement before* Roe v. Wade (New York: Oxford University Press, 2016), 198.

43   Faye D. Ginsburg, *Contested Lives: The Abortion Debate in an American Community*, updated ed. (Berkeley: University of California Press, 1998), 71, 104–7; Roger Neustadter, "'Killing Babies': The Use of Image and Metaphor in the Right-to-Life Movement," *Michigan Sociological Review*, no. 4 (1990): 76–83 ("symbolic entrepreneurs"); Janelle S. Taylor, "The Public Fetus and the Family Car: From Abortion Politics to a Volvo Advertisement," *Public Culture* 4, no. 2 (1992): 67–80; Cynthia Gorney, *Articles of Faith: A Frontline History of the Abortion Wars* (New York: Simon & Schuster, 1998), 99–106; Williams, *Defenders of the Unborn*, chapter 6.

44   Willke and Willke, *How to Teach*, 29.

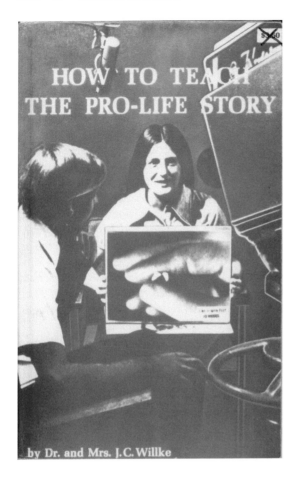

Figure 8.2. Cover of the Willkes' *How to Teach the Pro-Life Story*. The photo shows an activist on a TV set holding up a large photo of an adult hand with the "tiny human feet" of a fetus "at 10 weeks." Compare the embryonic feet in figure 8.1, this chapter. Dr. and Mrs. J. C. Willke, *How to Teach the Pro-Life Story* (Cincinnati, OH: Hayes, 1975).

but "little feet" worked by showing a part that was recognizable although clearly tiny. The adult hand hid the structures that made that fetus most different from a child (figure 8.2). Much evidence suggests that the strategy worked.[45]

Antiabortionists presented the pictures to enlarge the subject of concern and counter the assumption of gradual development. They argued that, genetically, life begins at fertilization, after which there was nowhere to draw the line. The Willkes agreed but began their slideshows at the end of the series to capture the "immediate visual judgment" of "the average uncommitted person." "Our job is to make that initial impression . . . 'That's a

---

45   Condit, *Decoding Abortion Rhetoric*, 79–80, 88–89; Williams, *Defenders of the Unborn*, 225.

baby.' If their initial impression is rather 'That's a glob,' then we've started in a hole." Having opened with "pictures of born premature babies, . . . we would show the eighteen-week *LIFE* Magazine cover, and ask, is this being human?" They then moved down the "age ladder . . . never giving . . . any . . . reason for changing the initial mindset," and selecting the photos that most "look like babies" (some in *Life* "look like fetuses"). They put up a last "visual at six weeks, and . . . *we'll show no visuals under six weeks* . . . because we feel that if we do, the audience may change their minds from their conviction that this is human life."[46]

The Willkes then paraded "war photos." Their *Life or Death* pamphlet and another by the Michigan Catholic Conference reproduced normal and dismembered development. As a pro-choice activist told anthropologist Faye Ginsburg after the defeated North Dakota referendum: "They distributed this color brochure with a picture of the fetus door-to-door in Fargo and the rest of the state . . . I got this absolutely tremulous woman who came to talk to me. You could see that her faith was really shaken."[47] Or, as the Willkes put it, "It is only . . . when they see that same age of baby dead that they recoil in horror at the reality of it all. . . . If this be shock, so be it. The pictures at M[y] Lai were also shock, but taught us something about war that words never could"—a reminder that this visual culture harks back to the use of photos of children in protests against the Vietnam War, nuclear testing, and nuclear power.[48] Although initially including African American spokespeople and deploying images of Black fetuses and babies, the "pro-life" movement became increasingly White as well as right-wing. Members likened it to struggles against the Holocaust and slavery, but in its supreme innocence the fetus, almost always male, displaced other rights demands.[49]

This imagery would prove hard to counter. Coat hangers, symbolizing backstreet abortions, were too chaste. Medical examiners' photos of women dead because of illegality could shock back, but risked pitting woman against fetus while projecting negative images of abortion, albeit as a legacy to

46 Willke and Willke, *How to Teach*, 6–11. Emphasis in original.

47 Ginsburg, *Contested Lives*, 71.

48 Willke and Willke, *How to Teach*, 11; Richard L. Hughes, "Burning Birth Certificates and Atomic Tupperware Parties: Creating the Antiabortion Movement in the Shadow of the Vietnam War," *The Historian* 68, no. 3 (2006): 541–58.

49 Carol Mason, *Killing for Life: The Apocalyptic Narrative of Pro-Life Politics* (Ithaca, NY: Cornell University Press, 2002); Williams, *Defenders of the Unborn*, 170–74; Holland, *Tiny You*.

overcome. The Statue of Liberty was perhaps the most potent image of the demand for choices other than motherhood.[50]

After *Roe*, providers made abortion one of the safest and commonest surgical procedures. The public fetus gained prominence in the backlash that made it one of the most controversial, too.[51]

"It Looked Like a Baby"

While Democratic opposition to abortion was strong in majority-Catholic areas, most registered Republicans supported legal access as late as 1976. Then antiabortionism split the New Deal coalition as part of a suburban rejection of civil rights and feminism and a populist revolt against medical and scientific elites. The fetus symbolized the antigovernment movement that brought Ronald Reagan to the presidency and conservative Christianity into national politics.[52]

The shape of things to come was dimly visible in a pivotal medico-legal drama, the 1975 trial of Kenneth Edelin, chief resident in obstetrics and gynecology at Boston City Hospital, for ending the life of a fetus he estimated at twenty-one to twenty-two weeks old.[53] The hospital provided most of the safe, legal abortions that *Roe* had made available to poor and African American women, but the Catholic nurses and doctors were uncomfortable with this. Antiabortionists received a tip-off about "babies in bottles" in the morgue; one came from a second-trimester abortion by Edelin about which colleagues were concerned. The termination was legal, but an assistant district attorney on the make charged Edelin with manslaughter for depriving "a baby boy" of oxygen after saline injections failed to expel the fetus and he removed it through a cut in the uterus.[54]

50 Condit, *Decoding Abortion Rhetoric*, 92–94; Suzanne Staggenborg, *The Pro-Choice Movement: Organization and Activism in the Abortion Conflict* (New York: Oxford University Press, 1991), 48–49; Gorney, *Articles of Faith*, 398–404; Laurie Shrage, "From Reproductive Rights to Reproductive Barbie: Post-Porn Modernism and Abortion," *Feminist Studies* 28, no. 1 (2002): 61–93.

51 Johanna Schoen, *Abortion after* Roe (Chapel Hill: University of North Carolina Press, 2015).

52 Williams, *Defenders of the Unborn*, chapter 9; Mary Ziegler, *After* Roe: *The Lost History of the Abortion Debate* (Cambridge, MA: Harvard University Press, 2015), chapter 6.

53 My account follows Dubow, *Ourselves Unborn*, chapter 3; Schoen, *Abortion after* Roe, chapter 2; and Jennifer Donnally, "The Edelin Manslaughter Trial and the Anti-Abortion Movement," *Massachusetts Historical Review* 20 (2018): 1–32.

54 Quoted in Dubow, *Ourselves Unborn*, 79, 84–85.

Edelin was convicted because the trial knotted together issues at the heart of the political transformation. Harvard trained, and the first African American to hold his position, he faced an all-White, non-college-educated jury mostly of Catholic men in a city riven by an attempt to desegregate the schools by busing. Although the guilty verdict was set aside on appeal, the trial had a chilling effect on abortions near viability and furthered the focus on the fetus, in part because the defense protected the seventeen-year-old high-school student and daughter of West Indian immigrants who had sought the termination. Antiabortionists' first significant victory since *Roe* showed what an incremental approach might achieve and the potential for using abortion to drive working-class voters into Republican arms. It also demonstrated the power of visual evidence.

Jurors' statements suggest that a photo of the normal fetus with fine, black curly hair, its face shriveled and skin wrinkled after sitting in formaldehyde for four months, helped to decide them that Edelin had done too little to save it. "We passed all the evidence around the table and everyone looked at each piece, but we paid a lot of attention to that picture," reported Anthony Alessi, a foreman for a phone company. "None of us had ever seen a fetus before. For all we knew, a fetus looked like a kidney. The picture was obviously of a well-formed baby, over 13 inches long." "It looked like a baby," said Liberty Ann Conlin, a homemaker married to a construction foreman.[55] The sight appears novel—the exhibits, books, films, and photo-essays notwithstanding—and shockingly familiar. The photo joined others on placards outside clinics, and the assumption hardened that if only everyone would see fetuses as babies, abortions would stop.

In 1976 the self-described "housewife" Ellen McCormack ran for the Democratic presidential nomination on an antiabortion ticket and qualified for federal matching funds to show TV spots.[56] Over an image of a late-stage fetus, with a heartbeat tracing across the screen and on the soundtrack, McCormack asked, "Did you know that the heart of an unborn baby begins to be formed at three weeks after conception? Did you know also that a million babies have their hearts stopped each year"—then the screen went dark and the heartbeat silent—"in a very painful way, by abortion?" McCormack appeared, and asked viewers, as she looked down to the baby she was holding, "Help me to keep these hearts beating" (figure 8.3).[57]

55 Quoted in Dubow, *Ourselves Unborn*, 102; on fetal images in courtrooms, further: Carol Sanger, *About Abortion: Terminating Pregnancy in Twenty-First-Century America* (Cambridge, MA: Belknap Press of Harvard University Press, 2017), 42–43.

56 Williams, *Defenders of the Unborn*, 225–29.

57 "Ellen McCormack: 1976 Campaign," Carrie Chapman Catt Center for Women and Politics, Iowa State University, https://www.youtube.com/watch?v=EN3h6auFSJw (last accessed May 27, 2023).

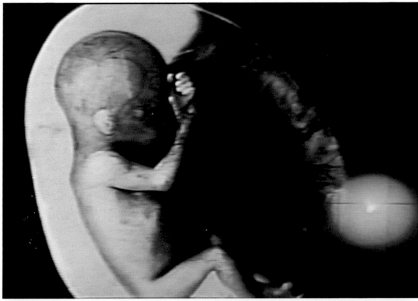
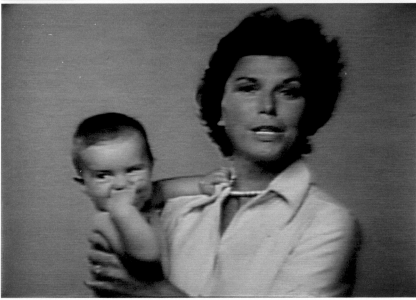

Figure 8.3. Ellen McCormack campaign ad, 1976, paid for by Pro-Life Action Committee, Bellmore, New York: (*top*) fetal image and spot of blue light representing heartbeat; (*bottom*) McCormack with baby, inviting its identification with the fetus. Screen captures (at 00:11 and 00:24) from videocassette at the Carl Albert Center, University of Oklahoma, P-329-01699, viewable at https://www. youtube.com/watch?v=LN7bYnQ4LMM.

That same year the Hyde Amendment outlawed federal funding of abortion.[58] As well as picketing clinics and harassing clients and staff, and blocking their construction, antiabortionists had since the late 1960s mimicked them with "crisis pregnancy centers" that entrapped women seeking an abortion or unsure about having one. While waiting for the result of a pregnancy test, they were shown pictures, models, and films of fetal development in a push to stop them "killing babies."[59]

Meanwhile legal rights expanded from redress for parents and child to the protection of the fetus as a person, especially from harms seen as coming from the pregnant woman herself. Women who had lost welfare support were blamed for their plight while rights were projected onto their fetuses. Women were prosecuted for "fetal abuse" and compelled into medical interventions. In a backlash against the antidiscrimination provisions of the Civil Rights Act of 1964, women were forced out of workplaces deemed unsafe for a potential fetus, notably battery and chemical factories, or pushed into sterilizations. Courts ultimately struck down many of these statutes, but alcohol and drug consumption and other behaviors were policed through laws targeting the poor, while advice books disciplined the middle class.[60]

Though not as central to these campaigns as to antiabortionism, visual images complemented the rhetoric. The opening sequence of the Emmy-winning WABC-TV documentary *The Littlest Junkie* (1973) dramatized the plight of addicted infants of heroin-using mothers by alternating a photo of a baby convulsed by withdrawal and Nilsson's image of a fetus. An American Cancer Society film against smoking while pregnant featured a sonogram.[61]

Such pictures gained ideological power as Americans began to produce and consume medical images on a vast scale, and obstetricians to use ultrasound far more than they had ever used X-rays. Following the movement

58 Mary Ziegler, *Abortion and the Law in America:* Roe v. Wade *to the Present* (Cambridge: Cambridge University Press, 2020), chapter 2.

59 Schoen, *Abortion after* Roe, chapter 5.

60 Johnsen, "Creation of Fetal Rights"; Cynthia R. Daniels, *At Women's Expense: State Power and the Politics of Fetal Rights* (Cambridge, MA: Harvard University Press, 1993); Rachel Roth, *Making Women Pay: The Hidden Costs of Fetal Rights* (Ithaca, NY: Cornell University Press, 2000); Elizabeth M. Armstrong, *Conceiving Risk, Bearing Responsibility: Fetal Alcohol Syndrome & the Diagnosis of Moral Disorder* (Baltimore: Johns Hopkins University Press, 2003); Janet Golden, *Message in a Bottle: The Making of Fetal Alcohol Syndrome* (Cambridge, MA: Harvard University Press, 2005). Dubow, *Ourselves Unborn* dates the change earlier and then sees more continuity.

61 Dubow, *Ourselves Unborn*, 135; Laury Oaks, "Smoke-Filled Wombs and Fragile Fetuses: The Social Politics of Fetal Representation," *Signs* 26, no. 1 (2000): 63–108.

of childbirth into hospital, they had constructed a fetal patient, and in the 1960s imaging technologies, including endoscopy, vied for attention. "Seeing with sound," used in about one-third of US pregnancies by the mid-1980s, achieved dominance thanks to its increasing capacity to make noninvasive images as it went from underwhelming graphs and sections to real-time "baby TV" in 3-D. Accelerating the experience of pregnancy and reducing the importance of birth as a threshold, "baby's first pictures" treated the fetus as if already an infant and the pregnant woman as if already a mother.[62] Ultrasound would provide the deadliest visual salvo in the abortion wars.

The Fetal Patient in a "Star Wars Weapon"

Ronald Reagan's election in 1980 gave antiabortionists an administration on their side. His surgeon general, the born-again-Christian pediatrician C. Everett Koop, had coauthored with the conservative Presbyterian theologian Francis Schaeffer a film series and book. *Whatever Happened to the Human Race?* toured the country in 1979 recruiting young evangelicals to the anti-abortion cause. The director, Schaeffer's son Franky, equated fetus and baby by intercutting clips from Claude Edelmann's film *Les premiers jours de la vie* (The first days of life, 1971) with footage of babies moving in a white space. Even at eighteen to twenty-five days, Koop insisted, "the baby can hardly be considered just another part of the mother's body." Then his descriptions of abortion techniques accompanied shots of one thousand baby dolls strewn across the landscape around the Dead Sea (figure 8.4). On the site of the city of Sodom, "the most humanly corrupt city on earth," those (White and Black) dolls represented "the slaughter of the innocents" that was still going on. Koop implied that viewers' eyes just needed to be opened, and the "evils of abortion" perpetrated by the "secular forces of humanism" could be overcome.[63]

---

62 Lisa M. Mitchell, *Baby's First Picture: Ultrasound and the Politics of Fetal Subjects* (Toronto: University of Toronto Press, 2001); Janelle S. Taylor, *The Public Life of the Fetal Sonogram: Technology, Consumption, and the Politics of Reproduction* (New Brunswick, NJ: Rutgers University Press, 2008); Malcolm Nicolson and John E. E. Fleming, *Imaging and Imagining the Fetus: The Development of Obstetric Ultrasound* (Baltimore: Johns Hopkins University Press, 2013).

63 Franky Schaeffer V, dir., *Whatever Happened to the Human Race?* (Muskegon, MI: Gospel Films, 1979), at Vision Video, 2010, https://www.youtube.com/watch?v=py02pQTyeTE, 20:00–29:36 (last accessed May 27, 2023); Gorney, *Articles of Faith*, 340–42; Mason, *Killing for Life*, 114–18.

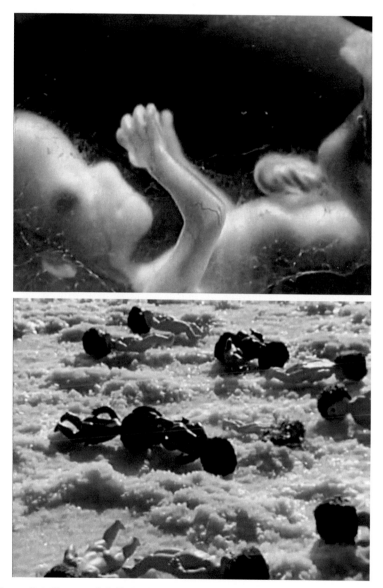

Figure 8.4. Fetus and dolls in the antiabortion movie *Whatever Happened to the Human Race?* (*top*) Fetal photo from the Edelmann film; (*bottom*) baby dolls representing aborted fetuses and salt of Sodom referring to the "evil" of saline abortion. Screen captures (at 21:58 and 25:30) from *Whatever Happened to the Human Race?* (Gospel Films, 1979), via Vision Video, https://www.youtube.com/watch?v=py02pQTyeTE.

A few days after his second inauguration, on January 22, 1985, the anniversary of *Roe v. Wade*, Reagan spoke from the Oval Office to the annual antiabortion march and referred to a twenty-eight-minute film, *The Silent Scream* (Jack Duane Dabner, 1984): "'For the first time, through . . . real-time ultrasound imaging, we're able to see with our own eyes . . . the abortion of a 12-week-old unborn child. . . . [I]f every member of Congress could see that [chilling documentation], they would . . . end the tragedy of abortion, and I pray that they will.'"[64] The footage had been commissioned in response to Reagan's claim—rebutted by the American College of Obstetricians and Gynecologists (ACOG)—that a fetus feels pain during an abortion. That was itself an attempt to reassert compassion after his first administration's withdrawal of benefits from people disabled by pain.[65]

The commissioner was the ob-gyn Bernard Nathanson, a renegade founder of the National Association for the Repeal of Abortion Laws who had directed a large abortion clinic before going over to the other side. The film framed him as a paternalistic authority figure who presented medical evidence, but he also narrated a morality play. Speaking to the camera, Nathanson lauded the "dazzling" technical advances that showed "abortion from the victim's vantage point. . . . And so . . . we are going to watch a child being torn apart, dismembered, disarticulated, crushed, and destroyed by the unfeeling steel instruments of the abortionist." Nathanson used plastic models to argue that there was no dramatic change at any developmental stage; he invoked the "second patient" as implying a subject doctors had sworn to preserve. Sitting beside a TV set, he took viewers through the three-minute, black-and-white, 2-D film-within-the-film. As the suction tip approached, the fetus underwent more "violent" movements. Nathanson pointed to the mouth, "wide open in . . . the silent scream of a child threatened imminently with extinction" (figure 8.5). Having drawn attention to the disappearance of parts as these were removed, he closed with the argument that women were victims, too, and that informed consent should include viewing such a movie. The hope was that the woman would "bond" with the fetus.[66]

Addressing the rally, the Southern Baptist televangelist Jerry Falwell agreed that, "As soon as we can show the pictures in prime time," like with "the starving children in Ethiopia, the big American heart will respond and say 'stop it!'" Ultrasound would let antiabortionists "vault over all the

64   Quoted in Dudley Clendinen, "President Praises Foes of Abortion," *New York Times*, January 23, 1985, A1, A15.

65   Dubow, *Ourselves Unborn*, chapter 5; Keith Wailoo, *Pain: A Political History* (Baltimore: Johns Hopkins University Press, 2014), 123–28.

66   Jack Duane Dabner, dir., *The Silent Scream* (Anaheim, CA: American Portrait Films, 1984); Petchesky, "Fetal Images," 265–67.

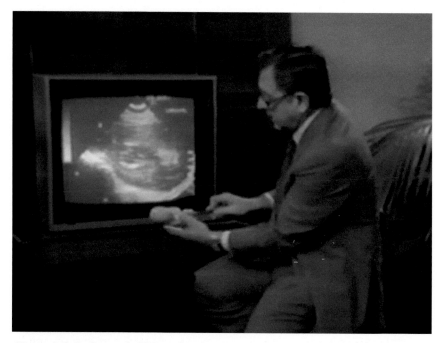

Figure 8.5. In front of a TV set showing an enlarged, manipulated film of real-time ultrasound, Bernard Nathanson demonstrates the actions of an abortionist using a magnified fetal model and a red pointer representing the suction tip. Screen capture (at 18:54) from *The Silent Scream* (American Portrait Films, 1984) via https://archive.org/details/BVL_0028.

1960-ish . . . bombast about women's rights and controlling one's own body. We now are . . . in the high-tech era and this is high-tech documentation." Invoking Reagan's rearmament program, Nathanson called it "a kind of Star Wars weapon for the pro-life movement."[67] The Right wanted nukes but no abortion; the Left wanted abortion rights not nukes. Was the focus on fetal extermination displacing the Right's bad conscience over its preparations for nuclear Armageddon?[68]

---

67 Clendinen, "President Praises Foes of Abortion"; Gilbert A. Lewthwaite, "Movie of Abortion Gives New Drama and Controversy to Issue," *Baltimore Sun*, February 19, 1985, 1A, 6A; Ginny Graybiel, "'Silent Scream' Pinches a Nerve in the Nation," *Pensacola News Journal*, March 10, 1985, 12, 22.

68 Zoë Sofia, "Exterminating Fetuses: Abortion, Disarmament, and the Sexo-Semiotics of Extraterrestrialism," *Diacritics* 14, no. 2 (1984): 47–59; Mason, *Killing for Life*.

The networks broadcast clips that evening, but the film, which was also screened across the United States via videotape and in 16 mm, sparked strong objections. Critics pointed out that most abortions were done earlier than twelve weeks. The ACOG debunked Nathanson's "inaccurate and dishonest" claims. The fetus showed "a reflex response that is too primitive to speak of in terms of pain"; still solid tissue, the lungs could not scream. Nathanson had omitted to say that the video was magnified and the models, too. He had exaggerated the dramatic effect by running the film "in very slow motion" before the suction catheter was placed and then returning to "regular speed."[69] Many newspaper articles still created an illusion of balance.[70] It was possible to accept both fetal personhood and abortion, but the argument was skewed by the insistent visual presence of the fetus.

Joining an intellectual movement to analyze popular culture and the culture of medicine, feminist activists and scholars began highlighting the visual power to exclude women from the picture.[71] Rosalind Petchesky wrote her essay and talked about it, notably after a screening at the annual "The Scholar and the Feminist" workshop at Barnard College in Manhattan on March 22, 1986. Petchesky noted "the more literal kind of rebuttal" but worked toward an analysis that would grasp how "people can simultaneously see behind the artifices and be moved by them."[72] Following the semiotician Roland Barthes, she decoded the video and ventured interpretations based on the "historical paradox of photographic images: their simultaneous power as purveyors of fantasy and illusion yet also of 'objectivist "truth."'"[73] Taking a longer view, and encompassing a wider range of media, historians

69   Dena Kleiman, "Debate on Abortion Focuses on Graphic Film," *New York Times*, January 25, 1985, B8; "A False 'Scream,'" *New York Times*, March 11, 1985, A18.

70   For example, Theresa Churchill, "'Silent Scream' Resounds in Area," *Decatur Herald and Review*, April 4, 1985, D1.

71   Ann Oakley, *The Captured Womb: A History of the Medical Care of Pregnant Women* (Oxford: Blackwell, 1984), chapter 7; Sofia, "Exterminating Fetuses"; Barbara Katz Rothman, *The Tentative Pregnancy: Prenatal Diagnosis and the Future of Motherhood* (New York: Viking, 1986), 111–15.

72   Recording at Barnard Center for Research on Women, "The Scholar and the Feminist XIII (Women's Images and Politics): Afternoon Session 17," parts 1 and 2, https://digitalcollections.barnard.edu/do/dd241718-5ad8-449c-b19b-85eea47ee5e5 (quotations from 1:14:20–55) and https://digitalcollections.barnard.edu/do/617522eb-3348-41a6-8bdd-aaacc5486ac1. Notes for Petchesky's talk at Barnard, as well as drafts of her essay and other materials, are at Smith College, Rosalind Petchesky Papers, SSC-MS-00639, Box 3.

73   Petchesky, "Fetal Images," 269.

would reconstruct how "woman's body" became a "public place" peopled with developing embryos and fetuses.[74]

For Petchesky, "The most disturbing thing about how people receive . . . the dominant fetal imagery, is their apparent acceptance of the image itself as an accurate representation of a real fetus. The curled-up profile, with its enlarged head and finlike arms, suspended in its balloon of amniotic fluid, is by now so familiar that not even most feminists question its authenticity (as opposed to its relevance)." But what Nathanson claimed as "the vantage point of the fetus" was in fact the view through the camera. An updated "abstract individualism," "effacing the pregnant woman and the fetus's dependence on her, . . . gives the fetal image its symbolic transparency, so that we can read in it our selves, our lost babies, our mythic secure past." This fetus was "a fetish," and if "a picture of a dead fetus is worth a thousand words," real-time sonograms brought stale photos to life in movies masquerading as medical evidence.[75] Abortion providers pictured fetuses differently (figure 8.6).

Some suggested that any effect of *The Silent Scream* depended on Nathanson's emotional commentary. One focus-group member said, "I'm an air traffic controller, and I gotta tell you, that might have been a fetus up there. . . . But it looked like a weather map to me."[76] Yet, as Petchesky observed, the film should not be isolated from the "contexts, media, and consciousnesses" which gave fetal images meaning. That was the basis from which she critiqued feminist essentialism, sought to grasp the appeal of fetal ultrasound to some women, and reflected on resonances between public and private.[77] A major context was an aesthetic assault on abortion.

Antiabortion activism escalated, fed by providers who had crossed the lines and the tiny proportion of women who regretted their abortions. With war photos and bottled bodies thrust into clients' faces outside besieged clinics, all had to confront the equation of fetal remains with murdered babies. In *Webster v. Reproductive Health Services* (1989) and *Casey v. Planned Parenthood* (1992), the Supreme Court reinforced government interest in protecting fetal life during pregnancy and encouraged state regulations to deter providers and clients. But, Reagan's failure to deliver nationally fed feelings of powerlessness in the face of what antiabortionists had learned to see as mass infanticide. This radicalized a few activists to bomb and murder.

74 Duden, *Disembodying Women* (quotations from the German title); and the research referenced in Buklijas and Hopwood, *Making Visible Embryos.*

75 Petchesky, "Fetal Images," 268, 270, 263.

76 Betty Cuniberti and Elizabeth Mehren, "Abortion Film Stirs Friend, Foe," *Los Angeles Times*, August 8, 1985, 1–3, 26–27, on 27.

77 Petchesky, "Fetal Images," 287.

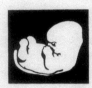
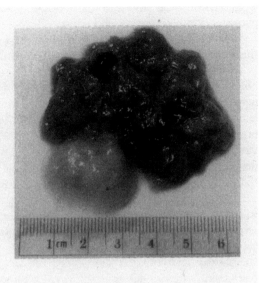

In contrast to the image of the nineteen-week fetus used by pro-Life rhetors, this photo shows the products of conception at eight menstrual weeks' gestation (weight 16 grams), The drawing of the cm bryo indicates its approximate appearance and size. Photo © 1989 by Warren Martin Hern

Figure 8.6. A counter to antiabortionist photos gives the scale and shows all products of conception; a standard textbook-type drawing focuses on the fetus but is reproduced to scale. Celeste Condit, *Decoding Abortion Rhetoric: Communicating Social Change* (Urbana: University of Illinois Press, 1990), 90; photo courtesy of Warren Hern (Boulder Abortion Clinic).

Found guilty of killing an abortion doctor and his bodyguard, a former Presbyterian minister asked that the sentencing judge watch a video such as *The Silent Scream*.[78]

"If There Were a Window"?

Fetal forms went everywhere. Americans saw them around clinics and—on billboards, bumper stickers, and trucks plastered with huge war photos—in the once-unlikely setting of the roads.[79] Embedded in conservative politics,

78　Schoen, *Abortion after* Roe, 145.

79　For example, Carol Sanger, "Seeing and Believing: Mandatory Ultrasound and the Path to a Protected Choice," *UCLA Law Review* 56 (2008): 351–408, on 406–7.

fetus icons summed up the "pro-life" story. "If there were a window on a pregnant woman's stomach, there would be no more abortions," went the saying, and there is vivid testimony to evidence "the conversion power of the fetus."[80]

As well as co-opting mainstream photos and films, pro-life businesses produced and sold their own. Inspired by seeing the "little feet" photo in a newspaper ad, Virginia Evers, a manufacturer of nationalist paraphernalia, churned them out as metal pins. One satisfied customer explained, "Clerks in stores, bank tellers, people in any crowd . . . inevitably ask what they are and it gives me a chance to impress a visual image on their minds that they will never forget."[81]

By the 1990s the director of a crisis pregnancy center reckoned, "If you can get a lady into an ultrasound room, then 90 percent will carry that baby to term."[82] Under the banner "A woman's right to know," informed-consent laws in about twenty states required those seeking an abortion to be given booklets detailing developmental stages of "the unborn child" and the alleged risks; some mandated that they be subjected to a real-time sonogram. The most coercive jurisdictions demanded a transvaginal procedure at stages when this produces a clearer picture, and that the image be placed in the patient's line of sight while they were made to listen to a description of what appeared on screen and to the heartbeat. These laws have forced people who do not wish to be pregnant to participate in a ritual associated with pregnancy. They produce portraits, those markers of personhood, which present the fetus as a grievable life. According to surveys, these ultrasounds have in fact changed few minds but may be experienced as distressing.[83] By contrast, most research participants who chose to see in a supportive environment the preabortion ultrasounds that staff used to determine the stage of gestation and normality reported a positive experience.[84]

---

80 Ginsburg, *Contested Lives,* 104 (quotations); Condit, *Decoding Abortion Rhetoric,* 79–82; Rayna Rapp, *Testing Women, Testing the Fetus: The Social Impact of Amniocentesis in America* (New York: Routledge, 1999), 127.

81 Quoted in Holland, *Tiny You,* 54.

82 Quoted in Holland, *Tiny You,* 128; further: Joanne Boucher, "Ultrasound: A Window to the Womb? Obstetric Ultrasound and the Abortion Rights Debate," *Journal of Medical Humanities* 25, no. 1 (2004): 7–19; Taylor, *Public Life,* chapter 2.

83 Sanger, "Seeing and Believing"; Ushma D. Upadhyay et al., "Evaluating the Impact of a Mandatory Preabortion Ultrasound Viewing Law: A Mixed Methods Study," *PLoS ONE* 12, no. 7 (2017): e0178871.

84 Studies from Canada and England: Ellen R. Wiebe and Lisa Adams, "Women's Perceptions about Seeing the Ultrasound Picture before an Abortion," *European Journal of Contraception and Reproductive Health Care* 14, no. 2

Imaging also provided the main justification for terminations. Ultrasound consultations were based on a contradiction: the main medical purpose of scans that make a pregnancy more socially real than a hormonal test has been to screen for the problems that crop up in a low percentage of cases, be they malformations or restricted growth. Unofficial, and in many countries illegal, use of ultrasound for sex selection has also resulted in abortion, usually of female fetuses. A technology that promoted fetal personhood thus helped to make pregnancy tentative, too.[85]

More remarkably, a group of independent abortion providers countered the barrage of stigmatization, harassment, and negative images by developing counseling strategies that include viewing fetuses while affirming the value of choice. From the 1990s some clinics offered clients the option of not just observing preabortion ultrasounds but also of seeing the fetal remains. Providers routinely checked that they had removed all "products of conception," work that could take an emotional toll, especially after dilation and extraction by dismemberment replaced saline instillation for the minority of second-trimester abortions. Having avoided sharing discomforting experiences from a justified fear that these would be weaponized against them, staff now responded to client demand. Supporting those who had grown up in the presence of the public fetus and with legal abortion, and so were more conflicted than the first generation to benefit from this, they created a safe space. Preparation for this "patient-centered pregnancy tissue viewing" includes being shown standard drawings and photos of remains at actual size first made for the purpose at a clinic in Toledo, Ohio, in 1993.[86]

Clients have appreciated the chance to view, even if not many take up the offer; interviews suggest that viewing made the experience harder for only a few. In first-trimester cases, the vast majority, service-users tended to be pleasantly surprised how small and non-babylike the fetal parts were.[87]

(2009): 97–102; Siân M. Beynon-Jones, "Re-Visioning Ultrasound through Women's Accounts of Pre-Abortion Care in England," *Gender and Society* 29, no. 5 (2015): 694–715.

85   Rothman, *Tentative Pregnancy*; Rapp, *Testing Women, Testing the Fetus*; Taylor, *Public Life*; Ilana Löwy, *Imperfect Pregnancies: A History of Birth Defects and Prenatal Diagnosis* (Baltimore: Johns Hopkins University Press, 2017).

86   Schoen, *Abortion after Roe*; Lena Hann and Jeannie Ludlow, "Look Like a Provider: Representing the Materiality of the Fetus in Abortion Care Work," in *Representing Abortion*, ed. Rachel Alpha Johnston Hurst (London: Routledge, 2021), 119–30.

87   Ellen R. Wiebe and Lisa C. Adams, "Women's Experiences of Viewing the Products of Conception after an Abortion," *Contraception* 80, no. 6 (2009): 575–77; Lena R. Hann and Andréa Becker, "The Option to Look: Patient-Centred Pregnancy Tissue Viewing at Independent Abortion Clinics in the

Women have had similar experiences of seeing "eggs" in the medical abortions up to nine weeks that are now about half of all terminations in the United States.[88] Providers and clients have felt more uncomfortable about viewing after second-trimester abortions. But some became convinced that seeing, and even touching, fetal remains helped both groups gain resilience. Abortion, where accessible, could offer simple relief. Yet sometimes, as had been established for miscarriage, stillbirth, and termination for fetal anomaly, grieving provided greater closure.[89] While controversial for how much it concedes, the practice resists leaving the visual field to either gruesome war photos or beautified icons.

Powers of Visual Culture

This chapter has historicized the public fetus, the rights-bearing already-baby made by circulation and copying in the United States between the late 1960s and 1990. I took a long view in order to highlight the specificity in time and space of a phenomenon that drew on prior imagery but also departed from it and was constructed variously earlier and later elsewhere. Recognizing this fetus as produced by antiabortionists but defined by their feminist critics, I have incorporated some of what has been learned historically and changed in practice since Petchesky's article. I have stressed the strategies and tactics through which proponents subverted the developmental series to project a baby back onto earlier stages, and even denied that these were fetuses at all.

Critiques have struggled with this icon, particularly when limited to debunking or trapped in the binary of woman or fetus. Pictures that associate abortion with responsible reproduction are up against the simple appeal, apparent naturalness, and political connections of the isolated fetus, and its reinforcement by the anticipatory visual practices adopted in embryology, obstetrics, and reproductive biomedicine. With their frequently decontextualized representations of development and sometimes voyeuristic gaze, these specialties enabled that fetus. They offer alternatives, too.

In a sign of antiabortionist and feminist reach, in 2003 the author of the leading developmental biology textbook set criteria for selecting a cover

---

United States," *Sexual and Reproductive Health Matters* 28, no. 1 (2020): 1730122.

88   On France: Elaine Gale Gerber, "Deconstructing Pregnancy: RU486, Seeing 'Eggs,' and the Ambiguity of Very Early Conceptions," *Medical Anthropology Quarterly* 16, no. 1 (2002): 92–108.

89   On miscarriage: Linda L. Layne, *Motherhood Lost: A Feminist Account of Pregnancy Loss in America* (New York: Routledge, 2003).

image of a human embryo to block appropriation "for antiabortion lobbying": that internal anatomy be included, that the stage precede the development of a human-looking face, and that "the umbilicus, amnion, and placenta" "be readily observable . . . to retain the embryo in its maternal (natural) context."[90] Illustrators can also insist on indicating the scale. Framing development within generational cycles might more routinely challenge the assumption of an obvious starting point. Acknowledging rates of wastage makes clear that most fertilized eggs never develop to term.[91] Ultrasound, supposedly an antiabortionist superweapon, provides countless indications for termination, and even fetal remains may be viewed in ways that support a decision to abort. Unshakable among large, powerful groups, the public fetus is here for the foreseeable future. It does not have the field to itself, even after *Dobbs*.

90 Scott F. Gilbert and Rebecca Howes-Mischel, "'Show Me Your Original Face Before You Were Born': The Convergence of Public Fetuses and Sacred DNA," *History and Philosophy of the Life Sciences* 26, no. 3–4 (2004): 377–94, 477–79.

91 Anne McLaren, "Where to Draw the Line?" *Proceedings of the Royal Institution of Great Britain* 56 (1984): 101–21; Freidenfelds, *Myth of the Perfect Pregnancy*.

Chapter Nine

Public Menstruation

Visualizing Periods in Art, Activism, and Advertising

Camilla Mørk Røstvik

Just like pregnancy, menstruation has a multifaceted visual history. Both bodily phenomena are linked to issues of stigma, hope, and fear, and bring with them visual signifiers that many will recognize. Both are connected to iconic images, such as those of Lennart Nilsson in the case of the fetus or Tampax advertising for periods. Furthermore, both bodily events produce "acceptable" and "unacceptable" visual signs. In the case of menstruation, the most obvious visual sign is blood, yet historically it has often been censored and thought of as taboo in terms of representation. So what can "the opposite" of pregnancy reveal about the "public fetus"? Are there similar attitudes toward the visual signs of both extremes of the menstrual cycle, or have the two previously hidden visual cultures parted ways, forming separate iconographies? The following analysis of menstrual signs in art and culture suggests that examining the public fetus in the context of the larger menstrual and reproductive cycle might reveal additional layers to its complex position in culture today.

Since the 1970s, visual representations of menstruation have increased, with the bulk of material still originating from commercial actors. Menstrual technology, especially disposable tampons and pads, is therefore often invoked in reference to menstruation, whether as part of a policy initiative or to illustrate a newspaper article. For instance, the same type of unused white tampon graced *Newsweek*'s 2016 cover story on menstrual activism, a consultation document for the Scottish government's Period Products (Free Provision) Bill in 2017, and a series of medical research articles in

Scientific American.[1] By contrast, art depicting menstrual themes remained focused on used products or blood, showing how public menstrual *bleeding* remained taboo, despite the increased visual representation of menstrual themes. In this, contemporary artists echo earlier product-centric menstrual artworks, such as Judy Chicago's *Red Flag* from 1971, in which the artist is photographed removing a bloody product from her vagina, boldly showing what menstrual product advertising did not dare reveal at the time.[2] Activists and scholars argue that the belief in a "technology fix" for all menstrual problems neglects the multifaceted experience of menstruation, and artists showing menstrual blood are therefore part of the continuous protest against the "menstrual concealment imperative."[3] As part of a broader visual landscape in which images of reproduction have become more normalized, menstrual images have begun following a similar trend, in which iconicity follows past invisibility. Unlike the proliferation of fetal images in public through Nilsson's iconic photographs, menstruation remains symbolized through products designed to hide it, but both visual cultures share a tendency toward sanitizing the body's diverse experiences.

In this chapter, I examine various iterations of public menstruation through examples from the arts, advertising, and popular discourse. First, we explore the works of four very different contemporary mixed-media artists who received both praise and condemnation for their menstrual creations in the 2010s: Rupi Kaur, Sarah Maple, Bee Hughes, and Liv Strömquist. In their works, these artists directly and indirectly reference the history of menstrual art making, begun in the 1960s and galvanized by the feminist

1   Abigail Jones, "The Fight to End Period Shaming Is Going Mainstream," *Newsweek*, April 20, 2016, cover image; "Ending Period Poverty Bill: A Proposal for a Bill to Ensure Free Access to Sanitary Products, Including in Schools, Colleges and Universities," consultation by Monica Lennon, MSP for the Scottish Parliament for Central Scotland (2017); Virginia Sole-Smith, "What Is the Point of a Period?," *Scientific American*, May 1, 2019: https://www.scientificamerican.com/article/what-is-the-point-of-a-period/ (last accessed April 21, 2023).

2   Camilla Mørk Røstvik, "Blood Works: Judy Chicago and Menstrual Art since 1970," *Oxford Art Journal* 42, no. 3 (2019): 335–53.

3   Chris Bobel, "Disciplining Girls through the Technology Fix: Modernity, Markets, Materials," in *The Managed Body: Developing Girls and Menstrual Health in the Global South*, ed. Chris Bobel (Cham: Palgrave Macmillan, 2019), 243–80; Jill Wood, "(In)Visible Bleeding: The Menstrual Concealment Imperative," in *The Palgrave Handbook of Critical Menstruation Studies*, ed. Chris Bobel et al. (Singapore: Palgrave Macmillan, 2020), 319–36.

movement in the 1970s.[4] I therefore examine a selection of these pioneering works in order to see whether the reception of public menstruation in art has changed or not. Next, we take another step back to examine what artists working in the twentieth and twenty-first centuries are grappling with in terms of larger menstrual themes, including menstrual stigma and the menstrual product industry. In order to understand how the notion of public menstruation became so controversial, it is necessary to examine the forces that rendered menstrual blood invisible in the first place, including the normalization of disposable menstrual products in the twentieth century, and the accompanying advertising. In addition, we examine critical responses to the "menstrual concealment imperative," exploring how feminist, environmental, economic, and queer critiques are referenced in artworks from the 1960s to the present.[5] Finally, I consider the differences between images of the public fetus and the menstrual cycle.

While menstrual art can be shocking, this article argues that these works invoke a much deeper and more complex dialogue with a longer history of menstrual commercialization, marketing, and activism.

Menstruation in Contemporary Art

Starting soon after the launch of social media platforms in the 2000s, artists used the new technology and publishing outlets like Instagram and Facebook to share their menstrual art directly with a wider international audience. Barred or censored from traditional gallery or exhibition spaces, menstrual (and other taboo) art had found an obvious—if complicated—venue in social media by the 2010s.[6]

In early spring of 2015, Indian Canadian photographer and poet Rupi Kaur published a series of self-portraits titled *Period* on the social media platform Instagram. Photographed by her sister Prabh, Kaur was shown in everyday situations while menstruating. The images featured very little blood, centering instead on parts of Kaur's body or the white, gauzy rooms in which she moved. One photograph featured the artist lying fully clothed in bed with a pink hot water bottle, facing up. In another, Kaur turns her

---

4   Chris Bobel, "'Our Revolution Has Style': Contemporary Menstrual Product Activists 'Doing Feminism' in the Third Wave," *Sex Roles* 54, no. 5 (2006): 331–45.

5   Wood, "(In)Visible Bleeding," 319–66.

6   Ben Luke, "Art in the Age of Instagram and the Power of Going Viral," *Art Newspaper*, March 27, 2019: https://www.theartnewspaper.com/2019/03/27/art-in-the-age-of-instagram-and-the-power-of-going-viral.

back to the viewer and curls up in a fetal position, revealing a small rust-red menstrual stain on her trousers. Both water bottle and stain were carefully arranged to appear as the central focus of the photograph, drawing the viewer's eye to the middle of the composition. Kaur's series was celebrated as an act of activism and bravery after Instagram stated that the work violated its rules for acceptable posts. Positive and negative analysis of this episode focused on the stain visible on Kaur's trousers, largely neglecting the rest of the series, and the careful composition, lighting, and style. In response to Instagram, Kaur wrote a post stating that the platform had proven her point: menstruation was worth making art about because it was still considered taboo.[7] The artist was both celebrated and harassed for her efforts, but Instagram reversed its decision and has since hosted many menstrual artworks and artists, making it a viable, free, and accessible exhibition space. As an example of public menstruation, Kaur's intervention underlines the ways in which menstrual artists have to fight for access to public forums, often breaking new ground and challenging censorship.

In the years surrounding this landmark and highly public event of menstrual censorship, other artists working on menstrual themes were confronted with similar issues of controversy, celebration, and dismissal of their work. In the large oil painting *Menstruate with Pride*, British-Muslim artist Sarah Maple painted herself in a white dress while bleeding in front of horrified, mostly adult, onlookers. The oil painting shows a defiant protagonist who is not ashamed, aware perhaps of the small girl who looks on with curiosity while another adult tries to shield her from an instance of public menstruation. The painting features a diverse group of people and shows Maple experimenting with one of many Muslim British identities she is known for in her work, blurring the ideas of "good" and "bad" Islamic womanhood, while transgressing the transnational and pan-cultural taboo against public menstruation.

Maple's self-portrait appeared in a series of feminist exhibitions, but the artist also received death threats and calls for censorship for this and other works. Like Kaur, Maple challenged censorship debates and harassment directly, speaking about it in the press.[8] *Menstruate with Pride* was in part made to revisit her own shame as a young menstruator, and to reimagine her first menstrual experiences as an adult who no longer felt embarrassed about bleeding. As one of the recipients of the prestigious Sky Arts awards, she

---

7   Rupi Kaur on Instagram (@rupikaur) wrote, "Thank you @instagram for providing me with the exact response my work was created to critique," March 24, 2015.

8   Nell Frizzell, "Artist Sarah Maple: 'I've Had Death Threats,'" *Guardian*, July 14, 2015: https://www.theguardian.com/artanddesign/2015/jul/14/sarah-maple-feminist-artist-photography.

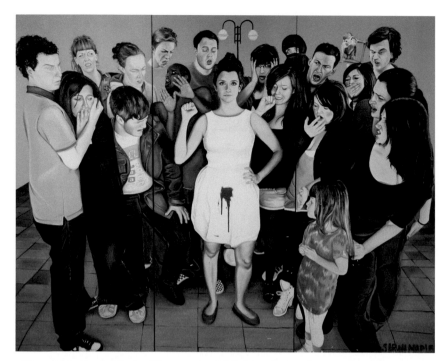

Figure 9.1. Sarah Maple, *Menstruate with Pride*, 2015. Oil on canvas. Photograph ©Sarah Maple.

has since become a better-known figure on the international art scene, while *Menstruate with Pride* remains her only menstrual-themed work. It is no accident, then, that the artist uses a photograph of herself standing directly in front of the painting as her CV image, prominently displaying it on her website and including it in interviews.[9] Like Kaur's work, Maple's menstrual painting managed to break taboos and challenge calls for censorship, leading to recognition by art institutions. Yet, Maple showed the painting actively in order for it to be part of the discourse surrounding her artistic success.

Around the same time, queer artists with an interest in menstrual themes faced barriers to public expression, this time concerning who has a right to talk about menstruation.[10] The fraught discussions around trans rights in

---

9   Sarah Maple, "About/CV," artist's website, https://www.sarahmaple.com/about (last accessed May 5, 2021).

10   Joan Chrisler et al., "Queer Periods: Attitudes toward and Experiences with Menstruation in the Masculine of Centre and Transgender Community,"

Britain soon included menstrual themes, such as the right to use certain bathrooms and the question of whether or not trans and nonbinary consumers should be included in menstrual product advertising and policy initiatives to provide free products in school and food banks. Around this time, nonbinary British mixed-media artist Bee Hughes began exploring the iconic form of the tampon, reimagining it as a life-sized, handheld clay sculpture. Their work was gathered together in the installation *Lifetime Supply*, where Hughes also began painting the clay objects in a rainbow of colors and organizing them in a grid to be photographed carefully from above. These small talismans nod to the LGBTQ flag but also serve as quiet reminders of the symbolic "icons" of menstruation and the ways in which tampons have come to represent menstruation in media, popular culture, and public debate. Reclaiming the tampon as a piece of multicolored sculpture (including bright red), Hughes suggests that we can free menstruation and even tampons from corporate symbolism and the habits of consumption. While Hughes's point was subtle, the debate about queerness and menstruation did not allow much space for multifaceted views on tampons, instead conceptualizing Hughes's and other queer artists' work on menstruation as activist statements. Queer artists with an interest in menstrual themes, including South African Zanele Muholi and American Cass Clemmer, were often questioned over their right to care about menstruation. While this criticism has its roots in transphobia, it also contributes to the overall censorship of public menstruation by attempting to prevent a group of people from engaging with this stigmatized topic. Like Kaur and Maple, however, Hughes managed to transgress calls for self-censorship, using a personal website, exhibitions in feminist and queer spaces, Twitter, and academia to circulate their work.[11]

In a similar move to that of artists who use the "public square" of social media to share menstrual work, a recent example of art showing menstrual blood in a physical public space reveals changing attitudes. In 2017, Swedish artist Liv Strömquist was invited to exhibit a series of menstrual artworks at various Stockholm Metro stations. While discreet advertising for menstrual products from the Swedish multinational corporation Essity had been visible at the stations before, this marked the first time that a noncommercial and blood-red depiction of menstruation appeared in this type of public space in Sweden. Provoking both celebration and condemnation, the artist proved

---

Culture, Health & Sexuality 18, no. 11 (2016): 1238–50.

11   Bee Hughes, artist's website, https://www.beehughes.co.uk/about (last accessed May 4, 2021).

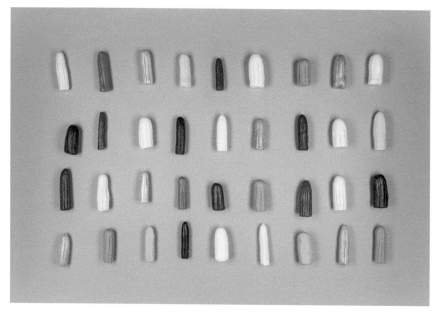

Figure 9.2. Bee Hughes, *Lifetime Supply*, 2017. Ongoing project seeking to create lifetime supply of unusable clay tampons. Photograph © Bee Hughes.

her point: menstruation is still a complicated topic to visualize in public.[12] At Slussen Station in Stockholm, Strömquist's line drawing of a figure skater visibly bleeding was accompanied by the statement "It's alright (I'm only bleeding)."[13] In claiming that this was indeed "alright," Strömquist was seen to blend the boundary between art and activism, and argued for the right to show menstrual themes and creative impressions of blood in public. Since then, the dissemination of menstrual images in public has grown substantially, not least through the increasingly realistic and artistic advertising campaigns from Essity and other corporations, suggesting that we are edging closer to the acceptance of visible menstruation.

While the works of Kaur, Maple, Hughes, and Strömquist are visually and thematically different, these artists all became interested in menstruation

---

12   Mike Classon Frangos, "Liv Strömquist's *Fruit of Knowledge* and the Gender of Comics," *European Comic Art* 13, no. 1 (2020): 45–69.

13   Interview with Strömquist about exhibition for Stockholm metro, titled *Nightgarden*, "Can Public Art Break the Taboo over Periods?" *Cultural Frontline*, 2 min., BBC Radio, first broadcast March 8, 2018, https://www.bbc.co.uk/programmes/p060h92j.

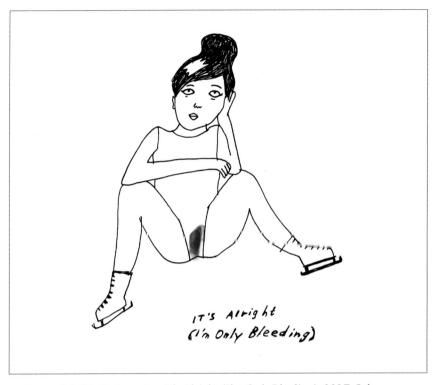

Figure 9.3. Liv Strömquist, *It's Alright (I'm Only Bleeding)*, 2017. Ink pen on paper, with red watercolor. © Liv Strömquist 2017. All rights reserved.

during a decade when menstrual activism increased across the globe. Thus they were in different ways markers of a proliferation of engagement from the general public in the 2010s, which intersected with large international activist campaigns to cut tampon tax, provide product ingredient information, "End Period Poverty," destigmatize menstrual health problems, and supply better menstrual health education.[14] There was also a visual component to the popularization of menstrual activism created by artists working

---

14   Malaka Gharib, "Why 2015 Was the Year of the Period, and We Don't Mean Punctuation," NPR.com, December 31, 2015: https://www.npr.org/sections/health-shots/2015/12/31/460726461/why-2015-was-the-year-of-the-period-and-we-dont-mean-punctuation; for a discussion of this claim, see Chris Bobel, introduction to Bobel et al., *Palgrave Handbook*, 1–9.

from within corporate structures.[15] The paint company Pantone launched "Menstruation Red" as part of their core collection (with the goal of "ending period stigma"), Scottish brewing company Brew Dog launched a "Bloody Good Beer" (profits went to the period poverty charity Bloody Good Period) featuring a pad and red colors, a menstrual-themed chocolate Easter egg sold out within days, and a series of increasingly realistic and artistic marketing campaigns from product manufacturers were launched around the world.

Artists like Kaur, Maple, Hughes, and Strömquist functioned as canaries in the coalmine for public menstrual debate, testing audiences' readiness to embrace or reject menstrual themes. For various and intersecting reasons, their works were both celebrated and attacked, and they were roundly dismissed as activism rather than art by the art world's institutional hierarchy. This, however, was not the first time artists interested in menstruation have faced the consequences of menstrual stigma in their practice. Rather, Kaur, Maple, Hughes, and Strömquist joined a long history of artists celebrated and ridiculed for making menstruation a public affair, actively invoking that history in their artistic practice.

Menstruation in Art History

Throughout the twentieth century, menstruators were usually invested in "passing" as nonmenstruating at all times.[16] Strong cultural norms about femininity ensured that menstrual blood was seldom seen in public.[17] The artists who began experimenting with menstrual themes and blood in the late 1960s therefore transgressed against "menstrual etiquette," challenging the rules of secrecy and crossing boundaries of good taste.[18]

---

15 Chris Bobel, *New Blood: Third-Wave Feminism and the Politics of Menstruation* (New Brunswick, NJ: Rutgers University Press, 2010), 113.

16 Lesley Hoggart and Victoria Louise Newton, "Hormonal Contraception and Regulation of Menstruation: A Study of Young Women's Attitudes towards 'Having a Period,'" *Journal of Family Planning and Reproductive Health Care* 41, no. 3 (2014): 210–15.

17 Lara Freidenfelds used archives and oral history to document the lived experience of menstruators from 1900 until the 1990s in *The Modern Period: Menstruation in Twentieth-Century America* (Baltimore: Johns Hopkins University Press, 2009).

18 Julie-Marie Strange, "The Assault on Ignorance: Teaching Menstrual Etiquette in England, c. 1920s to 1960s," *Social History of Medicine* 14, no. 2 (2001): 247–65. Strange draws on Sophie Laws's coinage of the term "menstrual

In much of their varied work, artists addressing menstrual themes in the 1960s and 1970s focused on making the taboo of menstrual blood visible.[19] Japanese artist Shigeko Kubota invoked menstrual themes in the infamous performance *Vagina Painting* (1965), in which she painted red paint across large sheets of paper using a paintbrush attached to her underwear. In the United States, Judy Chicago created works that centered on used menstrual products (1971–72), while her contemporary Carolee Schneemann collected and inserted her own menstrual fluids in *Blood Work Diary* (1972). Across the Atlantic, Judy Clark collected menstrual pads and exhibited them in a neat gridlike system (for the exhibition *Issues* in 1972), while Catherine Elwes freely bled in the durational performance piece *Menstruation* (1979).[20] In Scandinavia, Elsebet Rahlff (part of the radical collective Gruppe 66) created textile representations of the menstrual cycle in the controversial traveling exhibition *Common Life*, designed in part to inform audiences about sexual and reproductive health (1977). Throughout the Nordic countries, artists interested in feminist themes also embraced menstruation as a radical symbol of transgression, including it in exhibitions, public performance, and as part of collective protests.[21]

Collectively, these artists have little in common, and the only aspect linking their work was their interest (however brief) in menstrual themes. Nevertheless, they all faced various levels of self-censorship, institutional critique, and ridicule for daring to make menstruation public.[22] Outside of specific feminist art spaces and supportive art school environments, these works were not exhibited or made available for public viewing until decades later.[23] Most of these pioneering menstrual artists never returned to the theme, while the next generation of creators who gravitated toward menstruation in the 1980s and 1990s increasingly used menstrual art as a shock tactic for activist goals.[24] As a consequence, menstrual arts remained underground and countercultural for the rest of the century, circulating

etiquette" in *Issues of Blood: The Politics of Menstruation* (London: Palgrave Macmillan, 1990).

19   Ruth Green-Cole, "Bloody Women Artists," *Occasional Journal* (November 2015): https://enjoy.org.nz/publishing/the-occasional-journal/love-femi-nisms/text-bloody-women-artists#article (last accessed April 21, 2023); Bobel, *New Blood*.

20   Kathy Battista, *Renegotiating the Body: Feminist Art in 1970s London* (London: Bloomsbury, 2012).

21   Una Mathiesen Gjerde, "Blodig Alvor: Menstruasjonskunst i Skandinavia fra 1970 til 2015" (MA thesis, Copenhagen University, 2017).

22   Green-Cole, "Bloody Women Artists," 2.

23   Røstvik, "Blood Works," 335–53.

24   Bobel, *New Blood*, 128.

in small and welcoming spaces without fully penetrating the popular consciousness until much later.

The first wave of menstrual artists worked in a time before menstrual activism had entered public discourse in the late 1970s.[25] For this reason, their works were unusual and isolated examples of realistic menstrual representation in a culture where the marketing of commercial products dominated the visual landscape of menstruation. In order to understand why their works were seen as so controversial, we therefore need to examine what the status quo of menstrual representation had become by the late twentieth century.

Marketing Menstruation

The menstrual product industry has dominated the visual representation of menstruation for just over one hundred years. In the 1920s, companies first explored the idea of disposable pads and tampons, slowly growing their market and becoming the norm in terms of protecting clothing and women.[26] In the previous generations, homemade, natural, and washable options were often used, suggesting a culture in which visible menstruation was slightly more normal—if not acceptable. For instance, in Scandinavia, knitted pads were the norm until the entry of disposable pads in the early twentieth century. This marked a major shift from the semi-public creation and washing of menstrual technologies at home (and school) to a consumer habit largely kept private through discreet packaging practices and code words while shopping alone.[27]

25   Bobel, *New Blood*; Breanne Fahs, *Out for Blood: Essays on Menstruation and Resistance* (Albany: State University of New York, 2016); Breanne Fahs, "Menstrual Activism," in *The Wiley Blackwell Encyclopedia of Gender and Sexuality Studies*, ed. Nancy A. Naples (Malden, MA: Wiley-Blackwell, 2016); Chris Bobel and Breanne Fahs, "The Messy Politics of Menstrual Activism" in Bobel et al., *Palgrave Handbook*, 1001–18; Chella Quint, "From Embodied Shame to Reclaiming the Stain: Reflections on a Career in Menstrual Activism," *Sociological Review* 67, no. 4 (2019): 927–42.

26   Elizabeth Arveda Kissling, *Capitalizing on the Curse: The Business of Menstruation* (Boulder, CO: Lynne Rienner, 2006); Sharra L. Vostral, *Under Wraps: A History of Menstrual Hygiene Technology* (Lanham, MD: Lexington Books, 2008).

27   Anne Helene Kveim Lie, "Kvinnen som biologi: Menstruasjon i norsk medisin i annen halvdel av 1800-tallet," *Nytt Norsk Tidsskrift* 25, no. 3–4 (2011): 362–78; Camilla Mørk Røstvik, *Cash Flow: The Businesses of Menstruation* (London: UCL Press, 2022).

Early product manufacturers, like artists, faced an initial challenge of how to visualize and bring attention to menstrual themes. In contrast to artists, they could not alienate their viewers and potential consumers but nevertheless needed to draw some public attention to their new products. The balance between informing, enticing, and not offending was delicate, and shifted according to the public discourse surrounding menstruation. Like menstrual art and protest, menstrual product advertising was often censored, specifically by print, television, and other advertising standard institutions. In response, the industry learned from its mistakes and built a growing understanding of the acceptable and unacceptable ways to visualize and sell menstrual products.

National companies working in the first half of the twentieth century used different tactics to attract consumers without causing scandal. US companies dominated this early period, with brands such as Kotex (Kimberly-Clark), Tampax (Tambrands Inc., now Procter & Gamble), and Modess (Johnson & Johnson) experimenting with various styles and concepts. Modess hired painter Pruett Alexander Carter, who created campaigns featuring elegant White women in luxurious evening gowns and the mysterious slogan "Modess, because . . ." Once Jewish and African American women had proven to be enthusiastic consumers of the same products, tailor-made advertising campaigns were published in Jewish and Black publications, in the 1940s and 1960s respectively. Competing brand Kotex relied on discreet blue packaging to sell in stores, while its print advertising appropriated the language of first-wave feminism with allusions to emancipation and women's rights, and using the Flapper fashion of the 1920s to underline the product's suitability for dancing and physical activity.[28] Tampax followed suit, showing White women in red bikinis to demonstrate their product's suitability for swimming and tight clothing, with a promise that the product meant "a new day for womanhood" was on the horizon. In these ways, White middle-class aspirations of fashion, luxury, and sports activities were invoked in order to make menstrual products appear suitable rather than scandalous.

In Sweden, the old mill company Mölnlycke (today owned by Essity) used both feminist terminology and fashion to illustrate their Mimosept pad brand. As in the United States, print campaigns were often illustrated by artists, and focused on the beauty standards and middle-class aspirations of the time. Advertising featured women with pin-up proportions, wearing fashionable, tight clothing, and engaging in activities such as tennis and shopping. These images suggested that modern, elegant women would use disposable

---

28   Roseann M. Mandziuk, "'Ending Women's Greatest Hygienic Mistake':
      Modernity and the Mortification of Menstruation in Kotex Advertising, 1921–
      1926," *Women's Studies Quarterly* 38, no. 3–4 (2010): 42–62.

pads to conform to standards of good taste and femininity, while the text underlined that old-fashioned homemade pads were unhygienic and inappropriate. By midcentury, modernity and aspiration became implicit in the purchasing of menstrual products in the West.[29] And through the hiring of skilled illustrators, artists, copywriters, and photographers these commercial visual renderings came to dominate the menstrual visual culture more generally. Menstrual products were sold as aspirational and as part of modern hygiene habits, but not as luxuries—suggesting that this was a slice of feminine middle-class personal care that everyone could try.[30]

By the time the first generation of menstrual artists began using pads and tampons, the necessity of disposable menstrual products was rarely questioned; it had become a Western norm. In effect, menstrual blood was no longer seen in public, other than as an embarrassing "accident," or through rare and unusual menstrual artworks. While menstrual art from the 1960s onward was not seen by many people at the time, it was referenced by many early advocates of menstrual education and rights, who described their interaction with the work as a shock and a wake-up call. For activists, encounters with menstrual art made them reconsider the norms of menstrual concealment, which in turn made them question whether these norms were logical, or even harmful.[31]

Menstruation as Activism

Menstrual activism became more galvanized and solidified in the 1970s, and included active groups across the world, often associated with women's and reproductive rights activism.[32] The first books about menstrual culture and taboos by menstrual activists, scholars, and commentators aimed at the general public were published in the late 1970s, and often referenced encounters with menstrual art and its revolutionary effect on the writers and movement. In *The Curse: A Cultural History of Menstruation* (1976), the authors

29   Mandziuk, "'Ending Women's Greatest Hygienic Mistake,'" 42; Røstvik, *Cash Flow*, 57–80.

30   Jane Farrell-Beck and Laura Klosterman Kidd, "The Roles of Health Professionals in the Development and Dissemination of Women's Sanitary Products, 1880–1940," *Journal of the History of Medicine and Allied Sciences* 51, no. 3 (1996): 325–52.

31   Janice Delaney, Mary Lupton, and Emily Toth, *The Curse: A Cultural History of Menstruation* (Urbana: University of Illinois Press, 1976).

32   Bobel, "'Our Revolution Has Style,'" 331–32.

celebrated Judy Chicago and other artists' menstrual works as pioneering.[33] In *The Wise Wound*, also published in the late 1970s, art and poetry with menstrual themes were referenced as a radically different alternative to the dominant iconography of menstruation, which relied on euphemism and historic taboos.[34] Theoretical discussions about the invisibility of menstruation helped readers understand the visual aspects of menstrual stigma. Activist Sophie Laws conceptualized "menstrual etiquette" as a way to understand the self-policing and self-censorship of the visibly menstruating body.[35] In *Images of Bleeding: Menstruation as Ideology*, Louise Lander analyzed the damaging effect of product advertising and the commercial appropriation of menstrual blood itself, inviting the reader to question whether a better visual representation was even possible. And in Ann Treneman's explosive essay "Cashing In on the Curse: Advertising and the Menstrual Taboo," the industry was dissected and blamed for its use of stereotypes and sexism in visual pad and tampon marketing.[36] These writers felt deeply suspicious about the increased use of empowering language and visual representations of feminism in menstrual product marketing. Treneman summarized the problem in this way:

> The message is "Women are superior to men"—and what a seductive pitch it is! We emerge from reading this ad—our egos nicely massaged and our sense of humour tickled—feeling pretty good. It has gone beyond the area of many menstrual product ads. It only occasionally alludes to our burden, and presents Dr White as our bosom buddy who helps "make your life more bearable, whatever kind of periods you have to put up with." But with friends like these, we don't need enemies. For in addition to reinforcing the idea that our periods are a burden that we must hide, the doctor has just sold us the idea that the reason for our superiority is that we have been so successful in hiding our shameful secret![37]

Consumers like Treneman were critical toward the appropriation of feminism, providing important context about the long-standing blurred lines between consumer culture, advertising, and artistic creativity in the

---

33   Delaney, Lupton, and Toth, *Curse*, 275.
34   Penelope Shuttle and Peter Redgrove, *The Wise Wound: Menstruation and Everywoman* (London: Victor Gollancz, 1978).
35   Laws, *Issues of Blood*.
36   Louise Lander, *Images of Bleeding: Menstruation as Ideology* (New York: Orlando, 1988); Ann Treneman, "Cashing In on the Curse: Advertising and the Menstrual Taboo," published in *Spare Rib* and *The Female Gaze: Women as Viewers of Popular Culture*, ed. Lorraine Gamman (London: Women's Press, 1988).
37   Treneman, "Cashing In on the Curse," 22.

menstrual product industry. Collectively these books and thinkers asked: Why is everyone so frightened of visible menstrual blood? At the heart of their critiques was concern about the growth of corporate influence, and what they saw as a complicated promise of liberation through menstrual products. Many consumers agreed, especially in the years following the toxic shock syndrome (TSS) controversy of the late 1970s.[38] While menstrual activism and art remained underground, the TSS episode radicalized a new generation of menstrual product consumers, who questioned whether products were dangerous (and were informed of possible dangers in the new information leaflets inserted in tampon boxes after TSS), as well as why they were often taxed, uncomfortable, and expensive. In this way, TSS was a highly public instance of debate about menstruation, necessitated by the dangers posed to consumers. While tampon sales dipped momentarily, the norm of using disposable menstrual products (like pads) was maintained throughout the crisis.[39]

Throughout the late twentieth century, corporations listened to criticism and adapted their visual rhetoric. Increasingly, boundaries were broken by advertisers. During the 1990s, words such as "blood," "pad," and, ultimately, "menstruation" were included in marketing, often directly challenging advertising standards. Next, images began to change, featuring first blue liquid and then red.[40] While menstrual activists remained skeptical of these claims to transgress boundaries because the images were still rooted in commercial interests, the increased realism and detailed nature of menstrual advertising around the turn of the century nevertheless contributed to public discourse about the overall invisibility of menstruation. Like artists in the 1960s and 1970s, those growing up in the new millennium were initially prompted to make menstrual work because of the limitations of menstrual product advertising and what they saw as ridiculous representations of femininity, "hygiene," and products.[41] Their work questioned menstrual taboos, which they saw as deeply linked with the visual representation of menstruation. The relationship between advertisers, companies, activists, and artists thus remained interlinked, based on the underlying societal stigma against public menstruation.

---

38 Sharra L. Vostral, *Toxic Shock: A Social History* (New York: New York University Press, 2019); James K. Todd, "Toxic Shock Syndrome: Scientific Uncertainty and the Public Media," *Pediatrics* 67, no. 6 (1981): 921–23.

39 Freidenfelds, *Modern Period*, 227n22.

40 On the persistent use of water imagery in menstrual marketing from this time, see Røstvik, "Blood in the Shower: A Visual History of Menstruation and Clean Bodies," *Visual Culture and Gender* 13 (2018): 54–63.

41 Breanne Fahs, "Smear It on Your Face: Menstrual Art, Performance, and Zines as Menstrual Activism," in *Out for Blood*, 105–16.

Menstruation as Icon

Historically, decades or moments when menstruation was idealized through marketing, medicine, or symbolism have led to uneven progress.[42] In the twentieth century, it was argued that menstruation was, in turn, completely debilitating, perfectly normal, a threat to productivity, a symbol of femininity, a marker of reproductive capacity, linked to premenstrual syndrome and hysteria, deeply painful and difficult, and free from problems. These paradoxical and confusing messages have upheld myths about menstruation, illustrating how the combined biological and cultural nature of the menstrual cycle lends itself exceptionally well to stigmatization of those who menstruate.[43] Public menstruation threatens to collapse all these mythologies by simply revealing the core of the stigma and, in Strömquist's words, radically suggesting that visible menstrual blood in public is indeed "alright."

In the discussion following the circulation of works by Kaur, Maple, Hughes, and Strömquist, the question of what spaces are appropriate for public displays of menstruation was central. While advertising for menstrual products was already legal and possible in major public channels, artists had no equivalent guidebook, nor did the average menstruator. In the case of Strömquist, a discussion of the role of public art and the suitability of menstruation as an artistic subject was sparked by the Stockholm exhibition. Kaur's photographs, meanwhile, challenged social media platforms to reexamine their guidelines and change them. For Maple, questions about ethnic identity and femininity were posed, challenging the artist to defend her stance and refuse to be shamed for not conforming to societal pressure. And in the case of Hughes and other queer artists, the question of whether they should engage with menstrual themes emerged quickly and aggressively, leading the artists to defend their basic human rights. Each artwork thus posed the question: Is it okay to render menstruation public and, if so, who should do it and following what rules?

These complicated and unsolved questions are today also being invoked by advertisers, who continue to follow in the footsteps of artists who break visual menstrual boundaries. Essity's campaigns featuring real blood and Pantene's paint stunt would likely not have been possible without the pioneering work of artists who have addressed menstrual themes, beginning in the twentieth century. In fact, menstrual product companies and others who seek to benefit from the menstrual activism trend often partner with artists

---

42　M. Raftos, D. Jackson, and J. Mannix, "Idealised versus Tainted Femininity: Discourses of the Menstrual Experience in Australian Magazines That Target Young Women," *Nursing Inquiry* 5, no. 3 (1998): 174–86.

43　Lander, *Images of Bleeding*, 9.

working within and outside the advertising industry. Continuing the legacy of the pioneering advertisers of the 1920s, these creative professionals are tasked with treading the same fine line between enticing, informing, and including their potential consumers as those working on the hand-drawn illustrations of the past.

While artists and advertisers continue to challenge the "menstrual concealment imperative" visually, menstrual activists continue to advocate for basic rights, including the right to know what is inside products, fair pricing, and corporate responsibility when problems like TSS occur.[44]

Fundamentally, artists and activists working today are not just interested in menstrual iconography. To suggest that their only aims and requests are visual would be to do the field a disservice and play directly into advertisers' and companies' claims of boundary breaking through color coding alone. Rather, activists across the world identify the ways in which images are a means to an end, not the end in itself, which is to end menstrual stigma once and for all.

As for artists, menstruation remains a complicated topic—one still largely dismissed by the conventional art world and therefore best suited to alternative publication and exhibition outlets. Social media platforms, feminist art spaces, queer galleries, and public grants are examples of how artists can sidestep the censorship and surveillance of the art world.[45] There are perhaps no images of menstruation that have become as iconic as Lennart Nilsson's images of the human fetus. Nilsson's work foregrounded the reproductive body, whereas menstrual images (and menstrual blood) show a body that has not reproduced (in a specific month). The devaluation of child-free or childless women has made "not reproducing" an enticing topic for artists interested in stigma and taboos regarding gender, resulting in a menstrual image culture that is dominated by artistic interpretation that challenges this devaluation. While Nilsson's images exist in a medical framework and societal perspective that celebrates and fetishizes the mother and reproduction, menstrual imagery has been shared through commercial and creative means, divorcing the menstrual cycle somewhat from medicine's grip and celebrating the body beyond its reproductive capability. Whereas Nilsson's images quickly dominated the public's imagination of fetal iconography, menstrual

---

44   Jill M. Wood, "(In)Visible Bleeding: The Menstrual Concealment Imperative," *Palgrave Handbook*, 319–336.

45   For example, through the menstrual art exhibition curated by artist Jen Lewis for the Society for Menstrual Cycle Research conference in 2015, the *Syklus* exhibition of menstrual art in Norway in 2020, and the 2018 exhibition *Periodical* at the Being Human Festival in Liverpool, curated by Bee Hughes.

artworks and representations increasingly show a diverse set of menstrual experiences rather than one "beauty shot" of the cycle.[46]

Critical histories of the gendered body invite us to consider what it means when images of hitherto secret or unseen parts of the body are suddenly peeled open, dissected, explored, and utilized for profit or otherwise. Applying this question to the visual culture of menstruation reveals the ways in which public menstruation remains a transgressive force, yet to be fully accepted. While the examples of art by Strömquist, Kaur, Maple, and Hughes reveal the various and changing ways in which menstrual taboos operate in public today, they also show how questions first asked in the twentieth century remain unanswered. However, as in the case of the public fetus, corporate and activist ideas sometimes blend in unpredictable ways. As has been suggested by Lara Freidenfelds in the case of advertising menstrual products, corporations often followed the lead of consumers who wanted convenient ways to hide menstrual blood and subtle ads that would not feel embarrassing.[47] As such, the role of ordinary citizens in the visualization of both the fetus and menstruation blurs corporate-versus-activist boundaries, often bringing impulses of progressive and conservative visual culture together.

Public menstruation is indeed "alright," as long as it comes in an artistic, stylized form or within the confines of management through products. In the broader culture of images that reference the reproductive body, Nilsson's fetuses functioned in the same way—causing controversy, being utilized for different ideological means (especially in the case of abortion politics), while also helping clear the way for more public debates about the body. Similarly, images of menstruation—whether made by artists or advertisers—help set the stage for activists to be heard in the public realm without necessarily evidencing relaxed attitudes surrounding menstrual blood in real life.

---

46   On Nilsson, see Jülich, and Jülich and Björklund, this volume.
47   Freidenfelds, *Modern Period.*

Chapter Ten

From "Anatomical Specimen" to "Almost Child"

Pictures of Dead Fetuses in France

Anne-Sophie Giraud

In the summer of 2005, the discovery of the bodies of 351 dead fetuses kept in the "death chamber" of the Saint-Vincent-de-Paul Hospital in Paris triggered a massive scandal in France. Not only were the bodies stored in conditions deemed unacceptable, but the scandal was heightened by the fact that new ones were still being added to the collection. The hospital received numerous calls from parents. An administrative investigation conducted by a specialized government agency was initiated, the National Ethics Advisory Committee (Comité consultatif national d'éthique) was questioned, and the affair was brought to court. To many, it was a shock. The collection was ultimately removed, thereby exemplifying a general trend questioning the availability of human remains, especially fetal ones, their traceability, and their uses.[1] A similar controversy occurred in the early 1980s over the use of tissues from aborted fetuses for medical purposes.[2]

While the existence of such collections of dead fetuses and their use by medical professionals were very common in the nineteenth century, these cases reflect a deep shift relative to the social and legal status of the dead

---

1   On the history and fate of embryological collections, see Lynn M. Morgan, *Icons of Life: A Cultural History of Human Embryos* (Berkeley: University of California Press, 2009).

2   Françoise Fougeroux, "Utilisation de fœtus avortés et respect de la personne," in *Biomédecine et devenir de la personne*, ed. Simone Novaes, Collection Esprit (Paris: Seuil, 1981), 221–62.

fetus over the last thirty years. Such changes are visible in France but also in Europe, the United States, and Canada,[3] and they can be attributed to, among other factors, the rise of biomedical imaging technologies. Over time, the unborn has come to be perceived as a child-to-be at earlier and earlier stages of development.[4] As a result, the concept of the dead fetus as "waste" or even as an "anatomical specimen" has become disputed. In France, professionals have consequently begun to develop new rituals and practices since the 1980s, resulting in successive changes in the law in the 1990s and 2000s. Thus, this refusal to associate the dead fetus with "anatomical waste" has translated first into new management of its body: it is now dressed like a baby and buried as such.[5] It also can now legally be named and listed in public registers and in the family record book. In this regard, a particular practice has arisen whereby the dead fetus is photographed as a support for the memories of bereaved parents; images distinctly differ from those usually taken for autopsies. The dead fetus is shown as a child, fully dressed so as to hide its malformations. Mourning parents use these photographs to grieve, share them with their family and friends, and show them at public collective remembrance ceremonies and on the internet.

In this chapter, I will show that such practices are part of the emergence of the "public fetus" beyond the medical field but that these pictures nonetheless differ from those usually seen in the media.[6] First, they show dead fetuses, clearly without the appearance of life, but mostly presented as *living*. Second, they embody a singularized fetus with a name and a family, far from the medical specimen or the "universal" fetus usually represented. They are singularized in the sense that Luc Boltanski describes: depicted as singular,

---

3　For Europe, see "Les enfants nés sans vie" [Lifeless children], *The Senate Working Documents*, Comparative Law Series (Paris, Sénat, April 2008), and for Canada and the United States, see Linda L. Layne, *Motherhood Lost: A Feminist Account of Pregnancy Loss in America* (New York: Routledge, 2003).

4　Lynn M. Morgan and Meredith W. Michaels, eds., *Fetal Subjects, Feminist Positions* (Philadelphia: University of Pennsylvania Press, 1999); Nicole Isaacson, "The 'Fetus-Infant': Changing Classifications of 'in Utero' Development in Medical Texts," *Sociological Forum* 11, no. 3 (1996): 457–80; Layne, *Motherhood Lost*.

5　In France, "anatomical waste" is a legal category, defined as any "human fragments not easily identifiable," such as cysts, placentas, etc. (Art. R. 1335-1, Public Health Code, PHC). It is different from the "anatomical specimen," another legal category defined as any piece of human origin such as "organs or limbs, easily identifiable by a non-specialist" (Art. R. 1335-9, PHC). This distinction matters, as it translates into different practices, which I will deal with later.

6　For the term the public fetus, see chapter 12 in this volume.

unique, and irreplaceable individuals, and not only as members of a group as a whole.[7] They are not "life" in general, but a very specific life. They are named, dressed in a particular way, surrounded very often by personal possessions. It is then through an examination of the emergence of these new kinds of images that I will explore the transformations of the status of the dead fetus.

The chapter is based on a larger project conducted in France between 2009 and 2015. I began researching this topic precisely at the time of the last legal change concerning the dead fetus, making for an intense and rich context. The data consists of both ethnographic observations and semistructured interviews with sixteen professionals (health professionals—midwives, gynecologists, physicians, and so on—death care professionals, and association staff), and sixty-five bereaved individuals (sixty women and five men). All the bereaved people in the study have similar characteristics: they were involved in a process of "personifying" their deceased child, the vast majority were middle class, and all were White. I also conducted extensive ethnographic observations in two hospitals: the "Alpha" maternity ward in a small town in southern France, and the "Beta" maternity ward in Paris. Additionally, I observed two parent associations dedicated to pregnancy loss in southern France, numerous collective remembrance ceremonies, cemeteries for dead fetuses, and ordinary and private activities such as visits to the grave or care of a domestic altar dedicated to the child. Finally, I performed a document analysis, which included legal texts, data collected from websites, and newspaper articles.[8]

A brief note on terminology. The "unborn" is a social object, whose meaning and status depend on geographical, cultural, and historical contexts. That is why, as Deborah Lupton describes it, the terminology adopted to refer to the products of human conception is inevitably politically, emotionally, culturally—and I will add theoretically—charged. She uses "unborn" to refer to any type of organism produced from the union of human gametes, whether it is destined to become an infant or not, as she considers it the more "neutral" term.[9] Similarly in the parental context and the past, I adopt "unborn" to refer to the living product of the human conception still within the womb. I also adopt "deceased child" to refer to any fetus

---

7   Luc Boltanski, *The Foetal Condition: A Sociology of Engendering and Abortion* (Cambridge: Polity, 2013).

8   Anne-Sophie Giraud, "Les statuts de l'être anténatal: Un processus d'humanisation 'relationnel'; Assistance médicale à la procréation et mort périnatale" (Thèse de doctorat d'anthropologie sociale et ethnologie, Paris, EHESS, 2015).

9   Deborah Lupton, *The Social Worlds of the Unborn* (Basingstoke, UK: Palgrave Macmillan, 2013), 6.

that died *in utero* or newborn that dies shortly after birth. In these contexts, talking about "fetus" distorts the representations of some people who experienced pregnancy and its loss and distorts the past because in earlier periods what is now called a "fetus" was not even recognized as human.[10] I use the more technical medical term "fetus," and "dead fetus," in the legal and medical context as it is meaningful in these fields. I will not use the term "stillborn" as, according to the World Health Organization (WHO), it refers to a "baby who dies after 28 weeks of pregnancy" (or thirty weeks of amenorrhea [WA]).[11] Before thirty WA, it is known as a miscarriage or late fetal loss. Considering the legal context in France, where all fetuses after fourteen WA have the same legal status, talking about "dead fetuses" encompasses all the stages from this point to birth. In this chapter, I focus mainly on the case of the fetus which died *in utero* and not the child who died during or shortly after birth.

The Shrinking Category of Anatomical Waste

Since the 1990s, the legal status of the dead fetus and the treatment of its body have changed profoundly. The fetus increasingly tends to be personified. The Saint-Vincent-de-Paul Hospital scandal reveals the depth of these transformations, as it confronts practices now considered to be outdated, unnecessary, even unbearable, with a contemporary sensibility acknowledging the unborn as an almost child.

The law of January 8, 1993, marks the first legal step in this shift. Previously, along with fetuses who died in utero above twenty-eight WA, a child who was born alive and viable but died before being registered at the public office was not granted legal personhood (*personnalité juridique*). It was solely documented as a "lifeless child." With this law, the category of lifeless child was confined to the dead fetus alone, while newborns attested as viable and born alive by a medical certificate automatically acquire the legal status of "person," even if they pass away before being officially registered.[12] The law not only guarantees but mandates that persons must have a first

---

10   For a discussion, see Barbara Duden, "The Fetus on the 'Farther Shore': Toward a History of the Unborn," in Morgan and Michaels, *Fetal Subjects, Feminist Positions*, 13–25.

11   For a definition of stillbirth according to the WHO, see the organization's website, https://www.who.int/health-topics/stillbirth#tab=tab_1 (last accessed April 24, 2023).

12   Viability, that is, the capacity to live outside the womb, was established by the WHO in 1977 at twenty-two WA "with a lower limit of five hundred grams."

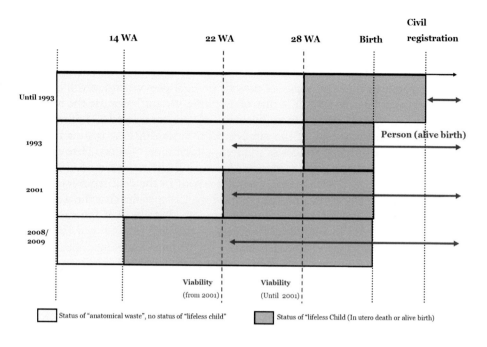

Figure 10.1. Changes in the legal status of the dead fetus in France.

name and a surname, that they must be recorded in the civil register and in the family record book, and that they must be given proper funerals.

But the 1993 law did not change the status of the dead fetus. The category of lifeless child was still limited to twenty-eight WA; below this threshold fetuses were considered "anatomical waste." As such, they were disposed of in a hospital incinerator, and operations on their bodies were not subject to regulation.[13] The treatment of lifeless children remained somewhat unclear, and as illustrated by the Saint-Vincent-de-Paul case, until the 2000s, there was only limited traceability. However, the category of lifeless child expanded in the 2000s to include increasingly early losses, starting at twenty-two WA in 2001,[14] then at fourteen WA in 2008 and 2009. Currently, any

---

13   Maryse Dumoulin and Anne-Sylvie Valat, "Morts en maternité: Devenir des corps, deuil des familles," *Etudes sur la mort* 119, no. 1 (2001): 77.

14   Circular No. 2001/576, November 30, 2001, and the Order of July 19, 2002, "on the registration and care of the bodies of children who have died before being declared at birth."

fetus that dies after fourteen WA —the legal limit of abortion in France until 2022 may be certified as a lifeless child. Below this fourteen WA limit, the dead fetus is considered anatomical waste.[15] Moreover, mainly as a result of the Saint-Vincent-de-Paul scandal, their traceability is now strictly respected.

Compared to the legal status of person, or legal personhood, the lifeless child status is intermediate: it is that of an "infra-person." First, terms such as "baby" or "child" may be used, but they only are considered as "compassionate" acknowledgment of the family's pain. Since 2021, it is now possible to grant a surname to lifeless children, establishing filiation. However, it is purely symbolic, as this inscription "has no legal effect" (law no. 2021-1576, December 6, 2021). Then, even if a record in the civil register provides a means to singularize the dead fetus,[16] the law specifies that the words "born," "birth," and "death" cannot be used to describe it.[17] Therefore, it is only registered in the "death" section of the civil register and family record book, and its inscription depends on the parents' preference. Legally, the dead fetus is considered by default to be an "anatomical specimen." If the couple does not want to organize a funeral, its body is disposed of like any other anatomical material: it is collectively and anonymously cremated according to a procedure that differs from the treatment of a legal person.[18]

Since the early 1990s, the limits that place the fetus in one or another of these categories—anatomical waste, anatomical specimen, deceased person, and, more importantly, lifeless child—have thus gradually shifted. The category of lifeless child has broadened, while that of anatomical waste has narrowed. Therefore, the dead fetus is considered to be an individual at earlier and earlier stages, rather than simply a part of the woman's body. In other words, it is perceived less as a fragment, or a residue, and more as an individual and a human being. This change is important from an anthropological point of view. Placing the dead fetus in the category of waste, anatomical specimen, or dead person, and even more so broadening the category of lifeless child, informs the representation of this being and its consequent treatment. Moreover, this shift indicates a change in the way medicine is expected to use products and elements of the human body. While the medical field

---

15   In 2022, the legal limit for abortion was extended from fourteen to sixteen WA (law no. 2022-295 of March 2, 2022, aimed at strengthening the right to abortion). This change did not seem to affect the boundary of the category of lifeless children.

16   Pierre Murat, "La Réforme de l'inscription à l'état Civil de l'enfant prématurément perdu: Entre progrès et occasion manquée," *Etudes Sur La Mort* 1, no. 119 (2001): 20.

17   The amended General Instruction on Civil Status of May 11, 1999.

18   Dominique Memmi, *La seconde vie des bébés morts* (Paris: Editions de l'Ehess, 2011).

once considered the tissues from abortion, pregnancy loss, and autopsy as medical property that could be collected without seeking people's consent, this began to change in the 1980s.[19] Scandals in France over the use of tissues from aborted fetuses and deceased persons are a case in point.[20] Medicine can no longer act as if it had full authority.

When Medical Professionals Make the Dead Fetus a "Child"

These legal changes are not the result of an explicit social demand on the part of bereaved couples but rather a consequence of a significant evolution in medical practices regarding the management of pregnancy loss.[21] Such practices, which tend to personify the dead fetus, strongly contrast with medical professionals' previous approach regarding pregnancy loss, described by activists as a "conspiracy of silence."[22]

Before the 1980s, when a woman gave birth to a dead fetus, she was placed under anesthesia or behind a surgical drape to prevent her from seeing the body, as recollected by Jeanne,[23] a psychologist from the Alpha maternity ward:

> When it was known that there was a fetal death in utero, the tendency was to sedate the mother for the time of the expulsion and to quickly remove the child. There were even times when the parents were not in the maternity ward.

Women who were to have a pregnancy loss, explained Jeanne, were indeed not considered as mothers-to-be, but as sick women. They were not hospitalized in the maternity ward but in gynecology services, as would have been the case for an abortion or an early miscarriage.[24] The death of a fetus, but also of a very early newborn, was mostly considered a

---

19   Morgan, *Icons of Life*, 197.
20   Fougeroux, "Utilisation de fœtus avortés"; Dominique Memmi, *La revanche de la chair: Essai sur les nouveaux supports de l'identité* (Paris: Éd. du seuil, 2014).
21   Memmi, *La seconde vie*.
22   Pierre Rousseau, "Psychopathologie et accompagnement du deuil périnatal," *Journal de gynécologie: Obstétrique et biologie de la reproduction*, no. 17 (1988): 285–94.
23   All names have been changed to preserve anonymity.
24   Alice Lovell, "Some Questions of Identity: Late Miscarriage, Stillbirth and Perinatal Loss," *Social Science & Medicine* 17, no. 11 (1983): 757.

"reproductive failure," rather than a "real death." Professionals advised women to forget it and attempt to have another child as soon as possible. It would have seemed unimaginable and simply cruel to present the fetus's body to the woman and even more so to ask her to give it a name. At the time, professionals believed that doing so would inhibit the couples' grieving process.[25] This attitude is partly explained by the lack of medical significance given to such events. Because involuntary termination of pregnancy is quite common (especially during the first trimester), the death of a fetus was considered a normal variation of the gestation process.[26] After delivery, the body was sent for a fetopathological examination when needed, and a funeral was held only exceptionally. The dead fetus was considered to have no other value than the potential medical information it bore. As Lynn Morgan observes for the United States, "The fetuses produced in the first half of the twentieth century were socially, morally, and qualitatively different from the fetuses of today."[27] This statement also applies to France. Neither the collection of fetal samples in the nineteenth century nor the treatment of the fetus as anatomical waste in the following century raised much ethical concern or debate. This is no longer the case.

The 1980s seem to have been a turning point in France, following an earlier trend from other countries such as the United Kingdom, where medical literature on perinatal bereavement has been published since the 1970s.[28] In France, this change was partly due to strong opposition of some professionals against the alleged "taboo on death," of which the "conspiracy of silence" surrounding pregnancy loss was just a part.[29] The development of biomedical imaging technologies also contributed to making the unborn

25 Marie-Ange Einaudi-De Siano, "Le décès périnatal: Vécu parental; Comprendre, décrire, améliorer," MA thesis, under the direction of Pierre Le Coz and Perrine Malzac, Université de la méditérannée, Aix-Marseille II (2008).

26 Linda L. Layne, "Breaking the Silence: An Agenda for a Feminist Discourse of Pregnancy Loss," *Feminist Studies* 23, no. 2 (1997): 292–93.

27 Morgan, *Icons of Life*, 200.

28 Joan Cameron, Julie Taylor, and Alexandra Greene, "Representations of Rituals and Care in Perinatal Death in British Midwifery Textbooks 1937–2004," *Midwifery* 24, no. 3 (September 2008): 335–43; Johan Cullberg, "Mental Reactions of Women to Perinatal Death," in *Psychosomatic Medicine in Obstetrics and Gynecology, 3rd Int. Congress* (London: Karger, 1972), 326.

29 Geoffrey Gorer, "The Pornography of Death," in *Death, Grief, and Mourning* (New York: Doubleday, 1955), 192–99; Rousseau, "Psychopathologie et accompagnement."

visible both as a child-to-be and as a "patient."[30] Thanks to such advancements, it is now possible to see the unborn alive and in movement. It can be heard, its heartbeat can be recorded, and it can even be the object of medical care.[31] Constructed as a child throughout pregnancy, should it die, it can no longer be reduced to a mere residue or the product of an abortion. Society, and medicine in particular, cannot continue to act as if nothing happened. "Creating" the unborn as a human that acts, suffers, and feels called for new rituals, especially when it came to death. Professionals, driven by a change in the paradigm of grieving in psychology (where seeing the materiality of the body would be necessary for mourning),[32] aim to restore the status of "child" that the unborn lost in dying. Seeing the corpse and recognizing it as a baby is now believed to be crucial to avoid pathological grieving.[33] Clarence, a pediatrician, explained:

> It is recommended to have procedures in place that humanize this child. For years, mothers were forbidden to see their dead baby because it could be difficult for them. Yet we realized, with the work of psychiatrists in particular, that this prevented them from mourning. So, we always suggest, without forcing it, that the mother sees the child. And some things are supposed to be organized, like asking the family whether they would like to participate in certain rituals at the birth, like bringing clothes, taking pictures, even though it may sound disturbing. . . . These are all things that help anchor the baby in humanity, in their personal history.

The old trend has been completely reversed and has, in fact, led to a voluntarist movement on the part of professionals who now strongly advise showing the dead fetus to the couple so that they may "grieve properly."[34]

Healthcare professionals, mainly midwives, have developed a humanized presentation of the dead fetus. Once named, cleaned, and dressed, it becomes a "child," making the bereaved couple "parents"—both statuses being linked. Women are now encouraged to give birth via vaginal delivery and to see their child. The women I interviewed claimed the delivery as proof that their child really existed and was not simply a product of miscarriage: "Because we hear that it was a simple curettage, that they evacuated him. No! No, I gave birth, it was a baby," said Justine, who lost her son

---

30 Morgan and Michaels, *Fetal Subjects, Feminist Positions*; Isaacson, "The 'Fetus-Infant'"; Layne, *Motherhood Lost*; Monica J. Casper, *The Making of the Unborn Patient: A Social Anatomy of Fetal Surgery* (New Brunswick, NJ: Rutgers University Press, 1998).

31 Isaacson, "The 'Fetus-Infant.'"

32 Memmi, *La seconde vie.*

33 Cullberg, "Mental Reactions of Women."

34 I personally take no position on the need to see the body or take photographs.

at twenty-eight WA after a medically terminated pregnancy due to a heart malformation.

After delivery, the dead fetus is sometimes directly presented to the parents but more often after being washed and dressed. Careful attention is paid to clothing, as it gives the dead fetus a childlike appearance as well as covering malformations. For instance, a cap will hide the absence of a skull in the case of anencephaly. Professionals systematically offer couples the opportunity to see the body at increasingly early stages, sometimes even at the limit of fourteen WA, as was the case for Angèle, who saw her daughter at this very early stage after a medically terminated pregnancy. There are thus very few constraints regarding the age or the appearance of the dead fetus.

The language employed is also important in this process. Professionals are careful not to use words such as "fetus," "miscarriage," or "expulsion." These terms are highly emotional, reflecting the status given to the dead fetus.[35] As mentioned before, the WHO recommends using "stillbirth" for a baby who dies after thirty WA.[36] Under this threshold, the death is considered a miscarriage. However, the definition of stillbirth is contested both by grieving parents and by some professionals who prefer a more "sensitive" definition, based on the parents' feelings, that recognizes the individuality of the dead fetus. As a neonatologist explained to me: "For the mother, whether she loses her baby in utero at 18 weeks, 19, 22, 24 or 30, it's the same. The suffering is not proportional to the number of weeks of amenorrhea." When the terms "miscarriage" or "abortion" are heard, this is a violent experience for parents, as was the case for Elodie. When she lost her daughter, a gynecologist told her she was having a miscarriage and that she was going to lose her fetus. By contrast, many professionals explain such experiences by speaking of the "baby" and of "birth." Some try to adjust their words to the patient, as Sarah, a midwife, explained to me:

> I'm adapting to their vocabulary, because it's really shocking if I ask, when was your miscarriage? So, if she tells me, "I've lost a baby," I'm going to try to adapt; I'm going to use her vocabulary instead.

Parents are also encouraged to name their child, to hold it in their arms, and to document it in their family record book. New theories regarding mourning suggest that material and concrete "traces" play an essential role in the objectification of the loss, and in the avoidance of pathological mourning.[37] Couples are therefore repeatedly encouraged to view their child at the hospital. As the protocol of the Alpha maternity ward reads: "When

---

35 Lupton, *Social Worlds of the Unborn*, 5.

36 But this definition is contested worldwide.

37 Memmi, *La seconde vie*, 16.

an induced abortion for medical reasons is conducted, the grieving process can only be based on a recognized reality of the child." Despite this injunction, some couples may refuse, for any number of reasons, to see the body, and some of them told me that they later regretted their decision, sometimes many years later. Many medical teams consequently insist on the importance of creating a "memory file" for the child. To this end, they may offer the parents a box containing different objects: footprints, handprints, a hospital ID bracelet, a cuddly toy, and clothes belonging to the child. They also encourage parents to create memories themselves with items related to the child, collected throughout the pregnancy: sonograms, clothes, pregnancy pictures, and photographs of the child itself. The latter are central to these memories.

From Medical to Remembrance Photographs, from Fetus to Child

With the development of imaging technologies, photographs have progressively replaced anatomical collections and wax models, now often considered obsolete.[38] Medical photography has become a common practice in a number of medical services—including to document a fetus's death. These images are for the exclusive use of medical personnel and anatomical pathologists and depict the dead fetus in a very specific manner: it is naked, not cleaned, often lying on its back with its limbs spread, so that malformations are clearly visible. The photograph is often taken with the body placed on a surgical drape or a tray, under crude lights. Such photographs are used as medical tools, informative with regard to abnormalities or the cause of death.[39] They constitute a key element of the death records.

But, as part of the new medical practices surrounding pregnancy loss, professionals have also started taking another kind of photograph. These are what I call "remembrance photographs," to differentiate them from the medical photographs. They are often presented by the actors involved, like all medical rituals around pregnancy loss, as being a simple return to mortuary practices of the past in order to reconnect with a relationship with death thought of as more virtuous and peaceful. From the nineteenth century until the 1950s in France—as well as in other European countries—remembrance photographs of the deceased were widespread. They were placed in family albums alongside the living and depicted both adults and children: but most prominently newborns. They were often taken after the child's death and, because of the scarcity of photographs, were frequently the sole image

---

38 Morgan, *Icons of Life*, 192.
39 Memmi, *La seconde vie*.

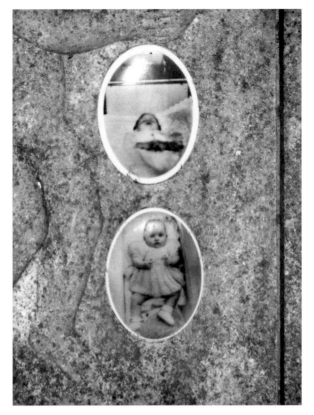

Figure 10.2. Photographs on a tombstone in a French cemetery of two children who died shortly after birth. Photo credit: Anne-Sophie Giraud.

kept by the family. In these images, the child is cleaned, combed, dressed in beautiful clothes, typically its baptismal gown. If some are clearly mortuary, depicting the child with closed eyes, lying in a cradle, others are more unsettling to a contemporary viewer. Eyes open, the child is held in its parents' arms or sits on a pillow in order to maintain an illusion of life.

Over time, with the development of photography and changes in attitudes toward death, these photographs became inappropriate, and the practice all but disappeared.[40] Both these earlier pictures and medical ones differ greatly from the "new" remembrance photographs: they do not represent

---

40   Marie-France Morel, "La mort d'un bébé au fil de l'histoire," *Spirale* 31, no. 3 (2004): 15.

the same being in the same way, they are not used in similar contexts (nor for the same purposes) and they involve different actors.

Firstly, under the guise of a simple return to the past, these new practices are actually quite contemporary and secular. Their aim is to not ensure the soul's access to heaven but rather to allow for "normal" grieving and, if anything, to accelerate the process.[41] There have also been very few representations of the fetus or even newborns who died soon after birth in the history of painting or photography outside the medical field, unlike those of young children and newborns.[42] Because pregnancy losses were quite common, and considered as a normal variation of the gestational process, in the past remembrance photographs depicted only "fully formed" children who lived for a few days or weeks. But those taken in hospitals since the 1990s depict either newborns who died immediately after birth or, in the vast majority of cases, fetuses that died in utero—sometimes as early as fourteen WA—before their face, skin, or limbs could come to resemble a newborn's. Professionals explained to me that there are very few constraints regarding the appearance of the dead fetus to be photographed. As mentioned, Angèle keeps a picture of her daughter Zoé, who died at fourteen WA. Zoé—who is smaller than Angèle's hand—is dressed in a sock cut into a tunic. If contemporary remembrance photographs now show fetuses who died in utero at a very early stage, photographs of dead newborns who passed away after birth are today relatively rare. Thanks to digital photography and especially camera phones, parents are now able to take pictures of their children while they are alive, and it is in this way that they want to remember them. These elements suggest that these are new and innovative practices and not "just" a return to the past, as it was first argued. They result from the general transformation of the status of the unborn: both parents-to-be and professionals have been portraying it as a child at progressively earlier stages. This shift is mainly due to the development of biomedical imaging technologies since the 1960s, which allowed fetal images to spread across the visual culture landscape and beyond the confines of the medical field.[43]

Second, unlike medical photographs, they are specifically intended for the bereaved couple and kept in their medical files, with the couple being informed that the photographs are there should they change their minds and want to see their child. Many of the interviewees did, in fact, take them

---

41   Memmi, *La seconde vie*.

42   Morel, "La mort d'un bébé."

43   Isaacson, "The 'Fetus-Infant'"; Rosalind Pollack Petchesky, "Fetal Images: The Power of Visual Culture in the Politics of Reproduction," *Feminist Studies* 13, no. 2 (1987): 263–92.

home.[44] In these photographs, not only is the dead fetus positioned to hide its malformations and blemishes but the pictures are often staged to present it socialized like a baby, in a cradle with cuddly toys. When no clothes can be found, frequently because of how small its body is, the dead fetus is swaddled in a bedsheet.

But because professionals are usually not well equipped, and because the photographs are frequently taken by busy midwives, their quality can be mediocre and the images blurry. The only photographs that Anne-Lise has of her daughter Gabrielle, taken by the hospital, are "cold" and "creepy," as she describes them:

> So the hospital asked if we wanted to see her, and we didn't, we had the choice, but they take photographs in any case to put them in the file, because after it's over. . . . So they took a picture. I'm not going to show you the photos because it's very hard to see a baby like this . . . They are not pretty, I can say that. She is laid out on a table, a grey table, partially covered by a sheet.

From what I observed, the pictures are sometimes simple Polaroids, or photographs printed on regular paper. That said, as these practices have become increasingly common in maternity hospitals, some have acquired better cameras, with a number of large maternity hospitals now using specialized photographers. Professionals, as well as associations, also encourage bereaved parents to take pictures themselves during their stay at the maternity hospital, allowing them to have better photographs. With the advent of camera phones, this has become easier for couples. Yet some people either forget or do not dare take a photograph in such a difficult moment. In other cases, the photographs can feel uncanny, as it can seem that the child depicted is not the same one they saw in the hospital. For instance, the colors may be different, its appearance can have changed hours after the birth, or the child pictured may differ from how they remember it.

In fact, these photographs taken by professionals are rarely used by parents, not only because of their poor quality but also because they portray a child that is not the one the parents would like to remember, or perhaps more importantly, not the one they want to show their relatives. When a child is born prematurely, it is covered with tubes and perfusions. When the child dies in utero, its color and appearance can differ from a viable one. The

---

44 Only sixteen (out of sixty-five people) did not pick up the photographs: five because there were no photographs, two because there was no available body, and three because their child was born alive and viable, and they had photographs from that time. Only four interviewees did not ask for the photographs, and the remaining two had made the request to the maternity hospital and were waiting for them at the time of the interview.

face and members are not well-formed, the skin color is reddish-blackish, and its appearance may be altered if the body has macerated in the womb. In such cases, steps can be taken to make the photograph more presentable, especially for a fetus that died at an early age, when the image may be overly graphic for family members. Parents may edit the photograph—for instance to change the color or the appearance of the skin—or even have portraits made so that the image can be more readily shared and the socialization of the child made easier. Drawings can also be used to reconstruct a certain image of the child. For example, Anne-Lise does not have any photographs of her daughter Gabrielle dressed. So, in order to retain a lucid memory of Gabrielle, she later asked an artist to draw the baby wearing the pajamas she had brought to the hospital. Other parents asked an artist to draw their child as an angel—the most commonly used symbol for pregnancy loss.

Making Children, Making Parents

The remembrance pictures (photographs and drawings) are used in many ways to "repair" situations created by pregnancy loss. Indeed, some people only have "virtual" memories of time shared with their child; if they saw its face at birth, they did so only briefly. Most of the interviewees are, in fact, afraid of forgetting it. Objects in general, and here specifically the pictures, thus play the role of "artificial memory," a substitute for memory, which is by nature fragile and defective.[45] For Meg, the pictures are the only things left of her son, Julien. They help her remember his face:

> I know I have very little about him, very few pictures, very little. So it's good for me that he has an identity. . . . I, I like to have the pictures because, there it is, I have a face.

In a sense twins of the loved one, pictures keep the memory of the child intact and make it present. "It felt good to look at the pictures. . . . It counteracts his absence. To see him, at least that was it. It keeps me from forgetting," says Suzy, who has many pictures of her son Jimmy displayed in her apartment. The picture becomes a physical support, without which the effective and lasting witness of a body and an existence would tend to return to oblivion.

Not only are pictures a means of seeing the dead child at a later date, but they can also, in some cases, be the only chance to see it as a complete entity, as it is usually presented dressed to the parents. Very few interviewees

---

45   Chiara Garattini, "Creating Memories: Material Culture and Infantile Death in Contemporary Ireland," *Mortality* 12, no. 2 (May 2007): 197.

saw their baby naked directly after delivery. Similarly, the pictures presented to couples usually do not show the body unclothed. Some interviewees expressed a feeling of lack in this regard. Morgane is one of them. She saw her daughter, Héloïse, shortly after birth, but she was already dressed. She regrets not daring to undress her. She wanted to see the baby in its entirety and to remember her as a whole being. To this end, she requested access to the medical photographs. Although the two types of photographs—medical and remembrance—usually remain strictly in their respective spheres, in some cases, the former are used by bereaved couples. Even if Morgane considers that they cannot be shown to everybody because they may be shocking (the umbilical cord is wrapped around Héloïse's neck and medical instruments are placed next to her), she needed to see her, and view the cause of the child's death—the umbilical cord that strangulated her:

> I need these photos to move forward. I cried, but almost out of relief. Because I saw that she really had the cord around her neck, and around the foot. I could see her naked, because I hadn't. I've seen her bum, her backside, the back of her head, when I hadn't even dared raise my daughter's hat. It's afterwards, I think, but I didn't even look to see if she had hair. I barely lifted her hat to see her little ears, but yes, it's weird to think, I'm not allowed to.

Fully seeing their naked child, especially when they did not see it at birth, was a way for interviewees to reassure themselves that they had given birth to a real baby, not a monster. For some, death and malformations can translate into a loss of personhood; the dead fetus is assimilated to an external element, barely human. During pregnancy, with the announcement of death or malformations, the unborn becomes "that," a "tumor" that needed to be removed. Sometimes many years later, people who did not see the body at the time may want to confirm that they actually had given birth to a child. In viewing the photographs, they could check all the elements that relate the dead fetus to humanity—its feet, its face, its nose, its fingers, and so on—proof that the bereaved parents gave birth to a "normal" child.

Pictures, clothes, or a prepared bedroom also help materialize the existence of a child that only existed in its mother's womb. They are evidence that the couple are parents; they embody both the status of child and of parent.[46] All the interviewees expressed the feeling that they are not acknowledged as "real" parents by their relatives. When the fetus dies in utero, it has no legal personhood. Thus it is not legally recognized as a child, nor is the

---

46   Maria Gudmundsdottir and Catherine A. Chelsa, "Building a New World: Habits and Practices of Healing Following the Death of a Child," *Journal of Family Nursing* 12, no. 2 (2006): 143–64.

couple recognized as its parents. The same lack of acknowledgment from extended family can occur when the child is born alive and viable but dies just after birth because the birth rites performed at the hospital are incomplete. The child is usually presented only to the couple and almost never to their relatives. Birth rites are typically completed with the return home and the presentation of the baby to the wider family, marking the definitive integration of the baby and the couple into their new roles of child, mother, and father.[47] These rites are what institutionalizes their status. When the death occurs shortly after birth, even if the child has legal personhood, because almost nobody saw the baby, neither its existence nor the status of being a parent is acknowledged by others. This is especially the case for people who have lost their first child. They have not yet legally and socially acquired the status of parents. This is what Carole, whose firstborn son died at twenty-six WA after a medically terminated pregnancy due to hydrocephaly, regrets:

> People do not recognize us as mothers. Not long ago my aunt and grandmother, speaking of my sister, said to me: "You will understand when you are a mother [. . .]." It hurts, because we consider ourselves to be mothers, and just because [my son] is not here doesn't mean that. . . . And then if I hadn't had other children after him, I would never have been a mother, I would never have been considered a mother. It's not normal.

Indeed, a social status can only be conferred to an individual by others through the rites of the kinship system of the society in which they live.[48] Although bereaved couples have enacted the procreative function, and in some cases have acquired the legal and symbolic status of parents, they cannot perform the latter as a means of showing their status and are thus not validated as parents by their social circles. In this regard, one mourning woman sadly expressed the following in a text dedicated to her son who died before birth: "I am the dead baby [son] of. . . . But I must not fool myself. I will never be the nephew, the cousin, the grandson of . . ." In this context, pictures are used as a way to complete birth rites by presenting the dead child to relatives. They are sometimes even shared on a birth announcement card, such as for a live newborn. Kept on a mobile phone, the photographs can also be shown more easily to relatives, family, friends, and other children.

> I wanted to show them that it wasn't a miscarriage that happened. It was a baby, that looks like this. It's in the back, I don't know if you can see? [She shows me the portrait of Clementine hanging on the wall behind her in the

---

47   Layne, *Motherhood Lost*, 60.

48   Marshall Sahlins, "What Kinship Is (Part One)," *Journal of the Royal Anthropological Institute* 17, no. 1 (2011): 2–19.

living room.] So, that's somebody! And I needed this, actually. I needed someone to identify her as my daughter. And not . . . we don't really know what." (Selma)

This is why Selma needed not only to show her family Clementine's pictures but also to hang up pictures of her daughter in the house, just as for her other living children. Displaying pictures is a way to normalize the dead child—presented along with the other children—and to anchor its presence in the domestic space. In some cases—where a room had not yet been prepared or the parents have put away the child's belongings—its presence within the family is materialized through a specific dedicated space, usually in the living room or bedroom: a domestic altar. Pictures often are the central part of this altar. Suzy's altar is, for example, organized around Jimmy's photograph and funeral urn. There she has placed all the objects that remind her of him: his cuddly toy, angels' figurines, drawings.

Finally, the pictures can be used and shown outside the family sphere, in public collective remembrance ceremonies and on the internet. Some interviewees explained this behavior as driven by a desire to normalize perinatal bereavement and pictures of dead babies and to break taboos surrounding these deaths. By sharing these images and their experiences, they wish to demonstrate that death is also part of life and pregnancy. Indeed, such actions form part of a larger social movement in France that aims to raise awareness of pregnancy loss and perinatal bereavement. This movement began in the United States in the 1990s, with the establishment of Pregnancy and Infant Loss Remembrance Day on October 15, and then spread to other countries, such as France, in the 2000s—although it has not yet been officially recognized by the French government. Numerous actions are organized on this day or the first weekend of October, such as "Angel remembrance ceremonies" (Fête des Anges), "Silent march for our angels" (Marche pour nos Anges) or the "Wave of lights." The sharing of pictures of dead fetuses contributes to this movement, creating a sense of community among bereaved parents. For instance, on the French-Canadian website Nos petits Anges au Paradis (Our little angels in heaven), a space is entirely dedicated to dead babies' pictures. Below each, a name is always mentioned, singularizing the child.

These communities and common spaces, off- and online, allow mourning parents to share their children's pictures without having to fear judgment or worry about shocking or offending anyone. Increasing numbers of pictures are also broadcast on more public platforms, such as YouTube. These websites participate in the spreading of images of dead fetuses that were previously not available to most people.[49] Yet such practices tend to

---

49   Lupton, *Social Worlds of the Unborn*, 90.

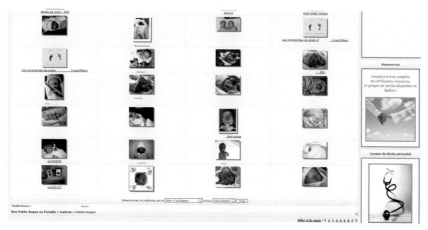

Figure 10.3. Screenshot of the "Little Angels" gallery from the Canadian website Nos petits Anges au Paradis (Our little angels in heaven), which was read by many grieving French parents at the time I conducted my fieldwork.

be limited, at least in France, to closed circles of relatives, or within the bereaved parents' community.

The Rise of the Singularized Dead Fetus

While the fetal body used to only be visible dead and after the termination of a pregnancy, biomedical imaging technologies have enabled showing it *alive* in its environment.[50] They do so even when the pictures are taken during procedures that could harm or kill it, as is the case for Lennart Nilsson's images.[51] They help to establish fetuses as "icons of life."[52]

In the context of the broad diffusion of images of the live unborn, images of dead fetuses with no appearance of life not only became scarce after the 1960s, but they became confined to very specific domains. Morgan categorizes them in three types.[53] The first consists of medical pictures, as discussed above, used by professionals, predominantly in the medical field. The

---

50   Isaacson, "The 'Fetus-Infant,'" 474.
51   Meredith W. Michaels, "Fetal Galaxies: Some Questions about What We See," in Morgan and Michaels, *Fetal Subjects, Feminist Positions*, 117–18.
52   Morgan, *Icons of Life*.
53   Morgan, *Icons of Life*, 197.

second concerns propaganda images used in antiabortion campaigns. They show deceased fetuses, very often dismembered, and focus on their most "human" parts, such as the hands and feet.[54] They are "trauma images" that aim to silence other discourses.[55] Such pictures are not, however, extensively used in French antiabortion campaigns, which tend to focus more on living fetuses, children, and pregnant women.[56] The third type of image comprises those used in crime reporting, when dead fetuses are found in inappropriate places such as toilets or trash bins. Morgan only briefly mentions dead fetuses' pictures taken for memorialization purposes and does not consider them to be a distinct category.[57] Yet I argue that they do form a fourth type in Morgan's framework—because they differ from the other types and because they serve a very specific purpose.

Remembrance photographs differ from images usually seen in the media, first because they do not have a real intention of showing the fetus alive. Even when the photographs show a newborn who died just after birth or close to full-term and looking quite similar to a sleeping baby, some details—such as marks of decomposition—make clear that it is dead. As for fetuses who died during earlier stages of gestation, despite the attempt to give them a child-like appearance, their halted development prevents them from fully looking like babies.[58] More importantly, the fetus depicted in the public space and in the medical field—either alive or dead—but also through earlier means of representing the unborn (wax models, prints, drawings), is desingularized. It is framed as a common "universal fetus." It has been reconfigured as a naturalized biological specimen, "free of its social trapping," a fetish of "life" itself, in a stand-alone manner that erases the woman who carries it.[59] It is the rise of the public fetus, disconnected from its physical and social environment, like an astronaut floating in space.[60] If biomedical imaging technologies have created the fetus as an "individual," separated from the

54   Petchesky, "Fetal Images."

55   For the notion of "trauma images," see Taylor, "Public Fetus and the Family Car," 74.

56   This is in part explained by differences in the legal definitions of abortion in France compared to the United States. The right to abortion in France is mainly focused on women's rights. See Jennifer Merchant, "Féminismes américains et reproductive rights/droits de la procréation," *Le mouvement social* 2, no. 203 (2003): 55–87.

57   Morgan, *Icons of Life*, 197.

58   Lupton, *Social Worlds of the Unborn*, 90.

59   Morgan, *Icons of Life*, 197. See also Janelle S. Taylor, *The Public Life of the Fetal Sonogram: Technology, Consumption, and the Politics of Reproduction* (New Brunswick, NJ: Rutgers University Press, 2008), 27–28.

60   Petchesky, "Fetal Images," 270.

woman, it remains a very universal one.[61] None of Lennart Nilsson's photographs or those used by antiabortion activists depict a singular fetus. They have no name, no filiation. They are always deinscribed from any specific history. Even when ultrasound images are shared in the intimate sphere by parents-to-be as the "first pictures" of their child, they are interchangeable due to their low visual quality.[62] It is impossible to differentiate one specific unborn from another. All of these images of fetuses, then, circulating in both medical and nonmedical contexts, are specimens. They are specimens of the human species, specimens of specific malformations, of gestational stages, of a life interrupted, specimens of life itself. And this is the very purpose of these images. By contrast, the remembrance images of dead fetuses that have spread in personal spheres and, increasingly, in the public domain, are always singularized.[63] The value of "person" is attached to them.

Far from the medical specimen or the "universal" fetus usually represented, these are singular individuals, loved by specific parents. Therefore, remembrance images aim to show that the dead fetus, the depiction is specific and unique, and that it should be accepted as its parents' child. They aim to memorialize the life of *this* being and not another one. And all this is possible because the fetus has already been singularized before its birth and at an earlier and earlier stage.

Conclusion

The analysis of these pictures reveals a profound transformation of the status of the dead fetus in France, as is also the case in most Euro-American countries. Far from anatomical specimen and anatomical waste, the dead fetus has been considered as a child at an increasingly early age and whose life must be recognized as unique and singular. The Saint-Vincent-de-Paul Hospital scandal illustrates this transformation by reflecting how old practices have become unbearable to contemporary observers. It is now considered

---

61   Marilyn Strathern, *Kinship, Law and the Unexpected: Relatives Are Always a Surprise* (Cambridge: Cambridge University Press, 2005), 20.

62   Rayna Rapp, "Real-Time Fetus: The Role of the Sonogram in the Age of Monitored Reproduction," in *Cyborgs and Citadels: Anthropological Interventions in Emerging Sciences and Technologies*, ed. Gary Lee Downey and Joseph Dumit (Santa Fe, NM: School of American Research 1997); Janelle S. Taylor, "An All-Consuming Experience: Obstetrical Ultrasound and the Commodification of Pregnancy," in *Biotechnology and Culture: Bodies, Anxieties, Ethics*, ed. Paul Brodwin (Bloomington: Indiana University Press, 2000).

63   Boltanski, *Foetal Condition*.

inappropriate and even unethical to collect fetal specimens, or to treat the human fetus as anatomical waste. A new management of pregnancy loss has developed, and with it, new images of the dead fetus that portray the latter as having a childlike appearance.

These images mostly remain within intimate circles but can be shared in specialized support groups. While they are scarce compared to those of living fetuses, they have slowly started to spread to the public sphere through activists' growing demands for recognition of perinatal bereavement. In this way, they contribute to the dissemination of dead fetal images, at earlier and earlier stages, beyond the medical field. If these pictures are part of the public rise of fetal images, they differ, however, from usual representations. Unlike them, remembrance pictures do not iconize the fetus as a generic embodiment of life itself but, on the contrary, aim to depict a singularized fetus, already a child, that has a name and a family.

Chapter Eleven

Reproducing Bodies in the Medical Museum

Pregnancy, Childbirth, and the Fetus on Display

Manon S. Parry

Over the last thirty years, medical museums previously used in medical research and education have opened up to a broadening public audience, attracting rising numbers of curious visitors, including many without any aspirations to a career in medicine. There is a wide variety of these institutions across Europe, with different collection strengths, a broad range of staffing levels and financial resources, and varying degrees of interreliance or independence from their founding medical institutions. Even so, they face some shared challenges as they invite general audiences to peer at historical collections previously closed to the public.

Among other historical items such as diagnostic tools, surgical implements, devices for treatment, and the personal effects of influential figures, the collections commonly include human fetuses, in the form of anatomical models, real skeletons, or jars of "wet specimens" made up of whole bodies or body parts. Such materials are a strong element of the appeal for a variety of visitors, although staff express rising anxieties about the motivations for seeking out such collections and the potential for negative reactions. In fact, at museums across Europe, such items are often subject to special restrictions for viewing. Some have been removed from display, and in a few instances, items considered too problematic to keep have even been destroyed.[1]

---

1   Fetal collections in Sweden and skulls in Belgium have been destroyed, and human remains derived from Nazi experimentation have been buried in Germany. See Tinne Claes and Veronique Deblon, "When Nothing Remains:

There are several intertwining reasons for the changing sensibilities around the public display of fetuses in medical museums, with the controversies surrounding the Body Worlds exhibitions of plastinated anatomies playing a prominent role. Launched in 1995 and visited by more than 44 million visitors worldwide, these exhibitions were widely criticized for including corpses suspected to come from executed prisoners who had not willingly donated their bodies.[2] After the introduction of consent-based donation process, critics continued to object to the sensationalized displays for posing subjects in "disrespectful" ways and making entertainment out of the exhibition of human remains.

Body Worlds (and the various other public anatomies their success has inspired), revive an older tradition of "popular" anatomical exhibitions that were open to the public for a fee from the late eighteenth century.[3] These exhibitions gave visitors a supposedly scientific rationale for looking inside the human body and gawping at models and specimens depicting grisly injuries, unusual deformities, and the ravages of venereal disease. By contrast, the closed collections of universities and medical schools, with access limited to students and medical professionals, were ostensibly less sensational and more educational, although they shared some features.[4]

While few popular collections have survived, university medical museums often retain numerous objects that blur the boundaries between science, art, and spectacle. Yet most are marketed to the public today in fairly circumspect ways, to differentiate these collections from Body Worlds and their imitators, and to justify the continuing display of objects that have been largely displaced from medical education.[5] The ethical and legal issues surrounding

Anatomical Collections, the Ethics of Stewardship and the Meanings of Absence," *Journal of the History of Collections* 30, no. 2 (2018): 351–62; Carola Azurduy Högström & Magnus Gelang, "Gallring av mänskliga kvarlevor," ("Thinning of Human Remains"), *Göteborgs Naturhistoriska Museum Årstryck* (2020): 67–80.

2   Gunther Von Hagens' BODY WORLDS, "Facts and Figures," n.d. https://bodyworlds.com/wp-content/uploads/2017/09/1498134149_bw_factsnumbers_chjun171.pdf (last accessed January 15, 2021).

3   Michael Sappol, *A Traffic of Dead Bodies: Anatomy and Embodied Social Identity in Nineteenth-Century America* (Princeton, NJ: Princeton University Press, 2004); Joanna Ebenstein, *The Anatomical Venus: Wax, God, Death & the Ecstatic* (New York: Distributed Art Publishers, 2016).

4   Rina Knoeff and Robert Zwijnenberg, eds., *The Fate of Anatomical Collections: The History of Medicine in Context* (Burlington, VT: Ashgate, 2015).

5   Yehia Marreez, Luuk Willems, and Michael Wells, "The Role of Medical Museums in Contemporary Medical Education," *Anatomical Sciences Education* 3, no. 5 (2010): 249–53.

the collection and exhibition of human remains drive additional concerns about what can be shown to the public, as well as requests for the repatriation of ancestors' remains and a broader call to address the colonial origins of museum collections in the narratives presented in exhibitions.

Yet within these debates, fetuses hold a special significance, and not only as human remains but also in the form of models made of wax or plaster. In Body Worlds, the partially dissected pregnant female cadavers displayed, with fetus visible in utero, provoked particular controversy. A sexualized display of a reclining pregnant woman, posed in the artistic style common to the depiction of the female nude in Western art, has drawn especially sharp criticism, and been labeled highly inappropriate for trivializing the "double tragedy" of their deaths.[6] Such objections reflect the particular culture of sentimentality surrounding pregnancy and childhood but also highlight a paradox in the representation of women in contemporary Western society. While female sexuality is widely displayed in mass culture, albeit usually according to the conventions of the male gaze, the intricacies of the female reproductive system and realistic depictions of the physical changes during pregnancy and childbirth are rarely represented. This imbalance has inspired a range of recent projects intended to address the resulting shame and stigma that surrounds female anatomy and reproductive functions, including popular publications, new research agendas, public health campaigns, and museum activities.[7]

As this edited collection attests, the human fetus is much more regularly depicted, although in heavily circumscribed ways. Feminist scholars have argued that representations commonly freeze moments of development and dynamic processes, privilege the fetus over the mother, and misrepresent death as life.[8] Medical museum fetuses can also be interpreted through this

---

6   Charleen M. Moore and C. Mackenzie Brown, "Experiencing Body Worlds: Voyeurism, Education, or Enlightenment?" Published online, n.p. The phrase "double tragedy" comes from von Hagens's own justification of the presentation of "The Reclining Pregnant Woman" as quoted by Moore and Mackenzie Brown.

7   Maya Dusenbery, *Doing Harm: The Truth about How Bad Medicine and Lazy Science Leave Women Dismissed, Misdiagnosed, and Sick* (New York: HarperOne, 2019); Jen Gunter, *The Vagina Bible: The Vulva and the Vagina: Separating the Myth from the Medicine* (New York: Citadel, 2019); Alexandra Topping, "Baby Loss Charities Call for Cultural Shift to Break Silence around Miscarriage," *The Guardian*, November 26, 2020, https://www.theguardian.com/uk-news/2020/nov/26/baby-loss-charities-call-for-cultural-shift-to-break-silence-around-miscarriage; Sarah Marsh, "World's First Vagina Museum to Open in London," *The Guardian*, November 15, 2019.

8   See chapter 12 in this volume.

lens. Even so, I make a case for the continued preservation and exhibition of these mesmerizing objects, but importantly, within a broader range of related items and perspectives to enrich the largely medical viewpoint usually on display.

What I aim to illustrate here, is that the anxieties surrounding these objects draw on a particularly complex set of problems, where claims of respect for the dead obscure irresolvable tensions between the rights of women and those of the unborn. Yet these collections also offer a unique opportunity to "de-sanitize" the "public fetus." As medical anthropologist and feminist science studies scholar Lynn Morgan has argued,

> Paradoxically, the cute, sanitized embryos and foetuses that that we know today are possible only because doctors, embryologists, anatomists, and scores of medical students once handled tangible dead embryos and foetuses, culling them from clots of miscarried tissue, transforming them into biological specimens, placing them in jars of formaldehyde, embedding them in paraffin, and cutting the specimens into thin slices for the production of embryological knowledge.[9]

Medical historians have examined these practices in detail, and in recent years, have looked more closely at the medical museums where these collections were stored and used for teaching and study.[10] As well as reconstructing the histories of lost collections, some of these studies examine surviving examples to uncover their origins and the techniques used to create them. Fetuses in these collections exceed the impact of the Nilsson photographs, by presenting visitors with the fetus in three dimensions, although they are no less mediated than his carefully staged and captioned images of embryological specimens, presented as if they revealed life in utero. In medical museum collections, both anatomical models and specimens of human remains have similarly undergone extensive manipulation to result in their presentable, preserved forms.[11]

---

9   "Strange Anatomy: Gertrude Stein and the Avant-Garde Embryo," *Hypatia* 21, no. 1 (Winter 2006): 15–34, 16.

10   Samuel J. M. M. Alberti and Elizabeth Hallam, eds., *Medical Museums: Past, Present, Future* (London: Royal College of Surgeons of England, 2013); Rina Knoeff and Robert Zwijnenberg, eds., *The Fate of Anatomical Collections: The History of Medicine in Context* (Burlington, VT: Ashgate, 2015); Hieke Huistra, *The Afterlife of the Leiden Anatomical Collections: Hands On, Hands Off* (New York: Routledge 2019).

11   See, for example, Marieke M. A. Hendriksen, "Casting Life, Casting Death: Connections between Early Modern Anatomical Corrosive Preparations and Artistic Materials and Techniques," *Notes and Records: The Royal Society Journal of the History of Science* 73, no. 2 (2019): 369–97.

I focus here on two types of artifact commonly found in these collections, beginning with human remains, especially those known by curators and visitors alike as "babies in bottles," before moving on to anatomical models, especially wax obstetrical models featuring a fetus in utero or in the process of being born.[12] The examples I consider are located in Vienna, Austria, a city with a long tradition of anatomical research and public displays of anatomical models and specimens.[13] My analysis draws on interviews with staff during site visits to these institutions, contextualized by four years of research into medical museums across Europe, as well as informal discussions with museum professionals during the decade I worked as a curator of exhibitions on the history of medicine.[14]

Although larger museums have sometimes undertaken studies into the audience perceptions of exhibitions, very little of this research is publicly available. Decisions about what can be shown and how are commonly made based on unproven assumptions about audience attitudes, the personal preferences of museum decision-makers, or anxieties about potential controversies. I offer this analysis as a step toward a wider recognition of the social relevance of such collections, arguing that they offer an important counterpoint to other representations of the fetus in mass culture, even though at first glance they appear to replicate some of the same problematic dynamics. Taking advantage of the "blood and guts" appeal of medical museums as a venue where the intricacies of bodily processes and the procedures of medical intervention can be explored in detail, these collections could be re-presented to powerfully address the complexities of reproduction as well as to deepen our understanding of the use of the bodies of women and children in the production of medical knowledge.[15]

---

12   Karin Tybjerg "From Bottled Babies to Biobanks," in Knoeff and Zwijnenberg, 263–78; Mark Brightside, "My Visit to the Vrolik Museum," Rarely a Brighter Side, August 27, 2015, https://marcbrightside.wordpress.com/2015/08/27/my-visit-to-the-vrolik-museum/.

13   Tatjana Buklijas, "Public Anatomies in Fin-de-Siècle Vienna," Medicine Studies 2, no. 1 (2010): 71–92; Anna Maerker, Model Experts: Wax Anatomies and Enlightenment in Florence and Vienna, 1775–1815 (Manchester: Manchester University Press, 2011).

14   The research project "Human Curiosities: The Social Relevance of Medical Museums," is funded by the Dutch Research Council (NWO) and will conclude with a book to be published in 2024.

15   On the value of the appeal of the gory aspects of medical museums, see Ken Arnold, Cabinets for the Curious: Looking Back at Early English Museums (London, UK: Routledge, 2005), 172. On the bodies of women and babies see Jenna M. Dittmar and Piers D. Mitchell, "From Cradle to Grave via the Dissection Room: The Role of Fetal and Infant Bodies in Anatomical

"Babies in Bottles"

Museum artifacts made with human remains invoke a complex array of legal requirements and ethical considerations. Most were gathered long before the development of the notion of "informed consent," and although it is difficult to trace the origins of many, it is clear from surviving evidence that some resulted from theft, colonial violence, or illegal experimentation.[16] Like ethnographic museums, which have faced particular criticism for their role in collecting, exhibiting, and ranking cultures in hierarchies of human progress, medical museums have received requests for the repatriation of remains that were stolen or attained by coercion under colonial regimes. In some of the cultures where these requests originate, there are strong prohibitions against any display of human remains.[17]

Medical collections also contain specimens whose exact origins are unclear but which were certainly preserved and presented to assert racial differences or to convey colonial legitimacy.[18] Historian Marieke Hendriksen has researched wet specimens of fetuses, decorated with beads and catalogued as "African" or "Asian," that can be found in three different Dutch museums and concludes that they were intended to fix ideas about race on colonial bodies and convey the wealth and global influence of the Netherlands during the so-called Golden Age of empire (figure 11.1).[19] Hendriksen makes a plea for more attention to this history in museum presentations of such

Education from the Late 1700s to Early 1900s," *Journal of Anatomy* 229, no. 6 (2016): 713–22; and "Equality after Death: The Dissection of the Female Body for Anatomical Education in Nineteenth-Century England," *Bioarchaeology International* 2, no. 4 (2019): 283–94.

16   Larissa Förster and Sarah Fründ, eds., "Human Remains in Museums and Collections: A Critical Engagement with the 'Recommendations for the Care of Humans Remains in Museums and Collections' of the German Museums Association," *Historisches Forum* 21 (2017).

17   Doreen Carvajal, "Museums Confront the Skeletons in Their Closets," *New York Times*, May 24, 2013, https://www.nytimes.com/2013/05/25/arts/design/museums-move-to-return-human-remains-to-indigenous-peoples.html.

18   Lisa O'Sullivan and Ross L. Jones, "Two Australian Foetuses: Frederic Wood Jones and the Work of an Anatomical Specimen," *Bulletin of the History of Medicine* 89, no. 2 (Summer 2015): 243–66. The authors of this article chose not to reproduce an image of the two fetuses they discussed, in keeping with Australian museum protocols for the representation and display of Indigenous human remains.

19   Marieke M. A. Hendriksen, "Aesthesis in Anatomy: Materiality and Elegance in the Eighteenth-Century Leiden Anatomical Collections" (PhD diss., Leiden University, 2012), chapter 5, and Marieke M. A. Hendriksen, *Elegant*

items, which instead are usually only accompanied by a short reference to their faraway origin, and, more rarely, with a brief explanation of their role in racial science. As she concludes, "These histories will be uncomfortable and confronting at times, but that does not outweigh the insights they offer."[20] For now, the formerly highly prized example at the Rijksmuseum Boerhaave, the country's national museum for the history of science and medicine, has been removed from display.[21]

Many fetal specimens were taken from vulnerable women, usually without their knowledge, although some were willingly donated to medical museum collections.[22] Like other types of human remains, their use has been affected by recent scandals over the medical mismanagement of bodies and body parts, such as the use of those donated for medical research for weapons testing by the military in the United States, and the retention of children's organs without the knowledge or permission of their parents in the UK.[23] In museums still affiliated with institutions that continue to collect human remains, decisions about display are thus informed by a need to preserve the public trust to ensure future donations of organs and cadavers for medical research. Medical Museion, Copenhagen, which displays a significant number of fetuses in their exhibition *The Body Collected*, opted not include

---

Anatomy: The Eighteenth-Century Leiden Anatomical Collections (Leiden: Brill, 2015).

20   Hendriksen, "Aesthesis in Anatomy," 163.

21   Interview with Bart Grob, curator, Rijksmuseum Boerhaave, October 1, 2019. A reconsideration of the representation of race in medical museums is underway, with major exhibitions devoted to the role of medicine in racial science developed by the German Hygienist's Museum in 2018 and Teknisk Museum in Oslo in 2018, as well as shifts in terminology and emphasis in the exhibition labels in other institutions, including the Boerhaave. I explore the role of medical museum collections in the history of racial science and their potential use in contemporary exhibitions elsewhere. See Manon S. Parry, "The Valuable Role of Risky Histories: Exhibiting Disability, Race, and Reproduction in Medical Museums," *Science Museum Group Journal* no. 14 (2021), https://journal.sciencemuseum.ac.uk/article/risky-histories/.

22   Sara Ray, "On Mothers and Monsters: Maternal Testimony, Monstrous Births, and Embryology, 1700–1849," Paper presented at the seminar series in body history, Utrecht University, November 7, 2018. See also Shannon Withycombe, *Lost: Miscarriage in Nineteenth-Century America* (New Brunswick, NJ: Rutgers University Press, 2018).

23   Royal Liverpool Children's Inquiry, *The Royal Liverpool Children's Inquiry Summary and Recommendations* (The Stationery Office, London UK, January 30, 2001); John Shiffman, "The Body Trade: Army Experiments," *Reuters Investigates*, December 23, 2016, https://www.reuters.com/investigates/special-report/usa-bodybrokers-industry/.

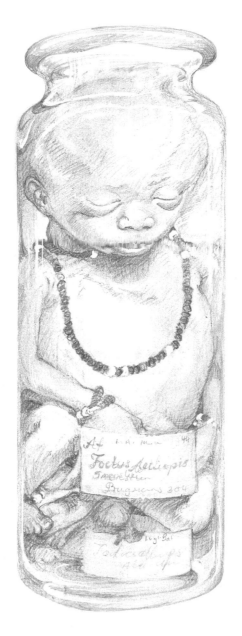

Figure 11.1. Illustration of a preparation from the eighteenth-century Leiden anatomical collections previously displayed at the Rijksmuseum Boerhaave, by Lisa Temple-Cox. Credit: Lisa Temple-Cox.

embryos with their feet cut off for this reason.[24] The idea that fetal specimens are particularly provocative is thus widely acknowledged within these institutions.

As a result, most museums impose strict restrictions on photography of these items, include warning signs about the display, or limit access to guided tours. Even so, an internet search for images of "medical museums" returns many visitor photographs of cabinets full of human remains, including "babies in bottles." Fetal specimens are also a ubiquitous element of media articles listing the world's "weirdest," or "most unique" tourist destinations.[25] These artifacts have thus become the iconic representation of the historical medical museum, symbolizing not just the transgression of the public seeing what was previously reserved for medical experts but also the particular taboo of dead fetuses on display, with the additional thrill produced by the unusual anatomies of some.

Framing medical museum collections in this manner undermines their credibility in two ways, first, by aligning them with the spectacle and voyeurism which the Body Worlds exhibitions trade in (and medical museums try in general to avoid), and secondly by invoking the history of the "freak show," in which human beings exhibited themselves or were coerced into exhibition for paying audiences, medical and nonmedical.[26] Human exhibits performed to display their unusual anatomies or as examples of particular "races," and some were also preserved in medical museums after their death.[27] The idea of publicly exhibiting living people for spectacle became socially unacceptable over the twentieth century and now the propriety of

---

24 Karin Tybjerg, "Curating the Dead Body Between Medicine and Culture," in *Curatorial Challenges: Interdisciplinary Perspectives on Contemporary Curating*, ed. Malene Vest Hansen, Anne Folke Henningsen, and Anne Gregersen (London: Routledge, 2019), 42.

25 Bryan Pirolli, "World's 10 Weirdest Medical Museums," *CNN*, December 10, 2014, https://edition.cnn.com/travel/article/world-medical-museums/index.html; Danielle Otteri,"Top 5 Museum Collections for the Morbidly Curious," *trip savvy*, June 26, 2019, https://www.tripsavvy.com/morbid-museum-collections-4037509.

26 Rosemarie Garland Thomson, ed., *Freakery: Cultural Spectacles of the Extraordinary Body* (New York: NYU Press, 1996).

27 The Mütter Museum in Philadelphia, for example, houses a cast and the livers of Chang and Eng Bunker, conjoined twins who toured the United States in the 1830s before marrying and retiring in the early 1840s. The Mütter Museum, "Exhibitions: Cast and Livers of Chang and Eng Bunker," n.d., http://muttermuseum.org/exhibitions/cast-and-livers-of-chang-and-eng-bunker/ (last accessed May 27, 2023).

staring at their remains in the cultural venue of the museum is also undergoing reevaluation.

However, it is common knowledge among medical museum staff that visitors often seek out fetuses among their collections. At the National Museum of Health and Medicine in Washington, DC, when conjoined twins were removed from exhibition during renovations, visitors (who often returned repeatedly to view them) asked when they would be back on display.[28] At the Narrenturm in Vienna, a geneticist encourages women awaiting results of prenatal testing to visit the collections of fetuses with a range of abnormalities.[29] At Medical Museion, Copenhagen, the new permanent exhibition installed in 2015 included fetal remains partly to address rumors that these collections had been hidden from the public. Despite the public clamoring to see them, visitors usually "go quiet" and are rarely unaffected by their encounter,[30] Curators report that women who have experienced a miscarriage or terminated a pregnancy due to the results of prenatal testing have been particularly moved by these collections and discuss their profound impact with staff.[31] These relatively "private" interactions between individual visitors, museum objects, and individual staff have gone on for years and form the basis for the conviction among some that they should remain on display.

However, strong opposition has been building in recent years. Growing awareness of the limitations of the medical model of disability, coupled with a drive to make museums more inclusive, has led to shifting approaches to the presentation of disability in some medical museums, notably in the United Kingdom where a series of research projects have helped drive forward this change.[32] Museums, like medicine more generally, have been criticized for an ableist view of disability as a medical problem in need of a cure and for fostering negative perceptions of disabled lives. Aside from wider criticisms of the presentation of people as medical "cases" and the display of unusual anatomies for the curious gaze of museum visitors, controversy has also

28 Alice Dreger, "Products of Conception," Bioethics Forum Essay, The Hastings Center, April 9, 2007, https://www.thehastingscenter.org/products-of-conception/.
29 On-site interview with Eduard Winter, Vienna, October 22, 2018.
30 Tybjerg, "Curating the Dead Body," 36.
31 See, for example, the remarks of National Museum of Health and Medicine director Adrienne Noe, quoted in Dreger, "Products of Conception." I have also been told of such experiences by tour guides and curators at several other medical museums in Europe and the United States.
32 Richard Sandell, Jocelyn Dodd, and Rosemarie Garland-Thomson, eds., *Re-Presenting Disability: Activism and Agency in the Museum* (London: Routledge, 2010).

raged over the exhibition of some human remains against the express wishes of the person they came from, or despite objections by their descendants.[33]

Fetuses with organs growing outside of the body, or those that developed with misshapen or missing limbs, are also implicated in the politics of abortion. As Dagmar Herzog has recently illustrated, the advance of disability rights since the 1970s has coincided with the use of prodisability rhetoric to limit abortion access.[34] All fetal specimens play a role, in fact, as they have been used for antiabortion propaganda and may be viewed by museum visitors as the product of abortion (although they are more likely to have resulted from the death of the mother during pregnancy, from miscarriage, or from the death of the fetus in utero or shortly after birth due to congenital abnormalities).[35] Although medical museums do not commonly declare a particular stance on contemporary abortion rights, their displays of fetuses are therefore deeply entangled in the issue.

In many venues, "cabinets of curiosities" are still on display, which contain fetuses with visible physical abnormalities such as a single eye, organs that grew outside of the body, or visible intersex genitalia forming a prominent part of these collections. The Narrenturm, for example, houses anatomy and pathology collections in a former asylum, built in 1784.[36] The circular building stores extensive collections on the upper floors, open to visitors on tours

---

33   See, for example, the controversy surrounding the display of the skeleton of Charles Byrne, a seven-foot-seven-inch man who performed in public exhibitions as the "Irish Giant" in the 1780s, in the Hunterian Museum in London. Byrne made specific arrangements to be buried at sea in a lead coffin to avoid being exhibited after his death, but surgeon John Hunter bribed the burial team to give him the body, which he then reduced to bone, hid for two years, and then exhibited. The skeleton was removed from display in the 2023 renovation of the Hunterian after years of public debate, although it will be retained in the collection for research. Royal College of Surgeons of England, "Statement on the skeleton of Charles Byrne from the Board of Trustees of the Hunterian Collection," January 11, 2023, https://www.rcseng.ac.uk/news-and-events/news/archive/statement-on-the-skeleton-of-charles-byrne/.

34   Dagmar Herzog, *Unlearning Eugenics: Sexuality, Reproduction, and Disability in Post-Nazi Europe* (Madison: University of Wisconsin Press, 2018).

35   Manon S. Parry, "Museums and the Material Culture of Abortion," in *Representing Abortion*, ed. Rachel Hurst (London: Routledge, 2020), 61–74, 65–66.

36   The collection of anatomical pathology in the Narrenturm is part of the Natural History Museum of Vienna. The building was established in 1784 as an asylum and was used for that purpose until 1869. After that the building was used for apartments for nurses and for workspaces used by craftsmen employed at the general hospital. The facility became a museum for pathology in 1971 and contains collections from different institutions. All of the

guided by the medical students, and displays thematic exhibitions on the ground floor. Amid the very crowded collections spaces (in the former patient rooms and offices of the old asylum), are five rooms containing approximately two thousand fetuses, from three different collections including the famous Semmelweiss hospital. They have many skeletons taken from the same fetuses also preserved as wet specimens, of conjoined twins, for example, as well as lots of examples of intersex anatomies. Little documentation about the mothers involved in these pregnancies has survived (unless they also died), but they do have records from the autopsies of the fetuses.

Curator Eduard Winter notes that female visitors who have come to the museum as part of their way of dealing with their own pregnancy losses often tell him about their experiences and that disabled people also come to show their families items in the collection. Pregnant women visit, curious about malformations in the womb, with some attending on the advice of a professor the museum collaborates with, who sends her patients to learn about the role of genetic testing in pregnancy. In general, audience reactions are quite positive, with most people appearing to be very interested in the history of medicine and the different pathologies displayed. Most of the complaints they receive are from visitors who wish they could see everything in the museum collection, which is not possible given the cramped conditions and lack of security in the upstairs rooms.

Negative reactions are rare. About once a year a young woman on a school visit will start crying in front of the fetuses with malformations, which Winter attributes to under-preparation by the teacher in charge of the group. In general, school staff use the museum's website and follow his guidance about planning for a class visit, and the visits usually go smoothly without such incidents. He estimates that about 5 percent of all visitors express "disgust," although he thinks many of these people come specifically to complain, as it is clear from the description of the museum online that the majority of the collection is made up of human remains and what kinds of objects the visitor will see. The only other negative reaction Winter recalls was when a woman volunteering there part-time to reorganize the library said that after she lost a child she could no longer work there.

These reactions raise a number of issues. For the minority expressing disgust, it is not clear what element generates this response—the existence or exhibition of body parts in specimen jars, the way any of them look, or the particular form of those with obvious malformations. Some medical museum curators have expressed concerns that young women may develop an exaggerated sense of the risks of life-threatening complications in pregnancy, for

information about the museum, unless otherwise cited, comes from an interview with curator Eduard Winter at the museum, October 22, 2018.

the fetus or themselves. This problem is compounded by the medicalization of childbirth in contemporary society, ableism and disability discrimination (plus the lack of resources for families with children with disabilities), and the limitations of genetic counseling, which often underestimate disabled people's quality of life. Yet, there are potential benefits among women who seek these collections out in order to process their own experiences of miscarriage or to inform their thinking about prenatal screening and the interpretation of the results.

One might assume that the more severe abnormalities displayed may deter women from continuing a pregnancy where prenatal screening identifies anything out of the ordinary about their fetus, but we actually do not know enough about visitor responses to draw this conclusion, as there has been very little systematic research done on audience reactions. Instead, curators' encounters with visitors viewing these collections, and the enduring fascination of diverse audiences, suggest that such displays offer a unique and often profoundly moving way to engage with issues of pregnancy loss and decisions about whether to have an abortion. This is especially pertinent given the lack of other venues to encounter nonromanticized representations of development from embryo to child given the cultural dominance of the floating fetus.

A final point to note here relates to the reaction of the woman who chose not to continue her work at the museum after the loss of her child. The majority of visitors encounter these collections with some advance knowledge of what they might see given their location within a medical museum and the widespread representation of these fetuses as an iconic item in such collections, and their reactions are overwhelmingly positive. It is clear, however, that other people will choose to avoid such museums or exhibitions. Occasionally, visitors will have an unexpected reaction and may regret their visit.

As this brief look at one collection shows, there is no universal consensus about what should be shown and who should see it.[37] The rising trend to remove fetuses from display therefore wrongly asserts a consensus where none exists. As Karin Tybjerg, curator at the Medical Museion in Copenhagen, argues regarding human remains in general, the issue of *whether* they should be exhibited "has overshadowed the question of *how* they should be exhibited."[38] In this way, the objects are assumed to have

---

37   See "Bringing Out the Dead," *Atrium: The Report of the Northwestern Medical Humanities and Bioethics Program* 1 (2005) for a wide array of perspectives on one collection, https://www.bioethics.northwestern.edu/docs/atrium/atrium-issue1.pdf.

38   Tybjerg, "Curating the Dead Body," 36.

an essential or embedded power, ignoring the role of the time and place in which they are seen, as well as the mode of display, in shaping the reactions of museum practitioners and of visitors.

Tybjerg goes on to argue that museums attempt to solve the problem ineffectively by decoupling the medical and cultural issues raised by these collections. The result is either a barely contextualized display of medical "cases" that dehumanize the people whose bodies are displayed and reduce them to problems in need of a cure, or an emphasis only on the troubling social issues the collections evoke, such as medical malpractice or the role of science in subjugating certain groups.[39] In my opinion, a better solution would be to experiment with new ways to exhibit these collections and to learn more from the visitors about the meanings they make of them.

Fetuses in Wax

Wax models are almost as provocative as human remains. In fact, as museums have taken up a renewed enthusiasm for exhibiting these items, similar questions are being raised about the origins of the models.[40] Historical models were based on the bodies of living people, sometimes incarcerated or otherwise subjugated for science, or exploited after death if burial was too expensive or they died in an institution such as a prison, poorhouse, or psychiatric facility. The models were typically made from observations of numerous dissected cadavers, although this is not obvious to an observer, who may assume they are looking at an exact replica of one individual.[41] Wax anatomies are some of the most elaborate renditions of the human body exhibited in medical museums today. Although a range of anatomical waxes of varying quality has survived, the most highly prized among museums originated in Italy in the eighteenth century.[42] Their impact depends heav-

---

39 Tybjerg, "Curating the Dead Body," 36.
40 Orla O'Donovan, "Wax Moulages and the Pastpresence Work of the Dead," *Science, Technology & Human Values* 46, no. 2 (2020): 231–53.
41 Thomas N. Haviland and Lawrence C. Parish, "A Brief Account of the Use of Wax Models in the Study of Medicine," *Journal of the History of Medicine and Allied Sciences* 25, no. 1 (1970): 52–75; Anita Guerrini, "Anatomists and Entrepreneurs in Early Eighteenth-Century London," *Journal of the History of Medicine and Allied Sciences* 59, no. 2 (2004): 219–39; Richard Barnett, "Lost Wax: Medicine and Spectacle in Enlightenment London," *Lancet* 372 (2008): 366–67.
42 Anna K. Maerker, *Model Experts: The Production and Uses of Anatomical Models at La Specola, Florence, and the Josephinum, Vienna, 1775–1814* (PhD diss., Cornell University, 2005).

ily on the skill of their maker, with the worst looking like clumsy copies of human flesh while the best appear as realistic as human remains and depict the body as if it were still alive. The way models show bodies and bodily processes in an eerily lifelike rendering of dead tissues and systems informs some of the concern about their display today.

Historically, artistic elements were central to anatomical modeling just as they were in anatomical illustration, including allegorical presentations of flayed human figures without their skin (mimicking the imagery of famous anatomist Andreas Vesalius), or symbols of mortality embedded in a scene.[43] The Anatomical Venus, a full-size female figure reclining on a velvet bed, blurred the lines of the sensual and the scientific. This naked woman, with long hair laid out on the pillow and wearing a necklace of pearls, looks off to one side as museum visitors "dissect" her body, with removable layers revealing a fetus in her womb. Scholars have argued that such models gave a scientific justification for gazing at (and within) the naked female body and connected "death, eroticism, and dissection."[44] Alongside the white-skinned figures that have survived, by the 1840s a "Moorish" Anatomical Venus later publicized as an "Abyssinian Venus" was also the highlight of a popular touring exhibition, capitalizing on the fashion at the time for examples of "exotic" bodies and exemplifying their sexualized presentation.[45]

An Anatomical Venus is the most popular object of the Josephinum Museum in Vienna, part of a stunning collection of nearly twelve hundred wax anatomical models, originally produced in Florence in the late eighteenth century, which is also when they were first displayed to the public at

---

43   Thomas Schnalke, *Disease in Wax: The History of Medical Moulage* (Berlin: Quintessence, 1995); Alan W. Bates, "Indecent and Demoralising Representations: Public Anatomy Museums in Mid-Victorian England," *Medical History* 52, no. 1 (2008): 1–22; Samuel J. M. M. Alberti, "Wax Bodies: Art and Anatomy in Victorian Medical Museums," *Museum History Journal* 2 (January 2009): 7–36; Michael Sappol, *Dream Anatomy* (Bethesda: National Institutes of Health, 2006).

44   Joanna Ebenstein, *The Anatomical Venus: Wax, God, Death & the Ecstatic* (New York: Distributed Art Publishers, 2016); Deanna Petheridge and Ludmilla Jordanova, *The Quick and the Dead: Artists and Anatomy* (Berkeley: University of California Press, 1997), 88.

45   Francesco Paolo de Ceglia, "The Importance of Being Florentine: A Journey around the World for Wax Anatomical Venuses," *Nuncius* 26 (2011): 83–108, 98. The models toured England and Scotland, America, and Central Europe, although it is not clear from the newspaper coverage of these exhibitions if this figure also included a fetus; see p. 101, n.73.

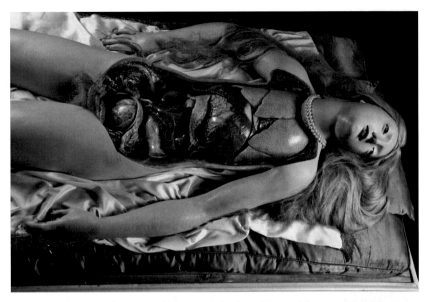

Figure 11.2. Anatomical Venus of the Josephinum Museum. Credit:
Josephinum – Ethics, Collections and History of Medicine, MedUni Vienna.

the museum.[46] The collection includes full-size complete human figures and
models of a wide array of internal organs and bodily systems, as well as the
largest group of obstetrical wax models in the world. The Anatomical Venus
is featured extensively in the museum's advertising and fundraising campaign to support a government-funded renovation (figure 11.2). When the
Rijksmuseum Boerhaave in Leiden in the Netherlands borrowed some of
the Josephinum collection for their installation, *Amazing Models*, the exhibition design and marketing materials highlighted the sexualized aspects of
this object by remaking her with a famous fashion model, apparently naked
under a silky sheet and digitally reconfigured to show half her face dissected
(figure 11.3). Neither publicity image features the fetus usually included in
an Anatomical Venus, presumably because this would have complicated the
presentation for contemporary viewers, who are not accustomed to seeing
sex and reproduction signified simultaneously in this way.

---

46   All information about the current activities of the museum, unless otherwise
      stated, are from an onsite interview with museum director Christaine Druml,
      October 22, 2018. Historical context is from Anna Maerker, "Florentine
      Anatomical Models and the Challenge of Medical Authority in Late-
      Eighteenth-Century Vienna," *Studies in History and Philosophy of Biological
      and Biomedical Sciences* 43, no. 3 (2012): 730–40.

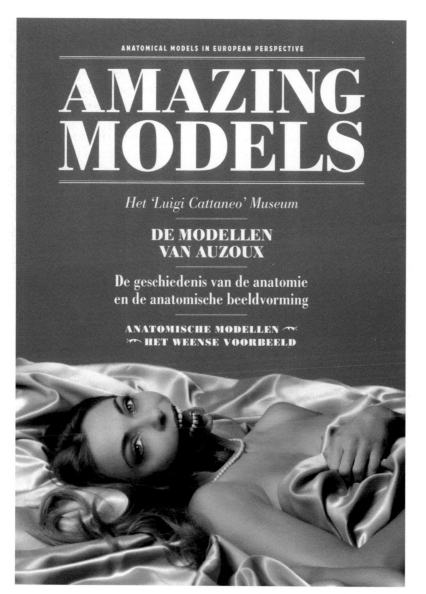

Figure 11.3. Marketing materials for the *Amazing Models* exhibition at Rijksmuseum Boerhaave, 2013. Credit: Rijksmuseum Boerhaave.

At the time of writing, the Joesphinum was closed for a €6 million renovation to restore the original building housing the collection, reinstate the main lecture hall, and expand the exhibition spaces. The reopened museum may allow more opportunities to publicly display the obstetrical models, but when I visited in 2018 these were exhibited in a separate room from the rest of the collections, only available to visit with a guide. Staff gave practical as well as more ideological reasons for this special treatment. On the one hand, the room is very crowded with fragile objects, housed in their original eighteenth-century glass cases, making it difficult, they suggest, to move safely around without potentially damaging the displays should they put objects down on the glass, press too heavily to take a closer look, or bump into the cases. A guided tour certainly makes it easier to safely navigate visitors around such a tight exhibit space.

However, other exhibition rooms were less crowded with artifacts. A simple solution then would be to add some of these items to those other spaces or swap out some of the displays so that the obstetrical material could be given more room. This would interfere with the organizing principle of the exhibitions, however, which kept the surviving collection in its original clusters. Perhaps the renovation will make it possible, in theory, to provide open access to the obstetrical collection. However, Christiane Druml, museum director, also wonders if these objects are really suitable to some audiences, saying perhaps they are a "bit drastic" for children and that visitors from some cultures might not want to see them. At the time of our tour, Druml was also president of the Austrian Bioethics Commission, reflecting and no doubt reinforcing her acute awareness of potential sensitivities around the public display of anatomies and the potential impact on medical research.[47] As we walked around this room together, she noted the graphic nature of the models and that some represented dangerous situations that were probably not survivable for either mother or child. She also commented that the details, such as pubic hair, might prove distracting to young visitors (figure 11.4).

The models mirror the techniques of anatomical illustration of the same era, focusing the viewer's attention on the uterus and the birth canal by "dismembering" the pregnant woman, cutting her off at the waist and the thighs.[48] As a result, the fetus is more dominant than the mother-to-be in all of the examples. Laid like the Anatomical Venus on soft cushion, they depict

---

47   Druml also serves as Chair on Bioethics of the Medical University of Vienna and former Member of the International Bioethics Committee of UNESCO (2008–2015).

48   Lyle Massey, "On Waxes and Wombs: Eighteenth-Century Representations of the Gravid Uterus," in *Ephemeral Bodies: Wax Sculpture and the Human Figure*, ed. Roberta Panzanelli (Los Angeles: Getty Research Institute, 2008): 83–107.

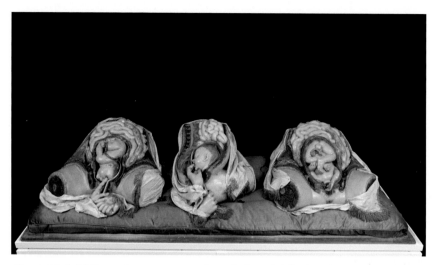

Figure 11.4. Eighteenth-century wax obstetrical model displayed at the Josephinum museum. Credit: Josephinum Museum—Ethics, Collections and History of Medicine, MedUni Vienna.

various types of fetal presentation in childbirth, as well as various interventions, with the hand or the forceps of the male physician sometimes inserted through the vagina. Depending on the moment or process illustrated, more or less of the external flesh is shown alongside the exposed inner activity. There are also models depicting conjoined twins and fetuses displaying obvious physical deformities. Druml concluded that the museum did not receive any negative reactions from visitors, although "from time to time a person will be a bit shocked, but as the objects and the display are so beautiful they are not usually taken aback." In her view, one important reason the institution does not attract controversy is because they have few human remains. The museum still prohibits photography, and staff emphasize the need to show respect for the people whose bodies were used in the making of these models.

In their discussion of postwar obstetrical waxworks at the Museum of Heath Care in Kingston, Ontario, titled "Delight or Disgust?" Marla Dobson and Emma Rosalind Peacocke describe "the primary concern surrounding these wax models as museum objects . . . [is] their display-ability as well as their positioning as potentially disgusting, graphic, and uncanny."[49]

---

49   Marla Dobson and Emma Rosalind Peacocke, "Delight or Disgust? The Afterlife of Anatomical Waxworks," *Museum & Society* 17, no. 3 (November 2019): 366.

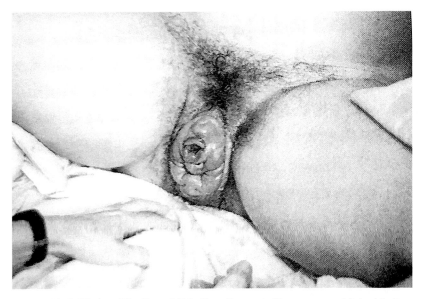

Figure 11.5. Birth at The Farm Midwifery Center in Tennessee, published in Ina May Gaskin's *Ina May's Guide to Childbirth* (New York: Bantam, 2003), a classic text celebrating homebirth and midwife assisted delivery. Credit: Ina May Gaskin.

The uncanny they refer to is the way the wax is modeled and painted to represent living flesh even though the state of dissection also presented would render the body (as if one body is depicted), dead. The "graphic" nature, echoing the comments of the Josephinum's director regarding the models in their collection, refers to the dissection in part but might be more associated with the depiction of childbirth and female genitalia.

It is this conjunction of the medical view and the traditionally male gaze (looking at female nudity), with the underrepresented image of uterus and vagina in the process of birthing, that appears to cause the most discomfort. While we commonly see fetuses safely ensconced in the womb, or babies shortly after birth, we very rarely encounter the image of a fetus leaving a woman's body through a vagina (figure 11.5). In fact, as they go on to reflect on the reactions their objects provoke, it is precisely this element of interaction—between female figure and medical practitioner, or female figure and fetus—that is the most shocking:

> The Winslow waxes appear as if alive and in motion; some even have a pair of gloved hands enacting a clinical intervention . . . in one waxwork, the vulva lies horizontally on the table, while an infant's hand reaches into the air from between the labia, as though emerging from another dimension. . . . Not

only do they depict female genitalia in stark detail, they show that genitalia violently exposed, often in a state of distress.[50]

They refer to "the violence of birth" as part of the power of these objects as museum artifacts. Although I have not seen the specific models they refer to, my experiences with the Josephinum examples and other medical museum collections suggest that such an interpretation is strongly influenced by present-day assumptions of the horror of childbirth in the past framed by an overwhelmingly medicalized approach today.

The lack of "graphic" realistic depictions of the processes of childbirth in contemporary culture lead audiences today to find encounters with such artifacts particularly confrontational. The medicalized narratives of childbirth common to European medical museums, but that are also a fundamental element of mass culture and dominate over nonmedical depictions, also reinforce the interpretation of such models as examples of painful and life-threatening events. This is not to say that these events were not traumatic (especially when they depict problematic situations in childbirth) but rather to emphasize that because audiences today cannot easily contextualize these representations within a wider array of representations of normal childbirth, they become particularly unnerving. In this way, then, like the fetuses of the previous section, these fetuses take on more significance because of the lack of a wider range of public images: in the case of the previous section, nonidealized floating fetuses, and in this case, of a fetus in the process of being born.

Other kinds of obstetrical models were also used in medical education, including full female figures, and as Kosmin discusses in her chapter in this volume, some were even designed to train attending physicians to notice the laboring woman's reactions to their interventions and to adjust their technique to avoid causing additional pain. Yet, surviving obstetrical mannequins are relatively rare compared to the array of images and models that instead depict only part of the female form during childbirth. Neither the mannequins nor these models do much to assert the role of the mother in this process. While they do freeze a process in a particular moment in time, in instances where the fetus is not simply lying in the womb but already moving into the birth canal or being manipulated by hand of forceps, the models convey a sense of motion: although by excluding the rest of the female figure, there is no sense that the pregnant woman herself is involved in such movement. Childbirth is happening to her, not by her.

With most of the female body excised from the scene, while the fetus is not floating it is the only "complete" human in the scene. Some anatomical models of pregnant women apparently did demonstrate links between mother-to-be and fetus, although they appear not to have survived in

---

50   Dobson and Peacocke, "Delight or Disgust?," 372.

museum collections. In 1733, for example, an exhibition in England included the figure of a woman who was eight months pregnant, with red liquid flowing between the mother and her fetus through glass tubes.[51] The model was the most famous exhibit in the early years of an infamous popular anatomical museum, Rackstrow's, which survived into the nineteenth century.[52]

Medical museum collections are dominated by practitioner perspectives, and their emphasis is mainly on disease and deformity. Although some anatomical models were intended to teach general anatomy rather than a disease or medical intervention, female models were *only* used to illustrate the reproductive system and primary and secondary sexual characteristics. Obstetrical models typically address a range of problems the physician might encounter among his patients, including an array of problems that might have ended with the death of the mother or fetus in earlier times. Other artifacts shown in these settings, including displays of different kinds of forceps and narrow or malformed female pelvises, contribute to the highly medicalized depiction of childbirth. As a result, museum visitors today encounter the female reproducing body as always in need of medical assistance.

While such displays are often framed as examples of the difficulties of the past in contrast to the achievements of modern medicine, such presentations do little to increase confidence in the potential for successful childbirth without extensive medical intervention. This is a missed opportunity to address the overuse of Cesarean section, the risks of PTSD following a difficult pregnancy or labor, and a supposed rising fear about childbirth among pregnant women.[53] A simple but successful addition to such displays, as seen at the German Hygiene Museum in Dresden, is a film of labor in progress where the activity of the laboring woman is obvious, and the emergence of her baby is also shown. This particular example is especially valuable as the birth is relatively straightforward, requires no medical intervention, the crowning and delivery of the baby is visible, and the reaction of the mother illustrates how positive the experience can be.

51   Francesco Paolo de Ceglia, "The Importance of Being Florentine: A Journey around the World for Wax Anatomical Venuses," *Nuncius* 26 (2011): 83–108, 84.

52   Ross MacFarlane, "Rackstrow's Museum," Wellcome Library, October 13, 2009, http://blog.wellcomelibrary.org/2009/10/rackstrows-museum/.

53   WHO/HRP, "WHO Statement on Caesarean Section Rates" WHO/RHR/15.02 (World Health Organization, 2015); Sharon Dekel, Caren Stuebe, and Gabriella Dishy, "Childbirth Induced Posttraumatic Stress Syndrome: A Systematic Review of Prevalence and Risk Factors," *Frontiers in Psychology* 8: 560 (April 2017); Maeve O'Connell, Patricia Leahy-Warren, Ali S. Khashan, and Louise C. Kenny, "Tocophobia: The New Hysteria?," *Obstetrics, Gynaecology & Reproductive Medicine* 25, no. 6 (2015): 175–77.

Conclusion

The medical museum fetus, whether human or model, has become an unusually highly charged object even within the context of all the other graphic, provocative, and sometimes disturbing items exhibited. As I have discussed here, some of the issues overlap with broader legal and ethical concerns regarding the collection and display of other human remains, including the colonial origins of some objects, the history of exploitation of the poor and prisoners for medical experimentation, the collection and display of people without their consent or against their express wishes, and the dehumanizing presentation of individuals as medical cases. An additional dimension is the particular cultural significance of the fetus within reproductive rights debates, coupled with silences about female sexuality and reproductive health in wider culture. Yet medical museums are a valuable platform in which all of these topics could be addressed, though they may need to augment collections and will have to shift approaches significantly in order to do so effectively.

As other chapters in this volume demonstrate, medical materials have had a significant role in constructing the public fetus and in obscuring the mother-to-be, and medical museums currently reflect a similar disproportionate emphasis. Even as they open up to admit general audiences, these venues continue to promote narrowly framed medicalized narratives, when healthcare professionals and their patients would benefit from a broader range of representations of experiences of pregnancy, fertility treatment, abortion care, and childbirth. Important objects have disappeared, and objects that do not fit into medicalized frameworks for women's reproductive health have also gone uncollected.[54] We are in danger of losing these histories and the materials that represent them.

Nonetheless, medical museums offer particular advantages. Fundamentally, they retain a high degree of cultural authority, even if they are, rightly, no longer perceived as neutral venues. Although the Nilsson photographs have been interpreted as having particularly persuasive power, artifact collections are also highly captivating, perhaps even more so, given that visitors can see "the real thing" in person, in three dimensions. Although the *Life* magazine photographs pretended to show living fetuses while deploying dead specimens to illustrate "The Drama of Life before Birth," such sleight of hand is impossible in the medical museum: here the role of dissection and preservation is broadly evident and is often part of the interpretive text explaining the origins and uses of the items on display.

---

54   See Kosmin in this volume.

288 &♦ MANON S. PARRY

While museum staff debate the motivation and consequences of enduring public interest in historical medical collections, the objects have taken up much of their attention, as if these artifacts are the source of the problem or the provocation. However, as the diverse responses among museum staff as well as visitors suggests, personal experiences, museum settings, and exhibition techniques, as well as broader social conventions, all inform a complex array of attitudes and reactions. Deeper consideration of different exhibition approaches to generate discussion and reflection would allow curators to explore their range of resonances among audiences and to develop new strategies for their display.

It would also be useful to collect and incorporate responses to the objects and issues exhibited. There has been very little research on audience reactions, and therefore many decisions about what can or should be shown are based on generalized assumptions about diverse audiences. While there is an increasing emphasis on broadening the perspectives on display—to incorporate nurses' views as well as those of doctors, or to bring in patient narratives where they can be found in historical sources—it is less common for medical museums to create new archival records from the recollections of visitors about their own experiences with particular medical issues or approaches, or about major events in the recent past. Asking visitors for their recollections of the personal impact of public fetus iconography would be valuable in better determining the role the imagery has played in private lives in the opinions and decisions of individuals. A final benefit of these shifts would be the integration of the experiences of women into the collections of medical museums to enable the preservation and exhibition of a wider range of perspectives on reproductive health.

Chapter Twelve

The Public Fetus

A Traveling Concept

Solveig Jülich and Elisabet Björklund

In the fall of 2022, the same year as *Roe v. Wade* was overturned in the United States, the film *Blonde*, directed by Andrew Dominik and based on Joyce Carol Oates's novel about Marilyn Monroe, premiered on Netflix. In the narrative, Monroe experiences two pregnancies: one that ends with a traumatic abortion and one that ends with a miscarriage. There is also a more ambiguous second abortion scene in the final part of the film. In all three cases, images showing computer-generated representations of embryos and fetuses floating inside a uterus are included. Most of them show a rosy, humanized, and almost fully grown fetus, presented in a style that clearly calls to mind Lennart Nilsson's famous photographs. In the sequence with the miscarriage, the fetus is also given a voice and can be heard talking to Monroe, asking her not to abort it.[1]

Blonde's representation of pregnancy, abortion, and the fetus quickly moved beyond film criticism to become a matter of concern in the wider cultural debate, where many—among them notable actors such as the Planned Parenthood—saw it as antiabortion propaganda.[2] This in itself clearly indicates the weight issues of representation are deemed to have in contemporary cultural discussions, not least in debates over reproductive rights.

---

1   Andrew Dominik, dir., *Blonde* (Beverly Hills, CA: Plan B Entertainment, 2022).

2   Rebecca Keegan, "Planned Parenthood: 'Blonde' Is 'Anti-Abortion Propaganda,'" *Hollywood Reporter*, September 30, 2022, https://www.hollywoodreporter.com/movies/movie-news/planned-parenthood-blonde-abortion-1235231175/.

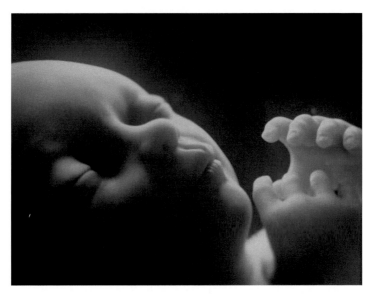

Figure 12.1. Screenshot of the talking fetus in *Blonde* (Plan B
Entertainment, 2022). Source: Netflix.

Interestingly, the importance of historicizing fetal images was also brought
forward. In an article in the *New York Times*, Amanda Hess argued that it
was ahistorical to think that Monroe would have imagined her fetus through
a mode of representation that emerged after her death, with Nilsson's images
in *Life* magazine in the mid-1960s. Hess ended her article by referring to
historian Barbara Duden's influential book *Disembodying Women: Perspectives
on Pregnancy and the Unborn*, written in the early 1990s:

> In her book "Disembodying Women," the medical historian Barbara
> Duden traces the public exposure of the fetus—and its rising cultural su-
> premacy—over the latter half of the 20th century. She calls this process
> "the skinning of woman." "Blonde" is also a movie about a woman be-
> ing flayed by the culture at large. First, by the Hollywood of her own era,
> which made her into a sex symbol. And now, by the Hollywood of ours,
> which has claimed to access her mind, only to serve up a recycled stock im-
> age of a magic fetus.[3]

The images of the fetus in *Blonde* and the responses they provoked illustrate two things: First, that the imagery of the universal fetus is a prevailing
element in our visual culture and so the pioneering work done by Duden

---

3   Amanda Hess, "The Empty Spectacle of Marilyn Monroe's Fantasy
     Fetus," *New York Times*, September 29, 2022, https://www.nytimes.
     com/2022/09/29/movies/marilyn-monroe-fetus-blonde.html.

and the other feminist scholars who first used the term "public fetus" in the 1980s and 1990s continues to be highly relevant. Second, that there is a high level of awareness of this way of representing the unborn, its problematic aspects, and the consequences that fetal images in public can have. Hence, Duden's groundbreaking *Disembodying Women* has been influential not only in the academic world but also in wider circles—it is still read and understood to be a central point of reference in the public discussion of visual culture, even though our visual culture has changed profoundly since the book was published in the 1990s.

In this volume, our aim has been to revitalize the discussion about the public fetus, thereby counteracting persistent ideas about the "universal" fetus. The depiction in *Blonde* indicates that there is still much to be done. As Hess points out, Marilyn Monroe's mental image of the fetus is not equivalent to the biological reality of any fetus at any time but rather an image that is dependent on a specific place and time. For many feminist and other scholars who have explored these historical constructions and the links between reproductive technologies, gender, and power, the concept of the public fetus has provided a useful configuration around which to build a theoretical framework. Even if the focus has mainly been on late twentieth-century visual culture, it has served as a reminder that fetal photographs, ultrasound images, and pictures of dead and bloody fetuses in antiabortion propaganda have not always been with us. But the concept of the public fetus also has a history that needs to be interrogated in order to sustain its critical edge and relevance in current scholarly discussions.

In this concluding chapter, we hence present a mini history of the public fetus concept and its journey over the past three decades. We demonstrate that from the very start, it has moved between disciplinary and national contexts in a way that, following Dutch cultural theorist Mieke Bal, allows it to be described as a "traveling concept." According to Bal, concepts are indispensable "tools of intersubjectivity" in that "they facilitate discussion on the basis of a common language" and offer "miniature theories." Concepts enable and determine how an academic community looks at, approaches, and constructs its objects of study. They are "the sites of debate, awareness of difference, and tentative exchange," the basis for meaningful agreement as well as productive disagreement. As such, concepts are not fixed; rather, they "travel" back and forth between disciplines and across various borders. Their meanings are constituted and transformed through these movements. Concepts only survive as long as scholars find them important to argue about and useful for analytical work.[4]

---

4   Mieke Bal, *Travelling Concepts in the Humanities: A Rough Guide* (Toronto: University of Toronto Press, 2002), 13, 22–25. See also the discussion on Bal's concept in Birgit Neumann and Ansgar Nünning, "Travelling Concepts as a Model for the Study of Culture," in *Travelling Concepts for the Study of*

In adopting the notion of the traveling concept, the aim of this concluding chapter is to examine crucial frameworks for the creation of the public fetus by feminist scholars in the late 1980s and early 1990s and highlight some of its subsequent uses and transformations. We ask several questions: How and when did this concept emerge? What borders and boundaries did it cross? In what ways have these movements infused the concept with new meanings? And how can it be developed to maintain its relevance?[5] The material consists of scholarly publications from a range of disciplines but largely in English. This is symptomatic of the present dominance of English-language concepts within many disciplines and fields of research in the humanities and social sciences. When adopted uncritically, a simple translation or transfer of concepts from the English may hinder rather than help to clarify theoretical ventures and the analysis of historical phenomena.[6] An overarching aim, then, is to provide insights that can make the public fetus concept useful in broader linguistic, cultural, and academic contexts.

To begin with, we discuss the work of Barbara Duden and Rosalind Petchesky, who coined the concept in the last years of second-wave feminism. Then we present scholarship that, beginning in the 1990s, extended the analysis of the public fetus to the "pregnant icon." Moreover, we highlight how historically oriented scholars challenged the implicit notion of newness in the adoption of the public fetus concept as well as the tendency to adhere to the "maternal erasure" theory. Finally, we summarize by discussing four distinct modes of travel, based on processes highlighted in the analysis. We conclude by suggesting that this attempt to develop a self-reflexive approach to the public fetus concept can help further interdisciplinary and transnational dialogues—starting with this volume.

Culture, ed. Birgit Neumann and Ansgar Nünning (Berlin: Walter de Gruyter, 2012), 3–4.

5   This chapter does not claim to offer a strict or comprehensive mapping of the movements of a concept. Even so, it draws on Neumann and Nünning's suggestion that four frameworks or "axes" should be included in the analysis of traveling concepts: (1) traveling between disciplines, (2) crossing national borders and cultures, (3) traversing historical time, and (4) traveling between academia and other domains of society. See their "Travelling Concepts," 11–14.

6   See Ulrike Hanna Meinhof, "Appendix: Audiences and Publics; Comparing Semantic Fields across Different Languages," in *Audiences and Publics: When Cultural Engagement Matters for the Public Sphere*, ed. Sonia Livingstone (Bristol: Intellect, 2005), 213.

The Public Fetuses of Duden and Petchesky

Any effort to trace the history of the concept of the public fetus necessarily starts from its component parts—"public" and "fetus." Adding to the complexity of these terms is not only that their meanings have changed and multiplied over time. Another important consideration is that they have different meanings in different languages, and thus varying relationships to other concepts. For instance, only English (or American English) appears to have a normative distinction between "public" and "audience," with positive or negative connotations respectively.[7] As for "fetus," it too has a rich and intricate etymological history. *Fetus* is a Latin word, meaning fruits of the earth, of trees, and of the body. However, according to Barbara Duden, no German dictionary of the eighteenth century mentions its use with today's meaning of a preperson or fetal subject. During the nineteenth century physicians started to adopt the term, but theologians stayed with the Greek word *embryo*. In light of this, she claimed that the public fetus is a historical novelty.[8]

In Duden's book *Disembodying Women*, published in English in 1993, she addressed the "modern woman" living in a rapidly shifting landscape of visual technologies and reproductive politics:

> I know that for her there is no way back to what pregnancy was. Pregnant or not, she lives in the age of the public fetus, the age in which birth has been reduced to the last stage in fetal development, in which death has become the cessation of "a life." There is no way back to the unborn below the horizon.[9]

With these ominous words, Duden invited readers to join her in a historical exploration of how the experiences of pregnant women had changed since the eighteenth century. In earlier times, pregnancy became known to a woman through "quickening," the first movement inside, felt and announced by her alone. But "in the course of one generation," Duden stated, women lost their "autonomous aliveness" and were no longer consulted as a source

---

7   Meinhof, "Appendix: Audiences and Publics," 215.

8   Barbara Duden, *Disembodying Women: Perspectives on Pregnancy and the Unborn*, trans. Lee Hoinacki (Cambridge, MA: Harvard University Press, 1993), 52–53. First published as *Der Frauenleib als öffentlicher Ort: Vom Missbrauch des Begriffs Leben* (Hamburg: Luchterhand-Literaturverlag, 1991). See also Barbara Duden, "The Fetus on the 'Farther Shore': Toward a History of the Unborn," *Fetal Subjects, Feminist Positions*, ed. Lynn M. Morgan and Meredith W. Michaels (Philadelphia: University of Pennsylvania Press, 1999), 13–25.

9   Duden, *Disembodying Women*, 55.

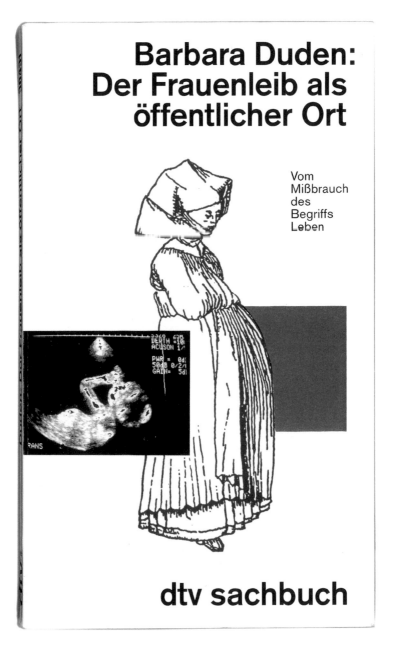

Figure 12.2. Front cover of German paperback edition of Barbara Duden, *Der Frauenleib als öffentlicher Ort: Vom Missbrauch des Begriffs Leben* (Munich: dtv, 1994.) Courtesy of dtv.

of privileged knowledge. Through visual technologies and prenatal diagnosis, the embodied experience of being pregnant had been transformed into a process to be managed within a biomedical framework: "life" displaced "aliveness," "the public fetus" replaced "the unborn."[10]

Duden traced this increasing visibility of the secrets of the womb back to the introduction of a new graphic technique in German anatomist Samuel Thomas Soemmering's visual representation of the unborn in 1799. She also emphasized the importance of the first uses of the stethoscope in the 1830s, the experiments with X-rays in obstetrics around 1900, as well as the advent of hormonal pregnancy tests in the 1940s. But the crucial moment was the publication of Swedish photographer Lennart Nilsson's extraordinary color pictures of the fetus, "looking like an astronaut in its transparent bubble," in *Life* magazine in 1965. In particular, the arrival of the fetal sonogram or ultrasound facilitated the pushing back of the visual horizon. According to Duden, the Nilsson photographs, together with ultrasound images, had been appropriated by antiabortion groups and through their wide dissemination in the media had come to represent "life."[11]

In several interviews and personal memoirs, Duden recalled how she became a historian of the human body and bodily perceptions with special attention to pregnancy.[12] She described two turning points in particular as decisive. First, in the late 1950s, her identical twin sister, Alexa, was diagnosed with a neurologic disorder and became "a case," one year before her untimely death at sixteen. This led Duden, like Michel Foucault and (her partner and collaborator) Ivan Illich, to start investigating the power of the medical gaze and the medicalization of health. But neither Foucault nor Illich addressed "the more fundamental issue of modern *disembodiment*." They and other medical historians, she argued, "have been reluctant to give flesh and blood to their 'histories': they have stopped short of the experienced body."[13]

---

10   Duden, *Disembodying Women*, 2, 110.

11   Duden, *Disembodying Women*, 14. See also Barbara Duden, "Quick with Child: An Experience That Has Lost Its Status," *Technology in Society* 14 (1992): 335–44.

12   Barbara Duden, "A Historian's 'Biology': On the Traces of the Body in a Technogenic World," *Historein* 3 (2001): 89–102; Barbara Duden, "'Ich wollte den Leuten immer unter die Haut,'" interview by Patrick Bauer, *Süddeutsche Zeitung Magazin*, December 19, 2016, https://www.sueddeutsche.de/panorama/barbara-duden-ich-wollte-den-leuten-immer-unter-die-haut-1.3295351?reduced=true; Barbara Duden and Imke Schmincke, "'Die Geschichtlichkeit der Körperwahrnehmung in der Tiefe ausbuchstabieren': Ein Interview mit Barbara Duden," *Body Politics* 7, no. 11 (2019): 41–54.

13   Duden, "Historian's 'Biology,'" 94–96.

Second, the search for a firsthand experience in the past led to an encounter with a "haggard widow" of the early eighteenth century, whose story Duden came to know through the diary of the woman's physician Dr. Storch. This source helped her develop an argument about the contingency of conception and pregnancy in the somatic experience of past generations of women. What today would be perceived as an abortion, miscarriage, or premature birth could then "be perceived as emitting bad blood, the birth of a mole, a moon-calf, as 'cleansing' of the womb, or as healthy flux against unhealthy stoppage." Women told doctors their stories of how they felt and knew that they were with child.[14]

Certainly, Duden's formative years as a historian overlapped with broader social and political tendencies. Studying at the Technical University Berlin during the turbulent 1960s, she became a pioneer in the women's movement. Decriminalization of abortion, safe contraceptives, and women's agency over childbirth stood at the forefront of the movement's concerns. Duden started researching and writing women's history and was one of the founders of the journal *Courage*, which played an important role for second-wave feminism in Germany.[15] In the late 1980s she acted as guest lecturer at several American universities, and in 1991 her dissertation, *The Woman Beneath the Skin: A Doctor's Patients in Eighteenth-Century Germany*, was published in English. Two years later, *Disembodying Women: Perspectives on Pregnancy and the Unborn* came out.[16] These pioneering works established Duden's position as "one of the foremost modern historians of the body."[17] In the Anglo-American context, it was the feminist theme of the public fetus that drew attention, and several journals published excerpts from *Disembodying Women*, in which she used examples from contemporary popular culture and especially Lennart Nilsson's photographs in *Life* in 1965 and 1990 to discuss the increasing significance of the objectified and politicized fetus (sometimes referred to as the "foetal icon").[18]

---

14 Duden, "Historian's 'Biology,'" 96–100; quotation from Duden, "Fetus on the 'Farther Shore,'" 16.

15 Duden, "Historian's 'Biology,'" 95; Duden, "'Ich wollte den Leuten immer unter die Haut,'" 48–49. *Courage* was published between 1976 and 1984.

16 Barbara Duden, *The Woman Beneath the Skin: A Doctor's Patients in Eighteenth-Century Germany* (Cambridge, MA; Harvard University Press, 1991). First published as *Geschichte unter der Haut ein Eisenacher Arzt und seine Patientinnen um 1730* (Stuttgart: Klett-Cotta, 1987); Duden, *Disembodying Women*.

17 Isabel V. Hull, "The Body as Historical Experience: Review of Recent Works by Barbara Duden," *Central European History* 28, no. 1 (1995): 73.

18 Barbara Duden, "Visualizing 'Life,'" *Science as Culture* 3, no. 4 (1993): 562–600 ("the foetal icon" is mentioned on 590); Barbara Duden, "The Fetus as

But Duden was not the first to write about the public fetus. In 1987, Rosalind Petchesky's paper "Fetal Images: The Power of Visual Culture in the Politics of Reproduction" was published in *Feminist Studies*.[19] As a political scientist and feminist theorist, Petchesky had long been involved in feminist activism and the struggle for reproductive and sexual rights. The same year, she had been hired as professor of political science and coordinator of women's studies at Hunter College in New York.[20] Her concern was that in the mid-1980s "the political attack on abortion rights moved further into the terrain of mass culture and imagery." While acknowledging that images had long been part of antiabortion rhetoric in the United States and Britain, she found that the conservative Reagan administration and the Christian right had accelerated their use of "pro-life" propaganda.[21]

To understand this major shift, Petchesky examined the 1984 video *The Silent Scream* (directed by Jack Duane Dabner, narrated by Bernard Nathanson, and produced in partnership with the National Right to Life Committee), which was aired on American television and purported to show real-time ultrasound imaging of a twelve-week-old fetus being aborted. However, it was not only supporters of antiabortion movements who responded to images of fetuses: "The 'public' presentation of the fetus

---

an Object of Our Time," *RES: Anthropology and Aesthetics* 25 (1994): 132–35.

19   Rosalind Pollack Petchesky, "Fetal Images: The Power of Visual Culture in the Politics of Reproduction," *Feminist Studies* 13, no. 2 (1987): 263–92. The exact wording of "the public fetus" occurs in only one passage (281). This overview of feminist debates on fetal subjects has profited from Georgina Firth, "Re-negotiating Reproductive Technologies: The 'Public Foetus' Revisited," *Feminist Review* 92 (2009): 54–71; and Bernice L. Hausman, "Public Fetuses," in *Health Humanities Reader*, ed. Therese Jones, Delese Wear, and Lester D. Friedman (New Brunswick, NJ: Rutgers University Press, 2014), 186–95.

20   Extensive documentation of Petchesky's work from 1959 to 2009 is kept in the Rosalind Petchesky papers, Sophia Smith Collection, SSC-MS-00639, Smith College Special Collections, Northampton, MA, US. Box 3 contains material on "US reproductive rights movement: 'Fetal Images,'" ca. 1980–2001, https://findingaids.smith.edu/repositories/2/top_containers/30609 (last accessed March 14, 2023). Petchesky narrates elements of her personal story in "JVP-NYC in Conversation with Transnational Feminist Rosalind Petchesky," Jewish Voice for Peace, YouTube, June 22, 2020, https://www.youtube.com/watch?v=kC6PNWOzPlc.

21   Petchesky, "Fetal Images." A shorter version was published in *Reproductive Technologies: Gender, Motherhood and Medicine*, ed. Michelle Stanworth (Cambridge: Polity Press, 1987). Also see Petchesky's important book *Abortion and Woman's Choice: The State, Sexuality, and Reproductive Freedom* (Boston: Northeastern University Press, 1984).

has become ubiquitous; its disembodied form, now propped up by medical authority and technological rationality, permeates mass culture. We are all, on some level, susceptible to its coded meanings."[22] In *The Silent Scream* but also in the science fiction blockbuster *2001: A Space Odyssey* (Stanley Kubrick, 1968) the fetus was portrayed as an autonomous individual and the pregnant woman as absent or peripheral. Petchesky traced this mode of picturing the fetus back to the early 1960s, but unlike Duden she did not explicitly mention Lennart Nilsson's photo-essays in *Life* (although it can be argued that she had these in mind). Instead, she discussed "Dramatic Photographs of Babies before Birth" in the competing magazine *Look*, a story promoting science author Geraldine Lux Flanagan's book *The First Nine Months of Life*, published in 1962.[23]

Duden and Petchesky also had somewhat different conceptions of the idea of the public fetus. The implicit notion of the public in Duden's discussion can be connected to Jürgen Habermas's classic discussion of the public sphere in *The Structural Transformation of the Public Sphere*, originally published in German in 1962 but translated into English in 1989 and hence a current work when she wrote *Disembodying Women*.[24] Duden's argument built on a separation between private and public and a historical analysis arguing that "the private"—reproduction, women's bodies, and the fetus—had become public in the twentieth century.[25] Like Habermas, Duden was strongly pessimistic toward changes in the public sphere and the development of new mass media in the twentieth century.

Petchesky, on the other hand, discussed the public fetus using the concept of visual culture, while also drawing on recent works on photography and film by scholars such as John Berger, Victor Burgin, and Annette Kuhn. Her discussion can thus be placed in the context of the diverse interdisciplinary field of visual culture studies that started to develop in the 1980s.[26] This

---

22 Petchesky, "Fetal Images," 281.

23 Petchesky, 268; Geraldine Lux Flanagan, "Dramatic Photographs of Babies before Birth," *Look* 26 (June 5, 1962): 19–23; Geraldine Lux Flanagan, *The First Nine Months of Life* (New York: Simon & Schuster, 1962). Flanagan's article and book are discussed in Solveig Jülich, "The Making of a Best-Selling Book on Reproduction: Lennart Nilsson's *A Child Is Born*," *Bulletin of the History of Medicine* 89, no. 3 (2015): 491–525.

24 Jürgen Habermas, *The Structural Transformation of the Public Sphere: An Inquiry of a Category of Bourgeois Society*, trans. Thomas Burger with the assistance of Frederick Lawrence (Cambridge, MA: MIT Press, 1989). Originally published as *Strukturwandel der Öffentlichkeit: Untersuchungen zu einer Kategorie der bürgerlichen Gesellschaft* (Neuwid/Berlin: Luchterhand, 1962).

25 Duden, *Disembodying Women*.

26 For discussions of the development of this field, see, for example, Margarita Dikovitskaya, *Visual Culture: The Study of the Visual after the Cultural Turn*

positioning implied a less suspicious stance toward the media. At the same time, like many of the scholars following her in the 1990s, her discussion centered on modern mass media (film, television), and images in commercial venues (billboards, shopping malls), which she understood as a powerful public visual culture influencing how reproductive technologies were used and how "private" pictures were interpreted.[27]

There were also other, perhaps more profound, differences between Duden and Petchesky. Both located a historical shift in the 1960s that led to an increasing public visibility of the autonomous fetus, the erasure of the embodied woman from the site of pregnancy, and the blurring of medical and cultural discourses in the spread of fetal imagery. They agreed that the rise of the public fetus had consequences for how women experienced their pregnancies, responded to anxieties about risks, or decided on abortions. But while Duden thought there was no way back to a "pure state," she seemed convinced that the only means to regain the intimate bodily experience of pregnancy was to resist the use of the new technologies of visualization. Petchesky, on the other hand, suggested that the scientific image of a fetus could be converted not only into a public object but also into a personal context. She noted that ultrasound imaging encouraged women and their families to bond with the child-to-be. Women are not just passive victims in the situation; reproductive technologies can also offer opportunities for empowerment.[28]

Still, there is no generalized experience to build feminist theory and practice upon, Petchesky argued. How different women see fetal images depends on many factors, including class, race, sexual preference, age, physical disability, and fertility history. In contrast to Duden's rather linear view of the popularization of science (despite drawing on Ludwik Fleck), she emphasized that images themselves come with no inherent objective qualities; they take on meaning from the particular circumstances of viewing, from talking about and using them, as well as from a larger visual culture.[29] To make a change, then, feminists should "restore women to a central place in the pregnancy scene." According to her, "we must create new images that recontextualize the fetus, that place it back into the uterus, and the uterus back into the woman's body, and her body back into its social space." With this and some other proposals, "both modest and utopian," Petchesky ended her article. After this publication, along with her extensive research, she founded the International Reproductive Rights

---

(Cambridge, MA: MIT Press, 2005); and Marquard Smith, ed., *Visual Culture Studies: Interviews with Key Thinkers* (Los Angeles: SAGE, 2008).

27   Petchesky, "Fetal Images."
28   Duden, *Disembodying Women*; Petchesky, "Fetal Images."
29   Duden, *Disembodying Women*; Petchesky, "Fetal Images."

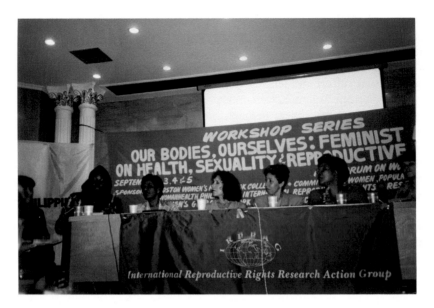

Figure 12.3. Rosalind Petchesky (in the middle) on an International Reproductive Rights Research Action Group (IRRRAG) panel at the Beijing Fourth World Women's Conference in September 1995. Other participants on the panel were (from left to right) Hajara Usman (Nigeria), Rajeswari Nagaraja (Malaysia), Amal Abdel Hadi (Egypt), Evelyne Longchamp (United States), and Cassia Carloto (Brazil). Courtesy of Rosalind Petchesky and with thanks to Smith College Special Collections.

Research Action Group (IRRRAG) in 1992, which consisted of seven national research teams that held conferences and published collaborative work in several languages.[30]

From the Public Fetus to the Pregnant Icon

Following Duden and Petchesky, several feminist scholars explored and debated aspects of the public fetus. Many focused on the representation of the fetus as an independent being in antiabortion propaganda as well as how

---

30   Petchesky, "Fetal Images," 286–87, quotation on 287. A book that grew out of IRRRAG's work, authored by Rosalind Pollack Petchesky and Karen Judd, was *Negotiating Reproductive Rights: Women's Perspectives across Countries and Cultures* (London: Zed, 1998).

this representational style spread to and was employed in other domains. Increasingly, images of women's pregnant bodies in a variety of public spaces came to occupy the center of feminist analyses of a changing media landscape. Most of these were preoccupied with and related to developments in the US context.

In an often-cited 1992 article, Janelle S. Taylor discussed an advertisement for the Swedish car company Volvo that featured a large black-and-white ultrasound image of a fetus to arouse longings for safety and protection. Below was a small color photograph of a Volvo. She saw this commercial use of ultrasound imagery as a consequence of its distribution in contemporary antiabortion materials. What characterized the public fetus, Taylor argued, was its value "as a universal abstraction, a representation of that which is supposed to be common to all fetuses—whether stages of development, 'humanity,' or a 'right to life.'" Yet, at the same time, it was designed to emphasize the uniqueness of each individual fetus carried by a woman.[31] In a later book, Taylor analyzed the making of the "fetishized public fetus" by investigating the technology of obstetric ultrasound that produced images of "life" and helped to shape their visual components, also drawing attention to the people who operated this technological apparatus.[32]

Still others investigated new biomedical technologies, including Monica Casper's ethnography of the making of fetal surgery and the unborn patient and Rayna Rapp's interviews with women who underwent genetic counseling and prenatal diagnosis. In addition, several studies explored how public health campaigns on smoking, alcohol, and drug use portrayed fetuses as vulnerable and endangered entities. The pregnant body was imagined as a risky environment that must be monitored and regulated in the interest of the unborn. Potential mothers were constructed as good, bad, normal, deviant, or even dangerous. The common starting point for these scholars was earlier discussions on public fetuses and antiabortion politics.[33]

---

31   Janelle S. Taylor, "The Public Fetus and the Family Car: From Abortion Politics to a Volvo Advertisement," *Public Culture* 4, no. 2 (1992): 67–80, quotation on 71.

32   Janelle S. Taylor, *The Public Life of the Fetal Sonogram: Technology, Consumption and the Politics of Reproduction* (New Brunswick, NJ: Rutgers University Press, 2008). On the fetishism of fetuses, see 27–29, quotation on 29.

33   Monica J. Casper, *The Making of the Unborn Patient: A Social Anatomy of Fetal Surgery* (New Brunswick, NJ: Rutgers University Press, 1998), 16–18; Rayna Rapp, *Testing Women, Testing the Fetus: The Social Impact of Amniocentesis in America* (New York: Routledge, 2000), 119–21; Laury Oaks, "Smoke-Filled Wombs and Fragile Fetuses: The Social Politics of Fetal Representation," *Signs* 26, no. 1 (2000): 63–108.

Feminist writings of the 1990s credited photographer Lennart Nilsson as having a huge influence. For Lauren Berlant, the publishing of "Drama of Life before Birth" in *Life* magazine in 1965 "initiated an entirely new scopic regime, a whole new calendar, and finally, a whole new voice for the American citizen."[34] In this and manifold other analyses, the focus was on the cultural construction of fetal autonomy and personhood in Nilsson's photographs. Through extreme enlargement and other advanced photographic techniques, the images of embryos and fetuses were made to look like the creation of life: a developing individual inside the womb. But in fact, as many observed, most of the pictures were taken of aborted, dead fetuses outside the maternal body—a paradox, considering that they had been appropriated for "pro-life" propaganda.[35]

On the verge of the new millennium the edited volume *Fetal Subjects, Feminist Positions* appeared. Acknowledging earlier work on the proliferation of fetuses in law, medicine, and popular culture, the editors, Lynn Morgan and Meredith Michaels, suggested that feminists still avoided talking about "fetal subjects" because this could play into the hands of anti-abortion activists. They urged a move beyond stable definitions of fetal personhood and arguments about the ethics of dependency in the maternal-fetal relationship. Instead, they invited analyses of the multiple social and cultural meanings attached to fetuses, pregnancy, and motherhood, across cultural and national borders.[36] The volume became a crucial reference for

34 Lauren Berlant, *The Queen of America Goes to Washington City: Essays on Sex and Citizenship* (Durham, NC: Duke University Press, 1997), 105–11, quotation on 105.

35 Sarah Franklin, "Fetal Fascinations: New Dimensions to the Medical-Scientific Construction of Fetal Personhood," in *Off-Centre: Feminism and Cultural Studies*, ed. Sarah Franklin, Celia Lury, and Jackie Stacey (London: HarperCollins Academic, 1991); Carol A. Stabile, "Shooting the Mother: Fetal Photography and the Politics of Disappearance," *Camera Obscura* 10, no. 28 (1992): 179–205; Valerie Hartouni, "Fetal Exposures: Abortion Politics and the Optics of Allusion," *Camera Obscura* 10, no. 29 (1992): 130–49 (Nilsson is discussed on 135); E. Ann Kaplan, "Look Who's Talking, Indeed: Fetal Images in Recent North American Visual Culture," in *Mothering: Ideology, Experience, and Agency*, ed. Evelyn Nakano Glenn, Grace Chand, and Linda Rennie Forcey (New York: Routledge, 1994), 126–27; Nathan Stormer, "Embodying Normal Miracles," *Quarterly Journal of Speech* 83, no. 2 (1997): 172–91.

36 Lynn M. Morgan and Meredith W. Michaels, "Introduction: The Fetal Imperative," in *Fetal Subjects, Feminist Positions*, ed. Lynn M. Morgan and Meredith W. Michaels (Philadelphia: University of Pennsylvania Press, 1999). See also Lynn M. Morgan, "Fetal Relationality in Feminist Philosophy: An Anthropological Critique," *Hypatia* 11, no. 3 (1996): 47–70.

multidisciplinary work, including studies showing how the fetus was interpreted in various cultures.[37]

At the same time, Petchesky's argument for redirecting feminist attention back toward the social visibility of the pregnant body as a counterpoint to the excessive use of fetal images and videos stimulated numerous writings. Hollywood cinema, with films such as *Rosemary's Baby* (Roman Polanski, 1968), offered ambiguous material, to say the least.[38] In Sandra Matthews and Laura Wexler's *Pregnant Pictures* the focus was on a selection of photographs from the twentieth century with a strong emphasis on the United States after World War II.[39] According to them, it was the diverse genre of instructional photographs, including the images in *Our Bodies, Ourselves* (1971) by the Boston Women's Health Book Collective, that for the first time targeted primarily female viewers and brought pregnant bodies into "the public sphere."[40] Yet it was not until the end of the twentieth century that a bigger change took place, they argued. Just like Lennart Nilsson's *Life* cover photograph in 1965 had won enormous attention, photographer Annie Leibovitz's picture of pregnant actress Demi Moore on the cover of *Vanity Fair* magazine in August 1991 started "a small revolution": The "fetal icon" was supplemented by the glamorous "pregnant icon." After initial resistance, a more relaxed attitude toward publicly picturing pregnancy in the United States followed, assisted by the breakthrough of in vitro fertilization (IVF). Importantly, for Matthews and Wexler, the new images of pregnancy had to be scrutinized, too, both for what they portrayed and for what they left out, notably people of color and the not-so-glamorous average experience of being pregnant.[41]

Several other feminist scholars writing in the early twenty-first century argued that the prolific representations of pregnancy and childbirth in

---

37   See, for instance, Tine Gammeltoft, *Haunting Images: A Cultural Account of Selective Reproduction in Vietnam* (Berkeley: University of California Press, 2014); Sharon R. Kaufman and Lynn M. Morgan, "The Anthropology of the Beginnings and Ends of Life," *Annual Review of Anthropology* 34, no. 1 (2005): 317–41; Gonçalo Santos and Suzanne Z. Gottschang, "Rethinking Reproductive Technologies and Modernities in Time and Space," *Technology and Culture* 61, no. 2 (2020): 549–58.

38   Katryn Valerius, "*Rosemary's Baby*, Gothic Pregnancy and Fetal Subjects," *College Literature* 32, no. 3 (2005): 116–35. See also the more recent work of Erin Harrington, *Women, Monstrosity and Horror Film: Gynaehorror* (Abingdon, UK: Routledge, 2018).

39   Matthews and Wexler, *Pregnant Pictures*, 1–2.

40   Matthews and Wexler, *Pregnant Pictures*, 151, 157–60.

41   Matthews and Wexler, *Pregnant Pictures*, 199, 211–12, quotation on 199. On the racialized subtext of the pregnant icon, see 218, 234.

social media, reality television, and television drama signaled the ending of the visual "taboo" of childbirth.[42] Across platforms such as YouTube and Instagram, women's sharing and participatory use of images of abortion, miscarriage, and the moment of crowning demonstrated that childbirth was "becoming routinely witnessed and represented in more graphic and public ways." According to Imogen Tyler and Lisa Baraitser, this heterogenous "field of 'maternal aesthetics' has transformed previous notions of beauty, taste and disgust around bodies and practices." They contextualized the rise of pregnancy's visibility within a neoliberal consumer culture but nevertheless envisioned that the new visual culture of birth could enhance women's empowerment and lead to the democratization of knowledge of pregnancy in its diversity.[43]

Finally, feminist scholars have moved beyond central traits in the analysis of the public fetus to develop the framework of reproductive justice. This perspective challenges former feminist discussions of reproductive rights and choice, which are understood as expressions of a Western liberal discourse ignoring power relations based on, for instance, race and class. Instead, as Rachel Alpha Johnston Hurst, the editor of *Representing Abortion*, has explained, "Reproductive justice centers on the interrelationship of reproduction with racism, colonialism, classism, ableism, homophobia, and transphobia, and offers expansive, creative inquiry into the politics of reproduction that exceeds 'choice.'" The volume consequently offers a collection of analyses of counter-images of abortion created by current writers, artists, and activists.[44]

Challenging Newness and the Maternal Erasure Theory

Since the 1990s, alongside the important work of feminist scholars, historically oriented studies on images of fetal and pregnant bodies have also been conducted. While often inspired by Duden's work, the historians of the late

---

42 Robyn Longhurst, "YouTube: A New Space for Birth?," *Feminist Review* 93 (2009): 46–63; Imogen Tyler, "Pregnant Beauty: Maternal Femininities under Neoliberalism," in *New Femininities: Postfeminism, Neoliberalism and Subjectivity*, ed. Rosalind Gill and Christina Scharff (Basingstoke, UK: Palgrave Macmillan, 2011), 21–36.

43 Imogen Tyler and Lisa Baraitser, "Private View, Public Birth: Making Feminist Sense of the New Visual Culture of Childbirth," *Studies in the Maternal* 5, no. 2 (2013): 1–27, quotations on 1 and 7. For a critical discussion, see Lauren Bliss, *The Maternal Imagination of Film and Film Theory* (Cham: Palgrave Macmillan, 2021), 143–52.

44 Rachel Alpha Johnston Hurst, "Representing Abortion," in *Representing Abortion*, ed. Rachel Alpha Johnston Hurst (London: Routledge, 2020), 5.

twentieth century seemed reluctant to directly engage with the concept of the public fetus, which had by then become closely associated with the contemporary abortion debate. This might be explained by a fear of anachronism. Significantly, severe criticism was directed against literary scholar Karen Newman, who, in her 1996 book *Fetal Positions*, reviewed antiabortion images in a longer historical perspective but missed the point that many of the early modern anatomical drawings and models represented *homunculi*, miniature humans, rather than the individual fetus.[45] Even so, several familiar themes reemerged. For instance, Atina Grossmann's and Cornelie Usborne's histories of the female body in Weimar-era Germany both emphasized the role of the public arena in making sexuality, abortion, and birth control issues of political relevance.[46]

Importantly, like Duden, these and other historians of reproduction have suggested a perspective on the proliferation of images of pregnancy and childbirth that goes further back in time than the emblematic 1960s photojournalism, the routinization of obstetric ultrasound imagery, and prenatal diagnosis. In addition, engagement with previously unexplored materials and contexts has uncovered a greater historical variety.[47] Although Sara Dubow's *Ourselves Unborn: A History of the Fetus in Modern America* was still restricted to a US context and relied heavily on an analysis on legal cases, she historicized the public fetus from the late nineteenth century through

---

45   Karen Newman, *Fetal Positions: Individualism, Science, Visuality* (Stanford, CA: Stanford University Press, 1996). For a critical discussion, see Duden, "Fetus on the 'Farther Shore,'" 21; and, more recently, Sebastian Pranghofer, "Changing Views on Generation: Images of the Unborn," in *The Secrets of Generation: Reproduction in the Long Eighteenth Century*, ed. Raymond Stephanson and Darren N. Wagner (Toronto: University of Toronto Press, 2015).

46   Atina Grossmann, *Reforming Sex: The German Movement for Birth Control and Abortion Reform, 1920–1950* (New York: Oxford University Press, 1995); Cornelie Usborne, *Cultures of Abortion in Weimar Germany* (Oxford: Berghahn, 2007).

47   Although not specifically addressing the concept of the public fetus, several recent edited volumes and special issues have argued for the benefits and constructive challenges of long-term perspectives on the history of reproduction. See in particular Nick Hopwood et al., "Introduction: Communicating Reproduction," *Bulletin of the History of Medicine* 89, no. 3 (2015): 379–405; Nick Hopwood, Rebecca Flemming, and Lauren Kassell, "Reproduction in History," in *Reproduction: Antiquity to the Present Day*, ed. Nick Hopwood, Rebecca Flemming, and Lauren Kassell (Cambridge: Cambridge University Press, 2018); Bettina Bock von Wülfingen, Christina Brandt, Susanne Lettow, and Florence Vienne, "Temporalities of Reproduction: Practices and Concepts from the Eighteenth to the Early Twenty-First Century," *History and Philosophy of the Life Sciences* 37, no. 1 (2015): 1–16.

the twenty-first.[48] In her research, Lynn Morgan added a historical perspective on today's politicized fetal imagery by examining how dead embryos and fetuses, collected by early twentieth-century embryologists at the Carnegie Department of Embryology in Baltimore, only later came to represent "icons of life."[49] Furthermore, Nick Hopwood's extensive research has deepened our understanding of the material, intellectual, and cultural work that underpinned and shaped the visual standards of modern embryology. In his book on 150 years of controversies surrounding the German evolutionist Ernst Haeckel's images of vertebrate embryos, he demonstrated an intricate relationship between change and continuity. Contrary to the emphasis on novelty in many histories of the public fetus, these old pictures were never completely forgotten or replaced but continued to live, spark interest, and innovate knowledge in different and unforeseen ways.[50]

Historians of reproduction have come to question the maternal erasure theory by way of revisiting arguments in Duden's work on body history. Rebecca Whiteley used this phrase to describe earlier interpretations of the images of in utero "birth figures" in early modern midwifery books, which took them as evidence of the irrelevance of the maternal body and the importance of fetal personification. Instead, she considered the birth figures as a manifestation of a complex and, to a modern eye, bewildering body culture: "To look at these images is to be confronted with what seem to us to be contradictions—images of medical practice, influenced by anatomy, that are also verdant and analogical, alchemical and humoral, even wondrous." This echoes Duden's call for understanding the specificity of past thinking and imagining of the pregnant interior.[51]

Shannon Withycombe has more broadly critiqued earlier feminist scholarship for simplistically dividing the past two hundred years of viewing pregnancy into two models: first the conception of pregnancy as illness and, second, its replacement by the view of the pregnant body as a container for the fetus (in other words, the maternal erasure theory). While she argued that the illness model was useful in understanding the increasing professionalization and medicalization of pregnancy and childbirth, it failed to capture

---

48   Sara Dubow, *Ourselves Unborn: A History of the Fetus in Modern America* (New York: Oxford University Press, 2011).
49   Morgan, *Icons of Life.*
50   Nick Hopwood, *Haeckel's Embryos: Images, Evolution, and Fraud* (Chicago: University of Chicago Press, 2015).
51   Rebecca Whiteley, "Figuring Pictures and Picturing Figures: Images of the Pregnant Body and the Unborn Child in England, 1540–c.1680," *Social History of Medicine* 32, no. 2 (2019): 241–66. Whiteley draws on Mary Fissell, *Vernacular Bodies: The Politics of Reproduction in Early Modern England* (Oxford: Oxford University Press, 2004).

the fluidity of pregnancy experiences in the nineteenth century. Through the examination of women's descriptions in personal correspondence and diaries, she aimed to reveal a variety of individual interpretations of pregnancy ranging from "a person in the making" to "a more nebulous object or an object that only became a person at birth." This emphasis on the embodied experience of pregnancy drew inspiration from Duden's writing.[52]

Historians' resurgent interest in Duden's work is intriguing. Tellingly, for Whiteley as well as Withycombe, it was *The Woman Beneath the Skin* rather than *Disembodying Women* that they found historically productive.[53] As we recall, both of these books were launched in English in the early 1990s, but it was *Disembodying Women* that became most important for feminist scholars in the United States writing about the negative effects of the new visualization technologies on women's autonomy and the appropriation of fetal images by antiabortion movements. The concept of the public fetus seemed to capture this transformative and urgent moment. However, its close link to abortion politics tended to direct historical investigation toward visual evidence of maternal erasure and fetal personhood. For historians such as Whiteley and Withycombe who were interested in pre–twentieth century periods, it seems as this focus became limiting. *The Woman Beneath the Skin* offered an opportunity to interrogate the history of pregnancy in novel ways. Yet their critical analyses continued to be framed by feminist research employing the concept of the public fetus.

Rethinking the Public Fetus

The concept of the public fetus has traveled far and wide. The journey has engaged multiple scholars, starting with Duden and Petchesky but also many others over time. For some researchers, it has become a sort of miniature theory. However, no strong consensus has materialized on how it should be defined or employed in historical analysis. To initiate and invite further clarification and discussion, four frameworks for understanding the public fetus as a traveling concept can be highlighted.

---

52 Shannon Withycombe, "Unusual Frontal Development: Negotiating the Pregnant Body in Nineteenth-Century America," *Journal of Women's History* 27, no. 4 (2015): 160–83, quotation on 173. See also Shannon Withycombe, *Lost: Miscarriage in Nineteenth-Century America* (New Brunswick, NJ: Rutgers University Press, 2019).

53 This is not to say that Duden's arguments in *The Woman Beneath the Skin* have not been criticized. For a review of the first English edition, see Thomas W. Laqueur, "Bodies of the Past," *Bulletin of the History of Medicine* 67, no. 1 (1993): 155–61.

First, the public fetus has been shown to cross academic boundaries and research fields. As an object of study, it has drawn together scholars from various disciplines, including political science, sociology, anthropology, philosophy, and history. Above all, it has fueled interdisciplinary work, especially in feminist theory and women's and gender studies but also in visual studies. Yet, as this volume demonstrates, more work across borders is needed to bring in fresh perspectives, approaches, and materials.

Second, the collection has highlighted that the concept's mobility across national and linguistic contexts has been fairly limited. More specifically, the journey has been constrained within American and European borders. This is problematic since "public fetus" means different things in different languages but also because geographical and cultural contexts operate in multiple ways: they are objects of investigation when exploring the rise of the public fetus, but at the same time they tend to affect how scholars look at the public fetus as an object of study. For instance, attention will be focused differently depending on variations in political systems, the role of religion, or national histories of power structures based on race, class, gender, sexuality, and ability. To offer more diversity in this respect, this volume covers a wide range of national contexts: Austria, Canada, Denmark, France, Germany, Italy, the Netherlands, Russia, Spain, Sweden, the United Kingdom, and the United States. Still, a large part of the world is missing.

Third, the public fetus concept has traveled over a relatively short period of time, from the late 1980s onward. Nonetheless, it has been loaded with cultural meanings and political importance and continues to be regarded as relevant, which emphasizes the need to examine broader frameworks. Therefore, fourth, this chapter has highlighted the movement of the public fetus concept between academia and other domains of society. Above all, we see how abortion politics in different countries has motivated scholars and activists to come together and sharpen their intellectual tools—for example, by employing the concept of the public fetus and the theoretical and historical discussions that came with it. Also of crucial importance for scholars writing about the public fetus are the reproductive and visual technologies that have been introduced during the past decades and their impact on conceptions of pregnancy, from color photography, ultrasound, and other methods of prenatal diagnosis, to digital imaging techniques and the changing media landscape of the internet and social media.

All in all, these movements between and across various contexts have widened the meaning of the public fetus concept and reshaped its use for academic analysis. The "public" has broadened to include "publics" and "audiences" as well as multiple "public spaces," and the blurring of the boundaries between "public" and "private." Similarly, "visual culture" has come to encompass more than "the media" in the traditional sense of twentieth-century mass media. Both the fetal icon and the pregnant icon have emerged as changing configurations of sociocultural meanings, discourses, practices, and affections. As this volume has further explored, the public fetus is no longer considered to be a product of the late twentieth century but rather connected to a long history that certainly includes the pregnant body.

In conclusion, this meta-analysis demonstrates the continued relevance of the public fetus as a concept, which we hope will stimulate fresh ideas about how to advance the discussion of the visual culture of pregnancy, past and present. This, we find, is essential to challenge the persistent presence of notions such as the "universal" fetus.

Selected Bibliography

The bibliography consists of secondary sources cited in the introduction and chapters. The emphasis is on titles in English.

Adams, Alice E. *Reproducing the Womb: Images of Childbirth in Science, Feminist Theory, and Literature*. Ithaca, NY: Cornell University Press, 1994.

Alberti, Samuel J. M. M. *Morbid Curiosities: Medical Museums in Nineteenth-Century Britain*. Oxford: Oxford University Press, 2011.

Alberti, Samuel J. M. M., and Elizabeth Hallam, ed. *Medical Museums: Past, Present, Future*. London: The Royal College of Surgeons of England, 2013.

Anemone, Anthony. "The Monsters of Peter the Great: The Culture of the St. Petersburg Kunstkamera in the Eighteenth Century." *The Slavic and East European Journal* 44, no. 4 (2000): 583–602.

Anker, Suzanne, and Sarah Franklin. "Specimens as Spectacles: Reframing Fetal Remains." *Social Text* 29, no. 1 (2011): 103–25.

Apple, Rima D. *Mothers and Medicine: A Social History of Infant Feeding, 1890–1950*. Madison: University of Wisconsin Press, 1987.

Armstrong, Elizabeth M. *Conceiving Risk, Bearing Responsibility: Fetal Alcohol Syndrome and the Diagnosis of Moral Disorder*. Baltimore: Johns Hopkins University Press, 2003.

Bal, Mieke. *Travelling Concepts in the Humanities: A Rough Guide*. Toronto: University of Toronto Press, 2002.

Ballestriero, Roberta. "Anatomical Models and Wax Venuses: Art Masterpieces or Scientific Craft Works?" *Journal of Anatomy* 216, no. 2 (2010): 223–34.

Bates, A. W. "'Indecent and Demoralising Representations': Public Anatomy Museums in mid-Victorian England." *Medical History* 52, no. 1 (2008): 1–22.

Battista, Kathy. *Renegotiating the Body: Feminist Art in 1970s London*. London: Bloomsbury, 2012.

Berlant, Lauren. *The Queen of America Goes to Washington City: Essays on Sex and Citizenship*. Durham, NC: Duke University Press, 1997.

Björklund, Elisabet. "The Most Delicate Subject: A History of Sex Education Films in Sweden." PhD diss., Lund University, 2012.

Blackwell, Bonnie. "*Tristram Shandy* and the Theater of the Mechanical Mother." *ELH* 68, no. 1 (2001): 81–133.

Bliss, Lauren. *The Maternal Imagination of Film and Film Theory*, Cham: Palgrave Macmillan, 2021.

Blizzard, Deborah. *Looking Within: A Sociocultural Examination of Fetoscopy*. Cambridge, MA: MIT Press, 2007.

Blumenfeld-Kosinski, Renate. *Not of Woman Born: Representations of Caesarean Birth in Medieval and Renaissance Culture*. Ithaca, NY: Cornell University Press, 1991.

Blyakher, L. Ya. *History of Embryology in Russia from the Middle of the Eighteenth to the Middle of the Nineteenth Century*. Washington DC: Al Ahram Center for Scientific Translations, 1982.

Bobel, Chris. "Disciplining Girls through the Technology Fix: Modernity, Markets, Materials." In *The Managed Body: Developing Girls and Menstrual Health in the Global South*, edited by Chris Bobel, 243–80. Cham: Palgrave Macmillan, 2019.

_____. *New Blood: Third-Wave Feminism and the Politics of Menstruation*. New Brunswick, NJ: Rutgers University Press, 2010.

Bock, Gisela, and Pat Thane. Introduction to *Maternity and Gender Policies: Women and the Rise of the European Welfare State*, edited by Gisela Bock and Pat Thane. London: Routledge, 1991.

Bock von Wülfingen, Bettina, Christina Brandt, Susanne Lettow, and Florence Vienne. "Temporalities of Reproduction: Practices and Concepts from the Eighteenth to the Early Twenty-First Century." *History and Philosophy of the Life Sciences* 37, no. 1 (2015): 1–16.

Boer, Lucas, Anna B. Radziun, and Roelof-Jan Oostra. "Frederik Ruysch (1638–1731): Historical Perspective and Contemporary Analysis of His Teratological Legacy." *American Journal of Medical Genetics Part A* 173, no. 1 (January 2017): 16–41.

Boltanski, Luc. *The Foetal Condition: A Sociology of Engendering and Abortion*. Cambridge: Polity, 2013.

Bondestam, Maja. Introduction to *Exceptional Bodies in Early Modern Culture: Conceptions of Monstrosity Before the Advent of the Normal*, edited by Maja Bondestam, 11–36. Amsterdam: Amsterdam University Press, 2020.

Boucher, Joanne. "Ultrasound: A Window to the Womb? Obstetric Ultrasound and the Abortion Rights Debate." *Journal of Medical Humanities* 25, no. 1 (2004): 7–19.

Brauer, Fae. "Eroticizing Lamarckian Eugenics: The Body Stripped Bare during French Sexual Neoregulation." In *Art, Sex and Eugenics: Corpus Delecti*, edited by Fae Brauer and Anthea Callen, 97–136. Aldershot: Ashgate, 2008.

Brown, Meg. "Flip, Flap, and Crack: The Conservation and Exhibition of 400+ Years of Flap Anatomies." *The Book and Paper Group Annual* 32 (2013): 6–14.

Buklijas, Tatjana, and Nick Hopwood. *Making Visible Embryos* (online exhibition), 2008–10, http://www.hps.cam.ac.uk/visibleembryos/ (last accessed May 6, 2023).

Bullough, Vern L. "The Development of Sexology in the USA in the Early Twentieth Century." In *Sexual Knowledge, Sexual Science: The History of Attitudes to Sexuality*, edited by Roy Porter and Mikuláš Teich. Cambridge: Cambridge University Press, 1994.

Butsch, Richard. "Audiences and Publics, Media and the Public Sphere." In *The Handbook of Media Audiences*, edited by Virginia Nightingale, 149–68. Malden: Wiley-Blackwell, 2011.

_____. *The Citizen Audience: Crowds, Publics, and Individuals*. New York: Routledge, 2008.

Carli, Roberto, and Elisa Mazzella. "Ophelia at the Museum: Venuses and Anatomical Models in the Teaching of Obstetrics between the XVIIth and XVIIIth Centuries." *History of Education and Children's Literature* 3, no. 1 (2008): 61–80.

Carlino, Andrea. *Paper Bodies: A Catalogue of Anatomical Fugitive Sheets 1538–1687*, trans. Noga Arikha. London: Wellcome Institute for the History of Medicine, 1999.

Carlyle, Margaret. "Artisans, Patrons, and Enlightenment: The Circulation of Anatomical Knowledge in Paris, St. Petersburg, and London." In *Bodies Beyond Borders: Moving Anatomies 1750–1950*, edited by Kaat Wils, Raf de Bont, and Sokhieng Au, 23–50. Leuven: Leuven University Press, 2017.

_____. "Phantoms in the Classroom: Midwifery Training in Enlightenment Europe." *KNOW: A Journal on the Formation of Knowledge* 2, no. 1 (2018): 111–36.

Carlyle, Margaret, and Brian Callender. "The Fetus in Utero: From Mystery to Social Media." *KNOW: A Journal on the Formation of Knowledge* 3, no. 1 (2019): 15–67.

Carter, Julian B. *The Heart of Whiteness: Normal Sexuality and Race in America, 1880–1940*. Durham: Duke University Press, 2007.

Casper, Monica J. *The Making of the Unborn Patient: A Social Anatomy of Fetal Surgery*. New Brunswick, NJ: Rutgers University Press, 1998.

Claes, Tinne, and Veronique Deblon. "When Nothing Remains: Anatomical Collections, the Ethics of Stewardship and the Meanings of Absence." *Journal of the History of Collections* 30, no. 2 (2018): 351–62.

Clark, Owen E. "The Contributions of J. F. Meckel, the Younger, to the Science of Teratology." *Journal of the History of Medicine and Allied Sciences* 24, no. 3 (1969): 310–22.

Cole, Catherine. "Sex and Death on Display: Women, Reproduction, and Fetuses at Chicago's Museum of Science and Industry." *Drama Review* 37, no. 1 (1993): 43–60.

Condit, Celeste Michelle. *Decoding Abortion Rhetoric: Communicating Social Change*. Urbana: University of Illinois Press, 1990.

Cooper Owens, Deirdre. *Medical Bondage: Race, Gender, and the Origins of American Gynecology*. Athens: University of Georgia Press, 2017.

Creadick, Anna G. *Perfectly Average: The Pursuit of Normality in Postwar America*. Boston: University of Massachusetts Press, 2010.

Dacome, Lucia. *Malleable Anatomies: Models, Makers, and Material Culture in Eighteenth-Century Italy*. Oxford: Oxford University Press, 2017.

_____. "Women, Wax and Anatomy in the 'Century of Things.'" *Renaissance Studies* 21, no. 4 (September 2007): 522–50.

Daniels, Cynthia R. *At Women's Expense. State Power and the Politics of Fetal Rights*. Cambridge, MA: Harvard University Press, 1993.

Dasgupta, Sayantani, and Shamita Das Dasgupta. "The Public Fetus and the Veiled Woman: Transnational Surrogacy Blogs as Surveillant Assemblage." In *Feminist Surveillance Studies*, edited by Rachel E. Dubrofsky and Shoshana Amielle Magnet, 150–68. Durham, NC: Duke University Press, 2015.

Daston, Lorraine, and Katharine Park. *Wonders and the Order of Nature, 1150–1750*. New York: Zone Books, 1998.

de Ceglia, Francesco Paolo. "The Importance of Being Florentine: A Journey around the World for Wax Anatomical Venuses." *Nuncius* 26, no. 1 (2011): 83–108.

De Rooy, Laurens. "A Cabinet Departs." In *Forces of Form*, ed. Simon Knepper, Johan Kortenray, and Antoon Moorman, 59–69. Amsterdam: Amsterdam University Press, 2009.

Dijck, José van. "Bodyworlds: The Art of Plastinated Cadavers." *Configurations* 9 (Winter 2001): 99–126.

_____. *The Transparent Body: A Cultural Analysis of Medical Imaging*. Seattle and London: University of Washington Press, 2005.

Dittmar, Jenna M., and Piers D. Mitchell. "From Cradle to Grave via the Dissection Room: The Role of Fetal and Infant Bodies in Anatomical Education from the Late 1700s to Early 1900s." *Journal of Anatomy* 229, no. 6 (2016): 713–722.

Doss, Erika, ed. *Looking at* Life *Magazine*. Washington, DC: Smithsonian Institution Press, 2001.

Doyle, Nora. *Maternal Bodies: Redefining Motherhood in Early America*. Chapel Hill: University of North Carolina Press, 2018.

Dubow, Sara. *Ourselves Unborn: A History of the Fetus in Modern America*. Oxford: Oxford University Press, 2011.

Duden, Barbara. "Anatomie der guten Hoffnung. Darstellungen des Unge-borenen bis 1799." Habilitationsschrift, Universität Hannover, 1993.

_____. *Disembodying Women: Perspectives on Pregnancy and the Unborn*, trans. Lee Hoinacki. Cambridge, MA: Harvard University Press, 1993.

_____. "The Fetus as an Object of Our Time." *RES: Anthropology and Aesthetics* 25 (1994): 132–35.

_____. "The Fetus on the 'Farther Shore': Toward a History of the Unborn." In *Fetal Subjects, Feminist Positions*, edited by Lynn M. Morgan and Meredith W. Michaels, 13–25. Philadelphia: University of Pennsylvania Press, 1999.

_____. "A Historian's 'Biology': On the Traces of the Body in a Technogenic World." *Historein* 3 (2001): 89–102.

_____. "Quick with Child: An Experience That Has Lost Its Status." *Technology in Society* 14, no. 3 (1992): 335–44.

_____. "Visualizing 'Life.'" *Science as Culture* 3, no. 4 (1993): 562–600.

_____. *The Woman Beneath the Skin: A Doctor's Patients in Eighteenth-Century Germany*, trans. Thomas Dunlap. Cambridge, MA: Harvard University Press, 1991.

Duden, Barbara, Jürgen Schlumbohm, and Patrice Veit, ed. *Geschichte des Ungeborenen: Zur Erfahrungs- und Wissenschaftsgeschichte der Schwangerschaft, 17.–20. Jahrhundert*. Göttingen: Vandenhoeck & Ruprecht, 2002.

Dwork, Deborah. *War Is Good for Babies and Other Young Children: A History of the Infant and Child Welfare Movement in England 1898–1950*. London: Tavistock, 1987.

Ebenstein, Joanna. *The Anatomical Venus: Wax, God, Death & the Ecstatic*. New York: Distributed Art Publishers, 2016.

_____. "Ode to an Anatomical Venus." *Women's Studies Quarterly* 40 (2012): 346–52.

Eberwein, Robert. *Sex Ed: Film, Video, and the Framework of Desire*. New Brunswick, NJ: Rutgers University Press, 1999.

Eisenberg, Ziv. "The Whole Nine Months: Women, Men, and the Making of Modern Pregnancy in America." PhD diss.: Yale University, 2013.

Epstein, Charlotte. *Birth of the State: The Place of the Body in Creating Modern Politics*. Oxford: Oxford University Press, 2020.

Ettinger, Laura E. *Nurse-Midwifery: The Birth of a New American Profession*. Columbus: Ohio State University Press, 2006.

Fahs, Breanne. *Out for Blood: Essays on Menstruation and Resistance*. Albany: State University of New York, 2016.

Firth, Georgina. "Re-negotiating Reproductive Technologies: The 'Public Foetus' Revisited." *Feminist Review* 92 (2009): 54–71.

Fissell, Mary. *Vernacular Bodies: The Politics of Reproduction in Early Modern England*. Oxford: Oxford University Press, 2004.

Frangos, Mike Classon. "Liv Strömquist's *Fruit of Knowledge* and the Gender of Comics." *European Comic Art* 13, no. 1 (2020): 45–69.

Franklin, Sarah. "Fetal Fascinations: New Dimensions to the Medical-Scientific Construction of Fetal Personhood." In *Off-Centre: Feminism and Cultural Studies*, edited by Sarah Franklin, Celia Lury, and Jackie Stacey, 190–205. London: HarperCollins Academic, 1991.

Freidenfelds, Lara. *The Modern Period: Menstruation in Twentieth-Century America*. Baltimore: John Hopkins University Press, 2009.

——. *The Myth of the Perfect Pregnancy: A History of Miscarriage in America*. Oxford: Oxford University Press, 2020.

Gaissinovitch, A. E. "C. F. Wolff on Variability and Heredity." *History and Philosophy of the Life Sciences* 12, no. 2 (1990): 179–201.

Gammeltoft, Tine. *Haunting Images: A Cultural Account of Selective Reproduction in Vietnam*. Berkeley: University of California Press, 2014.

Garb, Tamar. *Bodies of Modernity: Figure and Flesh in Fin-de-Siècle France*. London: Thames and Hudson, 1998.

Gerber, Elaine Gale. "Deconstructing Pregnancy: RU486, Seeing 'Eggs,' and the Ambiguity of Very Early Conceptions." *Medical Anthropology Quarterly* 16, no. 1 (2002): 92–108.

Ghanoui, Saniya Lee. "Translating Sex Culture: Transnational Sex Education and the U.S.–Swedish Relationship, 1910s–1960s." PhD diss., University of Illinois, Urbana-Champaign, 2021.

Gilbert, Scott F., and Rebecca Howes-Mischel. "'Show Me Your Original Face Before You Were Born': The Convergence of Public Fetuses and Sacred DNA." *History and Philosophy of the Life Sciences* 26, no. 3–4 (2004): 377–94, 477–79.

Ginsburg, Faye D. *Contested Lives: The Abortion Debate in an American Community*, updated ed. Berkeley: University of California Press, 1998.

Golden, Janet. *Message in a Bottle: The Making of Fetal Alcohol Syndrome*. Cambridge, MA: Harvard University Press, 2005.

Gorney, Cynthia. *Articles of Faith: A Frontline History of the Abortion Wars*. New York: Simon & Schuster, 1998.

Grob, B. W. J. "The Anatomical Models of Dr. Louis Auzoux: A Descriptive Catalogue." *Museum Boerhaave Communication* 305, no. (2004): 109–49.

Grossmann, Atina. *Reforming Sex: The German Movement for Birth Control and Abortion Reform, 1920–1950*. New York: Oxford University Press, 1995.

Guerrini, Anita. "Anatomists and Entrepreneurs in Early Eighteenth-Century London." *Journal of the History of Medicine and Allied Sciences* 59, no. 2 (2004): 219–39.

_____. "The Creativity of God and the Order of Nature: Anatomizing Monsters in the Early Eighteenth Century." In *Monsters & Philosophy*, edited by Charles T. Wolfe, 153–68. London: College Publications, 2005.

Habel, Ylva. *Modern Media, Modern Audiences: Mass Media and Social Engineering in the 1930s Swedish Welfare State.* Stockholm: Aura förlag, 2002.

Hagner, Michael. "Enlightened Monsters." In *The Sciences in Enlightened Europe*, edited by William Clark, Jan Golinski, and Simon Schaffer, 175–217. Chicago: University of Chicago Press, 1999.

Hallam, Elizabeth. *Anatomy Museum: Death and the Body Displayed.* London: Reaktion, 2016.

Hanson, Clare. *A Cultural History of Pregnancy: Pregnancy, Medicine and Culture, 1750–2000.* Basingstoke, UK: Palgrave Macmillan, 2004.

Haraway, Donna. *Modest_Witness@Second_Millennium.FemaleMan©_Meets_OncoMouse: Feminism and Technoscience.* New York: Routledge, 1997.

_____. "Teddy Bear Patriarchy." In *Primate Visions.* New York: Routledge, 1989.

Harrington, Erin. *Women, Monstrosity and Horror Film: Gynaehorror.* Abingdon, UK: Routledge, 2018.

Hartouni, Valerie. "Fetal Exposures: Abortion Politics and the Optics of Allusion." *Camera Obscura* 10, no. 29 (1992): 130–49.

Harvey, Elizabeth D. "'The 'Sense of All Senses.'" In *Sensible Flesh: On Touch in Early Modern Culture*, edited by Elizabeth D. Harvery. Philadelphia: University of Pennsylvania Press, 2003.

Hausman, Bernice L. "Public Fetuses." In *Health Humanities Reader*, edited by Therese Jones, Delese Wear, and Lester D. Friedman, 186–95. New Brunswick, NJ: Rutgers University Press, 2014.

Hendriksen, Marieke M. A. *Elegant Anatomy: The Eighteenth-Century Leiden Anatomical Collections.* Leiden: Brill, 2015.

Henig, Robin Marantz. *Pandora's Baby: How the First Test Tube Babies Sparked the Reproductive Revolution.* Boston: Houghton Mifflin, 2004.

Herzog, Dagmar. *Unlearning Eugenics: Sexuality, Reproduction, and Disability in Post-Nazi Europe.* Madison: University of Wisconsin Press, 2018.

Hobgood, Allison P., and David Houston Wood, ed. *Recovering Disability in Early Modern England.* Columbus: Ohio State University, 2013.

Holland, Jennifer. *Tiny You: A Western History of the Anti-Abortion Movement.* Berkeley: University of California Press, 2020.

Holz, Rose. "'Art in the Service of Medical Education:' The 1939 Dickinson-Belskie Birth Series and the Use of Sculpture to Teach the Process of Human Development from Fertilization Through Delivery." In *Visualizing the Body in Art, Anatomy and Medicine Since 1800: Models and Modeling*, edited by Andrew Graciano, 129–56. New York: Routledge, 2019.

_____. "The 1939 Dickinson-Belskie Birth Series Sculptures: The Rise of Modern Visions of Pregnancy, the Roots of Modern Pro-Life Imagery, and Dr. Dickinson's Religious Case for Abortion." *Journal of Social History* 51, no. 4 (2018): 980–1022.

Hooper-Greenhill, Eilean. *Museums and the Shaping of Knowledge*. London: Routledge, 1992.

Hopwood, Nick. *Embryos in Wax: Models from the Ziegler Studio*. Cambridge: Whipple Museum of the History of Science, 2002.

_____. *Haeckel's Embryos: Images, Evolution, and Fraud*. Chicago: University of Chicago Press, 2015.

_____. "A Marble Embryo: Meanings of a Portrait from 1900." *History Workshop Journal* 73 (Spring 2012): 5–36.

_____. "Producing Development: The Anatomy of Human Embryos and the Norms of Wilhelm His." *Bulletin of the History of Medicine* 74, no. 1 (2000): 29–79.

Hopwood, Nick, Peter Murray Jones, Lauren Kassell, and Jim Secord. "Introduction: Communicating Reproduction." *Bulletin of the History of Medicine* 89, no. 3 (2015): 379–405.

Hopwood, Nick, Rebecca Flemming, and Lauren Kassell, ed. *Reproduction: Antiquity to the Present Day*. Cambridge: Cambridge University Press, 2018.

Hopwood, Nick, Simon Schaffer, and Jim Secord. "Seriality and Scientific Objects in the Nineteenth Century." *History of Science* 48, no. 3–4 (September 2010): 251–85.

Huet, Marie-Hélène. *Monstrous Imagination*. Cambridge, MA: Harvard University Press, 1993.

Hughes, Lindsey. *Russia in the Age of Peter the Great*. New Haven, CT: Yale University Press, 1998.

Hughes, Richard L. "Burning Birth Certificates and Atomic Tupperware Parties: Creating the Antiabortion Movement in the Shadow of the Vietnam War." *The Historian* 68, no. 3 (2006): 541–58.

Huisman, Tim. "Resilient Collections: The Long Life of Leiden's Earliest Anatomical Collections." In *The Fate of Anatomical Collections*, edited by Rina Knoeff and Robert Zwijnenberg, 73–92. Burlington, VT: Ashgate, 2015.

Huistra, Hieke. *The Afterlife of the Leiden Anatomical Collections: Hands On, Hands Off*. New York: Routledge 2019.

Hull, Isabel V. "The Body as Historical Experience: Review of Recent Works by Barbara Duden." *Central European History* 28, no. 1 (1995): 73–79.

Hurst, Rachel Alpha Johnston, ed. *Representing Abortion*. London: Routledge, 2020.

Jordanova, Ludmilla. *Sexual Visions: Images of Gender in Science and Medicine between the Eighteenth and Twentieth Centuries.* Madison: University of Wisconsin Press, 1989.

Joyce, Kelly A. *Magnetic Appeal: MRI and the Myth of Transparency.* Ithaca, NY and London: Cornell University Press, 2008.

Jülich, Solveig. "Fetal Photography in the Age of Cool Media." In *History of Participatory Media: Politics and Publics, 1750–2000,* edited by Anders Ekström, Solveig Jülich, Frans Lundgren, and Per Wisselgren, 125–141. London: Routledge, 2011.

———. "Lennart Nilsson's *A Child Is Born*: The Many Lives of a Pregnancy Advice Book." *Culture Unbound* 7, no. 4 (2015): 627–48.

———. "Lennart Nilsson's Fish-Eyes: A Photographic and Cultural History of Views from Below." *Konsthistorisk tidskrift/Journal of Art History* 84, no. 2 (2015): 75–92.

———. "The Making of a Best-Selling Book on Reproduction: Lennart Nilsson's *A Child Is Born*." *Bulletin of the History of Medicine* 89, no. 3 (2015): 491–525.

———. "Picturing Abortion Opposition: Lennart Nilsson's Early Photographs of Embryos and Fetuses." *Social History of Medicine* 31, no. 2 (2018): 278–307.

———. "Televising Inner Space: Lennart Nilsson's Early Medical Documentaries on the Interior of the Human Body." In *Representational Machines: Photography and the Production of Space,* edited by Anna Dahlgren, Dag Petersson, and Nina Lager Vestberg, 149–69. Aarhus: Aarhus Universitetsforlag, 2013.

Jülich, Solveig, ed. *Medicine at the Borders of Life: Fetal Knowledge Production and the Emergence of Public Controversy in Sweden.* Leiden: Brill, 2024.

Kaplan, E. Ann. "Look Who's Talking, Indeed: Fetal Images in Recent North American Visual Culture." In *Mothering: Ideology, Experience, and Agency,* edited by Evelyn Nakano Glenn, Grace Chand, and Linda Rennie Forcey. 121–38. New York: Routledge, 1994.

Kaufman, Sharon R., and Lynn M. Morgan. "The Anthropology of the Beginnings and Ends of Life." *Annual Review of Anthropology* 34, no. 1 (2005): 317–41.

Keller, Eve. *Generating Bodies and Gendered Selves: The Rhetoric of Reproduction in Early Modern England.* Seattle: University of Washington Press, 2007.

———. "The Subject of Touch: Medical Authority in Early Modern Midwifery." In *Sensible Flesh: On Touch in Early Modern Culture,* edited by Elizabeth D. Harvey, 62–80. Philadelphia: University of Pennsylvania Press, 2003.

Kertzer, David I. *Sacrificed for Honor: Italian Infant Abandonment and the Politics of Reproductive Control.* Boston: Beacon Press, 1995.

Kinkel, Marianne. *Races of Mankind: The Sculptures of Malvina Hoffman.* Urbana: University of Illinois Press, 2011.

Kirby, David A. "Regulating Cinematic Stories about Reproduction: Pregnancy, Childbirth, Abortion and Movie Censorship in the US, 1930–1958." *The British Journal for the History of Science* 50, no. 3 (September 2017): 451–72.

Knoeff, Rina. "Touching Anatomy: On the Handling of Preparations in the Anatomical Cabinets of Frederik Ruysch (1638–1731)." *Studies in History and Philosophy of Science Part C: Studies in History and Philosophy of Biological and Biomedical Sciences* 49 (February 2015): 32–44.

Knoeff, Rina, and Robert Zwijnenberg, ed. *The Fate of Anatomical Collections: The History of Medicine in Context.* Farnham, Surrey; Burlington, VT: Ashgate, 2015.

Kooijmans, Luuc. *Death Defied: The Anatomy Lessons of Frederik Ruysch.* Leiden: Brill, 2011.

Kosmin, Jennifer. *Authority, Gender, and Midwifery in Early Modern Italy: Contested Deliveries.* Abingdon: Routledge, 2021.

———. "Modelling Authority: Obstetrical Machines in the Instruction of Midwives and Surgeons in Eighteenth-Century Italy." *Social History of Medicine* 34, no. 2 (2021): 509–531.

Kuhn, Annette. *Cinema, Censorship and Sexuality, 1909–1925.* London: Routledge, 1988.

Laqueur, Thomas W. "Bodies of the Past." *Bulletin of the History of Medicine* 67, no. 1 (1993): 155–161.

Laukötter, Anja. "Listen and Watch: The Practice of Lecturing and the Epistemological Status of Sex Education Films in Germany." *Gesnerus* 72, no. 1 (2015): 56–76.

Lawrence, Susan C. "Educating the Senses: Students, Teachers and Medical Rhetoric in Eighteenth-Century London." In *Medicine and the Five Senses,* edited by W. F. Bynum and Roy Porter, 154–178. Cambridge: Cambridge University Press, 1993.

Layne, Linda L. *Motherhood Lost: A Feminist Account of Pregnancy Loss in America.* New York: Routledge, 2003.

Leavitt, Judith. *Brought to Bed: Childbearing in America 1750 to 1950.* New York: Oxford University Press, 1986.

Lennerhed, Lena. "Taking the Middle Way: Sex Education Debates in Sweden in the Early Twentieth Century." In *Shaping Sexual Knowledge: A Cultural History of Sex Education in Twentieth Century Europe,* edited by Lutz D. H. Sauerteig and Roger Davidson, 55–70. London: Routledge, 2009.

Lieske, Pam. "'Made in Imitation of Real Women and Children': Obstetrical Machines in Eighteenth-Century Britain." In *The Female Body in Medicine and Literature*, edited by Andrew Mangham and Greta Depledge, 69–88. Liverpool: Liverpool University Press, 2011.

Livingstone, Sonia. "On the Relation between Audiences and Publics." In *Audiences and Publics: When Cultural Engagement Matters for the Public Sphere*, edited by Sonia Livingstone. Bristol: Intellect, 2005.

Longhurst, Robyn "YouTube: A New Space for Birth?" *Feminist Review* 93 (2009): 46–63.

Lukina, T. A. "Caspar Friedrich Wolff und die Petersburger Akademie der Wissenschaften." *Acta Historia Leopoldina* 9 (1975): 411–25.

Lupton, Deborah. *The Social Worlds of the Unborn*. Basingstoke: Palgrave Macmillan, 2013.

Lurie, Samuel, and Marek Glezerman. "The History of Cesarean Technique." *American Journal of Obstetrics and Gynecology* 189, no. 6 (2003): 1803–6.

Lynch, John. *What Are Stem Cells? Definitions at the Intersection of Science and Politics*. Tuscaloosa: University of Alabama Press, 2011.

Löwy, Ilana. *Imperfect Pregnancies: A History of Birth Defects and Prenatal Diagnosis*. Baltimore: Johns Hopkins University Press, 2017.

Maerker, Anna. "Anatomizing the Trade: Designing and Marketing Anatomical Models as Medical Technologies, ca. 1700–1900." *Technology and Culture* 54, no. 3 (2013): 531–62.

_____. *Model Experts: Wax Anatomies and Enlightenment in Florence and Vienna, 1775–1815*. Manchester: Manchester University Press, 2011.

_____. "Papier-Mâché Anatomical Models: The Making of Reform and Empire in Nineteenth-Century France and Beyond." In *Working with Paper: Gendered Practices in the History of Knowledge*, edited by Carla Bittel, Elaine Leong, and Christine von Oertzen, 177–92. Pittsburgh: University of Pittsburgh Press, 2019.

_____. "'Turpentine Hides Everything': Autonomy and Organization in Anatomical Model Production for the State in Late Eighteenth-Century Florence." *History of Science* 45, no. 3 (2007): 257–86.

Margócsy, Dániel. "A Museum of Wonders or a Cemetery of Corpses? The Commercial Exchange of Anatomical Collections in Early Modern Netherlands." In *Silent Messengers: The Circulation of Material Objects of Knowledge in the Early Modern Low Countries*, edited by Sven Dupré and Christoph Lüthy, 185–216. Berlin: Lit Verlag, 2011.

Marland, Hilary. "The '*Burgerlijke*' Midwife: The *Stadsvroedvrouw* of Eighteenth-Century Holland." In *The Art of Midwifery: Early Modern Midwives in Europe*, edited by Hilary Marland, 192–213. New York: Routledge, 1993.

Martin, Emily. "The Egg and the Sperm: How Science Has Constructed a Romance Based on Stereotypical Male-Female Roles." *Signs: Journal of Women in Culture and Society* 16, no. 3 (1991): 485–501.

Mason, Carol. *Killing for Life: The Apocalyptic Narrative of Pro-Life Politics.* Ithaca, NY: Cornell University Press, 2002.

Massey, Lyle. "On Waxes and Wombs: Eighteenth-Century Representations of the Gravid Uterus." In *Ephemeral Bodies: Wax Sculpture and the Human Figure,* edited by Roberta Panzanelli, 83–107. Los Angeles: Getty Research Institute, 2008.

_____. "Pregnancy and Pathology: Picturing Childbirth in Eighteenth-Century Obstetric Atlases." *The Art Bulletin* 87, no. 1 (2005): 73–91.

Matthews, Sandra, and Laura Wexler. *Pregnant Pictures.* New York: Routledge, 2000.

McGregor, Deborah Kuhn. *From Midwives to Medicine. The Birth of American Gynecology.* New Brunswick, NJ: Rutgers University Press, 1998.

McLeary, Erin, and Elizabeth Toon. "'Here Man Learns About Himself:' Visual Education and the Rise and Fall of the American Museum of Health." *American Journal of Public Health* 102 (July 2012): e27–e36.

McTavish, Lianne. *Childbirth and the Display of Authority in Early Modern France.* Aldershot: Ashgate, 2005.

Medina-Doménech, Rosa M., "'Who Were the Experts?' The Science of Love vs. Women's Knowledge of Love during the Spanish Dictatorship." *Science as Culture* 23, no. 2 (2014): 177–200.

Medina-Doménech, Rosa M. and Alfredo Menéndez-Navarro. "Cinematic Representations of Medical Technologies in the Spanish Official Newsreel, 1943–1970." *Public Understanding of Science* 14, no. 4 (2005): 393–408.

Messbarger, Rebecca. *The Lady Anatomist: The Life and Work of Anna Morandi Manzolini.* Chicago and London: University of Chicago Press, 2010.

_____. "The Re-Birth of Venus in Florence's Royal Museum of Physics and Natural History." *Journal of the History of Collections* 25, no. 2 (2013): 195–215.

Michaels, Meredith W. "Fetal Galaxies: Some Questions about What We See." In *Fetal Subjects, Feminist Positions,* edited by Lynn M. Morgan and Meredith W. Michaels, 113–32. Philadelphia: University of Pennsylvania Press, 1999.

Mirilas, Petros. "The Monarch and the Master: Peter the Great and Frederik Ruysch." *Archives of Surgery* 141, no. 6 (June 1, 2006): 602–606.

Mitchell, Lisa M. *Baby's First Picture: Ultrasound and the Politics of Fetal Subjects.* Toronto: University of Toronto Press, 2001.

Monti, Maria Teresa. "Epigenesis of the Monstrous Form and Preformistic 'Genetics' (Lémery-Winslow-Haller)." *Early Science and Medicine* 5, no. 1 (2000): 3–32.

Morcillo, Aurora G. *The Seduction of Modern Spain: The Female Body and the Francoist Body Politics.* Lewisburg, PA: Bucknell University Press, 2010.

Morgan, Lynn M. "Fetal Relationality in Feminist Philosophy: An Anthropological Critique." *Hypatia* 11, no. 3 (1996): 47–70.

_____. *Icons of Life: A Cultural History of Human Embryos.* Berkeley: University of California Press, 2009.

_____. "A Social Biography of Carnegie Embryo no. 836." *Anatomical Record Part B: The New Anatomist* 276, no. 1 (2004): 3–7.

Morgan, Lynn M., and Meredith W. Michaels, ed. *Fetal Subjects, Feminist Positions.* Philadelphia: University of Pennsylvania Press, 1999.

Moscucci, Ornella. *The Science of Woman: Gynæcology and Gender in England, 1800–1929.* Cambridge: Cambridge University Press, 1990.

Muigai, Wangui. "'Something Wasn't Clean': Black Midwifery, Birth, and Postwar Medical Education in *All My Babies.*" *Bulletin of the History of Medicine* 93, no. 1 (2019): 82–113.

Needham, Joseph. *A History of Embryology.* New York: Arno Press, 1975.

Neumann, Birgit, and Ansgar Nünning. "Travelling Concepts as a Model for the Study of Culture." In *Travelling Concepts for the Study of Culture*, edited by Birgit Neumann and Ansgar Nünning. 1–22. Berlin: Walter de Gruyter, 2012.

Neustadter, Roger. "'Killing Babies': The Use of Image and Metaphor in the Right-to-Life Movement." *Michigan Sociological Review*, no. 4 (1990): 76–83.

Newman, Karen. *Fetal Positions: Individualism, Science, Visuality.* Stanford, CA: Stanford University Press, 1996.

Nicolson, Malcolm, and John E. E. Fleming. *Imaging and Imagining the Fetus: The Development of Obstetric Ultrasound.* Baltimore: Johns Hopkins University Press, 2013.

Nye, Robert A. *Crime, Madness and Politics in Modern France: The Medical Concept of National Decline.* Princeton, NJ: Princeton University Press, 1984.

Oakley, Ann. *The Captured Womb: A History of the Medical Care of Pregnant Women.* Oxford: Blackwell, 1984.

Oaks, Laury. "Smoke-Filled Wombs and Fragile Fetuses: The Social Politics of Fetal Representation." *Signs* 26, no. 1 (2000): 63–108.

O'Donovan, Orla. "Wax Moulages and the Pastpresence Work of the Dead." *Science, Technology & Human Values* 46, no. 2 (2020): 231–53.

Oliver, Kelly. *Knock Me Up, Knock Me Down: Images of Pregnancy in Hollywood Films.* New York: Columbia University Press, 2012.

Olszynko-Gryn, Jesse, and Patrick Ellis. "'A Machine for Recreating Life': An Introduction to Reproduction on Film." *The British Journal for the History of Science* 50, no. 3 (September 2017): 383–409.

Ortiz-Gómez, Teresa, and Agata Ignaciuk. "The Fight for Family Planning in Spain during Late Francoism and the Transition to Democracy, 1965–1979." *Journal of Women's History* 30, no. 2 (2018): 38–62.

O'Sullivan, Lisa, and Ross L. Jones. "Two Australian Foetuses: Frederic Wood Jones and the Work of an Anatomical Specimen." *Bulletin of the History of Medicine* 89, no. 2 (Summer 2015): 243–266.

Packham, Catherine. *Eighteenth-Century Vitalism: Bodies, Culture, Politics.* New York: Palgrave Macmillan, 2012.

Panzanelli, Roberta, ed. *Ephemeral Bodies. Wax Sculpture and the Human Figure.* Los Angeles: Getty Research Institute, 2008.

Park, Katharine. *Secrets of Women: Gender, Generation, and the Origins of Human Dissection.* New York: Zone Books, 2006.

Park, Katharine, and Lorraine J. Daston. "Unnatural Conceptions: The Study of Monsters in Sixteenth- and Seventeenth-Century France and England." *Past & Present* 92, no. 1 (1981): 20–54.

Parry, Manon S. *Broadcasting Birth Control: Mass Media and Family Planning.* New Brunswick, NJ: Rutgers University Press, 2013.

_____. "The Valuable Role of Risky Histories: Exhibiting Disability, Race, and Reproduction in Medical Museums," *Science Museum Group Journal* no. 14 (2021), https://journal.sciencemuseum.ac.uk/article/risky-histories/.

Petchesky, Rosalind Pollack. *Abortion and Woman's Choice: The State, Sexuality, and Reproductive Freedom.* Boston: Northeastern University Press, 1984.

_____. "Fetal Images: The Power of Visual Culture in the Politics of Reproduction." *Feminist Studies* 13, no. 2 (1987): 263–92.

Petchesky, Rosalind Pollack, and Karen Judd. *Negotiating Reproductive Rights: Women's Perspectives across Countries and Cultures.* London: Zed, 1998.

Pick, Daniel. *Faces of Degeneration: A European Disorder, c. 1848–c. 1918.* Cambridge: Cambridge University Press, 1989.

Quint, Chella. "From Embodied Shame to Reclaiming the Stain: Reflections on a Career in Menstrual Activism." *Sociological Review* 67, no. 4 (2019): 927–42.

Ramsey, Morag. *The Swedish Abortion Pill: Co-producing Medical Abortion and Values, ca. 1965–1992.* Uppsala: Acta Universitatis Upsaliensis, 2021.

Rapp, Rayna. *Testing Women, Testing the Fetus: The Social Impact of Amniocentesis in America.* New York: Routledge, 1999.

Reagan, Leslie J. *When Abortion Was a Crime: Women, Medicine, and Law in the United States, 1867–1973.* 1997; Oakland, CA: University of California Press, 2022.

Reed, James. *From Private Vice to Public Virtue: The Birth Control Movement in American Society Since 1830.* New York: Basic Books, 1978.

Reill, Peter Hanns. *Vitalizing Nature in the Enlightenment.* Berkeley: University of California Press, 2005.

Rich, Adrienne. *Of Woman Born: Motherhood as Experience and Institution.* New York: Norton, 1976.

Richardson, Ruth. *Death, Dissection, and the Destitute.* Chicago: University of Chicago Press, 2001.

Roe, Shirley A. *Matter, Life, and Generation: Eighteenth-Century Embryology and the Haller-Wolff Debate.* Cambridge: Cambridge University Press, 1981.

Røstvik, Camilla Mørk. "Blood in the Shower: A Visual History of Menstruation and Clean Bodies," *Visual Culture and Gender* 13 (2018): 54–63.

———. "Blood Works: Judy Chicago and Menstrual Art since 1970." *Oxford Art Journal* 42, no. 3 (2019): 335–53.

———. *Cash Flow: The Businesses of Menstruation.* London: UCL Press, 2022.

Roth, Rachel. *Making Women Pay: The Hidden Costs of Fetal Rights.* Ithaca, NY: Cornell University Press, 2000.

Rothman, Barbara Katz. *The Tentative Pregnancy: Prenatal Diagnosis and the Future of Motherhood.* New York: Viking, 1986.

Sahlins, Marshall. "What Kinship Is (Part One)." *Journal of the Royal Anthropological Institute* 17, no. 1 (2011): 2–19.

Sandell, Richard, Jocelyn Dodd, and Rosemarie Garland-Thomson, ed. *Re-Presenting Disability: Activism and Agency in the Museum.* London: Routledge, 2010.

Sanger, Carol. *About Abortion: Terminating Pregnancy in Twenty-First-Century America.* Cambridge, MA: Belknap Press of Harvard University Press, 2017.

Santesmases, María Jesús. "Circulating Biomedical Images: Bodies and Chromosomes in the Post-eugenic Era." *History of Science* 55, no. 4 (2017): 395–430.

———. "Women in Early Human Cytogenetics: An Essay on a Gendered History of Chromosome Imaging." *Perspectives on Science* 28, no. 2 (2020): 170–200.

Santos, Gonçalo, and Suzanne Z. Gottschang. "Rethinking Reproductive Technologies and Modernities in Time and Space." *Technology and Culture* 61, no. 2 (2020): 549–558.

Sappol, Michael. *Dream Anatomy.* Bethesda, MD: National Institutes of Health, 2006.

_____. *A Traffic of Dead Bodies: Anatomy and Embodied Social Identity in Ninteenth-Century America*. Princeton, NJ: Princeton University Press, 2002.

Schaefer, Eric. *"Bold! Daring! Shocking! True!" A History of Exploitation Films, 1919–1959*. Durham, NC: Duke University Press, 1999.

Schnalke, Thomas. *Diseases in Wax: History of the Medical Moulage*, trans. Kathy Spatschek. Carol Stream, IL: Quintessence Publishing.

Schoen, Johanna. *Abortion after* Roe. Chapel Hill: University of North Carolina Press, 2015.

Shrage, Laurie. "From Reproductive Rights to Reproductive Barbie: Post-Porn Modernism and Abortion." *Feminist Studies* 28, no. 1 (2002): 61–93.

Smith, Marquard, ed. *Visual Culture Studies: Interviews with Key Thinkers*. Los Angeles: SAGE, 2008.

Smith, Mark M. *Sensing the Past: Seeing, Hearing, Smelling, Tasting, and Touching in History*. Berkeley and Los Angeles: University of California Press, 2007.

Sofia, Zoë. "Exterminating Fetuses: Abortion, Disarmament, and the Sexo-Semiotics of Extraterrestrialism." *Diacritics* 14, no. 2 (1984): 47–59.

Stabile, Carol A. "Shooting the Mother: Fetal Photography and the Politics of Disappearance." *Camera Obscura* 10, no. 28 (1992): 179 205.

Staggenborg, Suzanne. *The Pro-Choice Movement: Organization and Activism in the Abortion Conflict*. New York: Oxford University Press, 1991.

Stanworth, Michelle, ed. *Reproductive Technologies: Gender, Motherhood and Medicine*. Cambridge: Polity Press, 1987.

Stephanson, Raymond, and Darren N. Wagner, ed. *The Secrets of Generation: Reproduction in the Long Eighteenth Century*. Toronto: University of Toronto Press, 2015.

Stephens, Elizabeth. "Venus in the Archive: Anatomical Waxworks of the Pregnant Body." *Australian Feminist Studies* 25, no. 64 (2010): 133–45.

Stormer, Nathan. "Embodying Normal Miracles." *Quarterly Journal of Speech* 83, no. 2 (1997): 172–91.

Strange, Julie-Marie. "The Assault on Ignorance: Teaching Menstrual Etiquette in England, c. 1920s to 1960s." *Social History of Medicine* 14, no. 2 (2001): 247–65.

Strathern, Marilyn. *Kinship, Law and the Unexpected: Relatives Are Always a Surprise*. Cambridge: Cambridge University Press, 2005.

Strassfeld, Benjamin. "A Difficult Delivery: Debating the Function of the Screen and Educational Cinema through *The Birth of a Baby* (1938)." *Velvet Light Trap*, no. 72 (Fall 2013): 44–57.

Taylor, Janelle S. "The Public Fetus and the Family Car: From Abortion Politics to a Volvo Advertisement." *Public Culture* 4, no. 2 (1992): 67–80.

_____. *The Public Life of the Fetal Sonogram: Technology, Consumption, and the Politics of Reproduction.* New Brunswick, NJ: Rutgers University Press, 2008.

Thomson, Rosemarie Garland ed. *Freakery: Cultural Spectacles of the Extraordinary Body.* New York, NY: NYU Press, 1996.

Tybjerg, Karin. "Curating the Dead Body Between Medicine and Culture." In *Curatorial Challenges: Interdisciplinary Perspectives on Contemporary Curating,* edited by Malene Vest Hansen, Anne Folke Henningsen, and Anne Gregersen, 35–50. London: Routledge, 2019.

_____. "From Bottled Babies to Biobanks." In *The Fate of Anatomical Collections: The History of Medicine in Context,* edited by Rina Knoeff and Robert Zwijnenberg, 263–278. Farnham, Surrey; Burlington, VT: Ashgate, 2015.

Tyler, Imogen. "Pregnant Beauty: Maternal Femininities under Neoliberalism." In *New Femininities: Postfeminism, Neoliberalism and Subjectivity,* edited by Rosalind Gill and Christina Scharff, 21–36. Basingstoke: Palgrave Macmillan, 2011.

Tyler, Imogen, and Lisa Baraitser. "Private View, Public Birth: Making Feminist Sense of the New Visual Culture of Childbirth." *Studies in the Maternal* 5, no. 2 (2013): 1–27.

Usborne, Cornelie. *Cultures of Abortion in Weimar Germany.* Oxford: Berghahn, 2007.

Valerius, Katryn. "*Rosemary's Baby,* Gothic Pregnancy and Fetal Subjects." *College Literature* 32, no. 3 (2005): 116–35.

Vicedo, Marga. *The Nature and Nurture of Love: From Imprinting to Attachment in Cold War America.* Chicago: University of Chicago Press, 2014.

Vogel, Klaus. "The Transparent Man: Some Comments on the History of a Symbol." In *Manifesting Medicine: Bodies and Machines,* edited by Robert Bud, Bernard S. Finn, and Helmuth Trischler. 31–62. Amsterdam: Harwood Academic, 1999.

Wagner, Corinna. "Replicating Venus: Art, Anatomy, Wax Models, and Automata." *19: Interdisciplinary Studies in the Long Nineteenth Century* 24 (2017): 1–27, https://doi.org/10.16995/ntn.783.

Weingarten, Karen. "From Maternal Impressions to Eugenics: Pregnancy and Inheritance in the Nineteenth-Century U.S." *Journal of Medical Humanities* 43 (2020): 303–17.

Wellmann, Janina. *The Form of Becoming: Embryology and the Epistemology of Rhythm, 1760–1830,* trans. Kate Sturge. New York: Zone Books, 2017.

White, Suzanne. "'Mom and Dad' (1944): Venereal Disease 'Exploitation.'" *Bulletin of the History of Medicine* 62, no. 2 (Summer 1988): 252–70.

Whiteley, Rebecca. *Birth Figures: Early Modern Prints and the Pregnant Body.* Chicago: University of Chicago Press, 2023.

———. "Figuring Pictures and Picturing Figures: Images of the Pregnant Body and the Unborn Child in England, 1540–c.1680," *Social History of Medicine* 32, no. 2 (2019): 241–66.

Williams, Daniel K. *Defenders of the Unborn: The Pro-Life Movement before Roe v. Wade.* New York: Oxford University Press, 2016.

Wilson, Adrian. *The Making of Man-Midwifery: Childbirth in England, 1660–1770.* Cambridge, MA: Harvard University Press, 1995.

Wilson, Emily K. "Ex Utero: Live Human Fetal Research and the Films of Davenport Hooker." *Bulletin of the History of Medicine* 88, no. 1 (2014): 132–60.

Withycombe, Shannon K. "From Women's Expectations to Scientific Specimens: The Fate of Miscarriage Materials in Nineteenth-Century America." *Social History of Medicine* 28, no. 2 (2015): 245–62.

———. *Lost: Miscarriage in Nineteenth-Century America.* New Brunswick, NJ: Rutgers University Press, 2019.

———. "Unusual Frontal Development: Negotiating the Pregnant Body in Nineteenth-Century America." *Journal of Women's History* 27, no. 4 (2015): 160–83.

Wood, Jill. "(In)Visible Bleeding: The Menstrual Concealment Imperative." In *The Palgrave Handbook of Critical Menstruation Studies*, edited by Chris Bobel et al., 319–36. Singapore: Palgrave Macmillan, 2020.

Zaretsky, Natasha. *Radiation Nation: Three Mile Island and the Political Transformation of the 1970s.* New York: Columbia University Press, 2018.

Ziegler, Mary. *Abortion and the Law in America: Roe v. Wade to the Present.* Cambridge: Cambridge University Press, 2020.

———. *After Roe: The Lost History of the Abortion Debate.* Cambridge, MA: Harvard University Press, 2015.

Contributors

Elisabet Björklund is associate professor in film studies at Lund University. Her research is focused on sexuality and reproduction in Swedish film and television history, and she is coeditor, with Mariah Larsson, of *Swedish Cinema and the Sexual Revolution: Critical Essays* (2016) and *A Visual History of HIV/AIDS: Exploring the Face of AIDS Film Archive* (2019). Currently, she is working on a research project on reproduction in Swedish television in the 1950s, 1960s, and 1970s, funded by the Swedish Research Council.

Jessica M. Dandona earned her PhD from the University of California at Berkeley in art history, with a specialization in nineteenth-century French art and visual culture. She is currently professor of art history in the Liberal Arts Department at the Minneapolis College of Art and Design. Dr. Dandona's book *Nature and the Nation in Fin-de-Siècle France: The Art of Emile Gallé and the Ecole de Nancy* was published by Routledge in 2017. Her current book project, *The Transparent Woman: Medical Visualities in Fin-de-Siècle Europe and the United States, 1880–1900*, examines the visual culture of medicine at the end of the nineteenth century.

Anne-Sophie Giraud is research fellow at the Center of Social Anthropology in Toulouse (LISST-CAS, CNRS). Her previous research investigated the changing status of embryos and fetuses in France and the constitution of personhood during reproduction, with a focus on fetal death and reproductive technologies. She is currently working on a research project about human intervention in procreation (preimplantation genetic diagnosis, prenatal diagnosis, late termination of pregnancy) in France.

Rose Holz received her PhD in history from the University of Illinois at Urbana-Champaign. Currently, she is professor of practice at the University of Nebraska-Lincoln, where she serves as associate director of the Women's & Gender Studies Program. Her teaching and research focuses on the history of sexuality and reproduction in America, with particular emphases on the medical and commercial provision of birth control, the history of Planned Parenthood, and more recently the use of art to teach the process of in utero development. She is the author of *The Birth Control Clinic in* *a Marketplace World* (2012). Her work has also appeared in the *Journal of Social History*, *American Historian*, and *Visualizing the Body in Art, Anatomy, and Medicine: Models and Modeling* (2019), edited by Andrew Graciano.

Nick Hopwood is professor of history of science and medicine in the Department of History and Philosophy of Science, University of Cambridge. He is the author of *Embryos in Wax* (2002) and *Haeckel's Embryos: Images, Evolution, and Fraud* (2015), which won the Levinson Prize of the History of Science Society; coeditor, most recently, of *Reproduction: Antiquity to the Present Day* (2018); and cocurator of the online exhibition *Making Visible Embryos* (2008). He is writing two books: *The Embryo Series: Seeing Human Development before Birth* and *The Many Births of the Test-Tube Baby*, the latter supported by a Leverhulme Major Research Fellowship.

Solveig Jülich is professor of history of science and ideas at Uppsala University. Her research focuses on late nineteenth- to early twenty-first-century histories of reproduction, and history of medical imaging and media culture. She has published articles on the historical trajectories of Swedish photographer Lennart Nilsson's images of embryos and fetuses in journals such as the *Bulletin of the History of Medicine* and *Social History of Medicine*. She is coeditor of the volumes *Knowledge in Motion: The Royal Swedish Academy of Sciences and the Making of Modern Society* (Makadam, 2018) and *Communicating the History of Medicine: Perspectives on Audiences and Impact* (Manchester University Press, 2020), and editor of *Medicine at the Borders of Life: Fetal Knowledge Production and the Emergence of Public Controversy in Sweden* (Leiden: Brill, 2024).

Jennifer Kosmin is assistant professor of history at Auburn University in Auburn, Alabama. Her research focuses on the intersections of medicine, anatomy, gender, knowledge production, and cultural understandings of the body in early modern Italy. Her first book, *Authority, Gender, and Midwifery in Early Modern Italy: Contested Deliveries* (Routledge, 2021), traces the emergence of midwifery schools and hospital maternity wards in eighteenth-century northern Italy. She is currently working on a project that considers late eighteenth-century debates about nature and artifice.

Manon S. Parry is professor of medical and nursing history at VU Amsterdam and associate professor of public history and American studies at the University of Amsterdam. She was previously curator in the History of Medicine Division of the National Library of Medicine, National Institutes of Health, Maryland, where she curated gallery and online exhibitions with budgets ranging from $14,500 to $3 million on a wide range of topics, including global health and human rights, disability in the American Civil War, and medicinal and recreational drug use. Her research focuses on health communication in historical perspective, including the monograph *Broadcasting Birth Control: Mass Media and Family Planning* (Rutgers University Press, 2013). She is currently completing a book titled *Human Curiosities: Engaging with Medical Museums*, on the social relevance of medical heritage and changing exhibition trends.

Sara Ray received her PhD in the history and sociology of science from the University of Pennsylvania. Her research examines the entwined histories of anatomical collecting, pregnancy, embryology, and disability in the eighteenth and early nineteenth centuries. Ray's work has been supported by the Council for European Studies, the Science History Institute, the Fulbright Program, and the Descartes Centre for the History and Philosophy of the Sciences and the Humanities at Utrecht University. She holds an MA in museum anthropology from Columbia University and currently works at the Science History Institute.

Camilla Mørk Røstvik is associate professor in history at the University of Agder. She is honorary lecturer in medicine at the University of Aberdeen and honorary research fellow in art history at the University of St. Andrews. She earned her PhD in art history from the University of Manchester and has been a postdoctoral fellow at the University of St. Andrews and University of Leeds. Røstvik was a Leverhulme Early Career Research Fellow in the School of Art History at the University of St. Andrews. In 2018 she established the Wellcome Trust–funded Menstruation Research Network UK. Her first book, *Cash Flow: The Businesses of Menstruation since 1970* was published by UCL Press, and her next book, *The Painters Are In: The Visual Cultures of Menstruation*, is forthcoming with McGill-Queen's University Press in 2024.

María Jesús Santesmases is research professor at the Instituto de Filosofía, Consejo Superior de Investigaciones Científicas (Spanish National Research Council; CSIC), in Madrid. Her research deals with post–World War II biology and biomedicine, women scientists, and gender. She has published on the history of biochemistry and molecular biology, and is currently developing projects on the early practices of human cytogenetics and gender and on gender, women, and antimicrobials from the 1970s onward.

Index

Printed in the United States
by Baker & Taylor Publisher Services